Most analytic writing sucks the life out of its subject—not so this luminous book, which makes reading itself a psychoanalytic experience. Jade McGleughlin's lively collection of essays demands losing one's way, demonstrating that in risking sovereignty what's gained is true living. With a fierce heart and a queer intelligence, McGleughlin inducts us into powerful forms of practice. When standing in the spaces is not enough, she helps us find the courage to fall through them into a world and a way of seeing illuminated by the harrowing wonder and the beauty of sheer being. McGleughlin's expansive intellectual reach bridges not only European and American psychoanalytic traditions but also social theory, philosophy, personal reflection, and art. Here is an analytic writer for the urgency of our moment, showing us how intensely personal landscapes are suffused with social import and how inhabiting vulnerability is the soul of good politics, vibrant practice, and embodied being.

Francisco Gonzalez, *Psychoanalytic Institute of Northern California*

Jade McGleughlin gives us a psychoanalytic book for our time, offering a new and impactful vision of psychoanalytic thinking and praxis. In the nexus of the ontological and the intersectional, the personal and the political, McGleughlin spells out a unique vision of psychoanalysis where the analyst's non-sovereignty and inevitable interpenetrative entanglements capture and transform absence, trauma, and the negative in the reality of the non-represented and non-verbal.

Working "beyond countertransference," McGleughlin finds a space to work in the unknowable while knowing something. Old categories of sameness, difference, race, and gender and nothing less than patient-and-analyst dissolve and reconfigure as McGleughlin transports us to her consulting room, her world, and her art.

Unafraid to imbricate her personal life and struggles with utterly compelling, sometimes unsettling, and always profound clinical stories, McGleughlin draws on her own art, transformational movies, novels, and photography to create a unique bricolage of what it means to be a clinician in today's world.

Robert Grossmark, PhD, ABPP, *New York University Postdoctoral Program in Psychotherapy and Psychoanalysis*

McGleughlin's writing often begins with a jolt, rendering us dizzied and upended. When we get back on our feet, we realize that we've entered a unique psychic country, one where ontology meets a different kind of intersubjective core. The usual referents of an ontological analysis, playing and reverie, don't always capture how far she has been able to go in experiencing and identifying with her patient's experience.

With a gift for moving back and forth between raw experience and theory, McGleughlin has found ways to have a creative experience of living something together with her patient and with us. Her art is in remaining curious, finding and refinding new elements of her patient and herself.

I locate McGleughlin's unique interest combining the social, relational, and ontological strands of psychoanalysis in her capacity to keep us moving inside experiences of reverie (the patient and analyst in her mind) and the actuality of patient and analyst as objects. Her writing captures the essence of psychoanalysis as something in private, in public, a rare gift that is on display in this highly creative and generous writing.

Stephen Cooper, *Clinical Professor of Psychiatry, Columbia University; Supervising and Training Analyst, The Boston Psychoanalytic Society and Institute* and *Columbia Center for Psychoanalytic Training and Research*

Delicate, stalwart, electrifying, and true, McGleughlin charges spaces so spare that psychoanalyst and patient inhabit them "in the negative," in a quiet that honors Otherness without superordination. McGleughlin insists that the analyst, as an implicated subject in the historically raced and gendered surround, must risk "necessary vertigo," a not-knowing that thoroughly destabilizes while it also contains. A politically savvy frame emerges from the negative harkening back respect without presumption. Notes on being accrue in often subtle, sometimes bold, and always meaningful gestures that have the precision of artist Agnes Martin's keenest brush strokes.

Stephen Hartman, PhD, *Joint Editor-in-Chief, Psychoanalytic Dialogues*

Joining Jade McGleughlin in her tender, admittedly futile, and nevertheless relentless attempts to connect with the human essence, you will suddenly, incomprehensibly, find access to what was previously unimaginable. With McGleughlin you learn how to love the most silent and withdrawn souls, and find ways to keep yourself company through the heartbreak. Her paintings carry us through that which cannot be named. Weaving the deeply personal and its socio-political context, McGleughlin's is a feminist-queer project, paradoxically using language to break apart its structures of colonization. Use this book: linger with it, teach it—this book will change you.

Orna Guralnik, PsyD, *New York University Postdoctoral Program in Psychotherapy and Psychoanalysis*; *Couples Therapy*, Showtime

McGleughlin has produced a rare gem, an experimental psychoanalytic book, and illuminated the conventions that limit psychoanalytic practice. The capacious reach, artistry, and playing that builds this book opens onto considerations of that which is hard to speak: trauma, the negative, nonbeing, non-belonging, the ineffable. Go for the content, but stay for the play.

Ken Corbett, PhD, *New York University Postdoctoral Program in Psychotherapy and Psychoanalysis*

This book, in a way that is novel and unsettling and deeply engaging, offers a number of radical new ideas for psychoanalytic work. Throughout her writing, McGleughlin makes a case for enigma, uncertainty, gaps in knowing and thinking and speaking for analyst, analysand, and reader. Reading the book brings us into the practice she is theorizing, allowing uncertainty and silence, in ourselves, in the writing, and in the clinical encounters, to work their way into minds and hearts. A book that enacts what it also teaches. A profound experience.

Adrienne Harris, *New York University Postdoctoral Program in Psychoanalysis and Psychotherapy, The New School for Social Research*

Clinical Storytelling, Art and the Problems of Being

In a series of overlapping clinical essays—sometimes highly personal, sometimes bristling with theory, sometimes employing experimental writing—Jade McGleughlin upends the ways we tell a psychoanalytic story.

Tracing the evolution of her thinking, the collection grapples with the problem of engaging patients when verbal representation fails. To do this, McGleughlin takes us inside some of her richest, most surprising encounters with patients who have suffered severe trauma, leading to a breach in the experience of self. McGleughlin imagines how to meet patients in the breach. She then brings us along, requiring the analyst's intense personal struggle to find and share the patients' experiences of liminality, of terror, of nonexistence—to tolerate the vertigo of deep engagement with the other. Rather than leading with authority and the illusion of an autonomous self, McGleughlin offers storytelling that mirrors the work; her enactive writing dares to replicate the unsettling experience of the breach and invites readers to experience not only seeing but being seen.

Drawing from film, literature, and art, including her own paintings, as well as extensive clinical experience, this book is essential reading for all psychoanalysts, psychotherapists, and anyone wanting to understand how communication in a clinical space can transcend the verbal.

Jade McGleughlin is past president, psychoanalyst, and faculty member of the Massachusetts Institute for Psychoanalysis.

Relational Perspectives Book Series

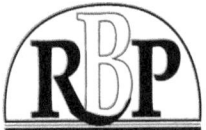

The Relational Perspectives Book Series (RPBS) publishes books that grow out of or contribute to the relational tradition in contemporary psychoanalysis. The term *relational psychoanalysis* was first used by Greenberg and Mitchell[1] to bridge the traditions of interpersonal relations, as developed within interpersonal psychoanalysis and object relations, as developed within contemporary British theory. But, under the seminal work of the late Stephen A. Mitchell, the term *relational psychoanalysis* grew and began to accrue to itself many other influences and developments. Various tributaries—interpersonal psychoanalysis, object relations theory, self psychology, empirical infancy research, feminism, queer theory, sociocultural studies and elements of contemporary Freudian and Kleinian thought—flow into this tradition, which understands relational configurations between self and others, both real and fantasied, as the primary subject of psychoanalytic investigation.

We refer to the relational tradition, rather than to a relational school, to highlight that we are identifying a trend, a tendency within contemporary psychoanalysis, not a more formally organized or coherent school or system of beliefs. Our use of the term *relational* signifies a dimension of theory and practice that has become salient across the wide spectrum of contemporary psychoanalysis. Now under the editorial supervision of Adrienne Harris and Eyal Rozmarin, the Relational Perspectives Book Series originated in 1990 under the editorial eye of the late Stephen A. Mitchell. Mitchell was the most prolific and influential of the originators of the relational tradition. Committed to dialogue among psychoanalysts, he abhorred the authoritarianism that dictated adherence to a rigid set of beliefs or technical restrictions. He championed open discussion, comparative and integrative approaches, and promoted new voices across the generations. Mitchell was later joined by the late Lewis Aron, also a visionary and influential writer, teacher and leading thinker in relational psychoanalysis.

Included in the Relational Perspectives Book Series are authors and works that come from within the relational tradition, those that extend and develop that tradition, and works that critique relational approaches or compare and contrast them with alternative points of view. The series includes our most distinguished senior psychoanalysts, along with younger contributors who bring fresh vision. Our aim is to enable a deepening of relational thinking while reaching across disciplinary and social boundaries in order to foster an inclusive and international literature.

A full list of titles in this series is available at https://www.routledge.com/ Relational-Perspectives-Book-Series/book-series/LEARPBS.

Note

1 Greenberg, J., and S. Mitchell. 1983. *Object Relations in Psychoanalytic Theory*. Cambridge, MA: Harvard University Press.

Clinical Storytelling, Art and the Problems of Being

The Analyst's Necessary Vertigo

Jade McGleughlin

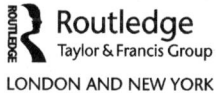
Routledge
Taylor & Francis Group

LONDON AND NEW YORK

Designed cover image: Vertigo © Jade McGleughlin, Oil on Canvas 16x20

First published 2024
by Routledge
4 Park Square, Milton Park, Abingdon, Oxon OX14 4RN

and by Routledge
605 Third Avenue, New York, NY 10158

Routledge is an imprint of the Taylor & Francis Group, an informa business

© 2024 Jade McGleughlin

British Library Cataloguing-in-Publication Data
A catalogue record for this book is available from the British Library

ISBN: 978-1-032-67033-1 (hbk)
ISBN: 978-1-032-67032-4 (pbk)
ISBN: 978-1-032-67034-8 (ebk)

DOI: 10.4324/9781032670348

Typeset in Times New Roman
by Apex CoVantage, LLC

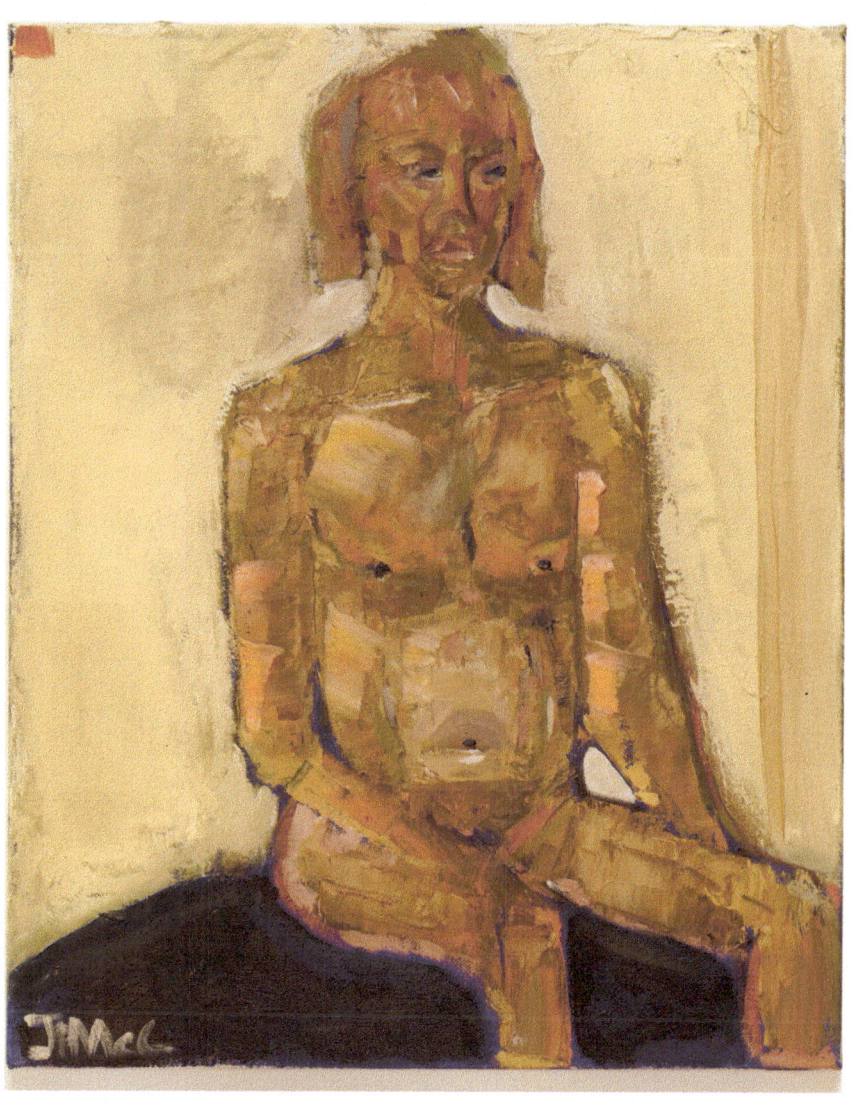

Vertigo © Jade McGleughlin, Oil on Canvas 16x20

For my mother

Contents

Acknowledgments   *xvii*
Preface   *xxii*

Introduction: on being a bricoleur   1

PART 1
The analyst's necessary vertigo (2011)   21

1 The analyst's necessary vertigo (2008/2011)   25

2 Love letter to a patient or the raw story *(2001)*   41

3 Afterword(s) on writing: we always tell it slant—clinical
   stories create truths, not describe them (2020)   67

4 Afterword(s) on technique: necessary reach (2009)   72

5 Two case vignettes: how Sarah helped me help Troy
   and (almost) Christina (2014)   83

PART 2
The breach   91

6 Do we find or lose ourselves in the negative? (2015)   95

7 Answering gestures: further thoughts on "Do we find
   or lose ourselves in the negative?" (2015)   117

8 "When you are in the cellar, am I dead?": understanding
   the limits of empathy and the power of otherness through
   the film *Hiroshima mon amour* (2020)   127

9 Interlude with life and death: eulogy to my stepfather (2016)   143

10 White empathy (2020)   147

PART 3
The problem of telling the story of another   173

11 The promise of radical relationality in Elena Ferrante's
    novels (2015)   181

12 Transgender imagining and the danger of normative
    theory (2019)   199

13 Thinking outside the Oedipus box (2021)   226

14 Translation: an alternative developmental mother
    story (2020)   237

PART 4
The negative   245

15 The analyst's necessary nonsovereignty and the generative
    power of the negative (2019)   251

16 The impossibility of meaning (2019)   275

   Bibliography   *296*
   Index   *313*

Acknowledgments

I wanted to write a book to accompany me. Because I am lonely. Not the kind of lonely that is met by more good people—I have many. A truly extraordinary sweetie whose world-changing holds me and pushes me up and out, and whose name I still want to shout from every rooftop 40 years later; two grown children with whom I share keen intellectual camaraderie and so much pleasure; a warm and loving community. Two best friends, a best girl gang, sometimes another. I could list more: a queer movement, a movement for racial justice, a psychoanalytic institute. So many groups. Too many groups. A steady bridge game, an art practice, walls full of portraits I make to keep me company, a garden, a perfect beach I visit, a lot of orange, platform shoes, a swell house. I don't lack people or things, occupations or place. But none of it levels up against the loneliness that comes as a condition of being this human, any human. And so I am also grateful for the beautiful smart people who have allowed me to find home in their minds. To find home in the mind of another is transformative (Spezzano 2007).

I start with Ann, without whom I might never have thought of myself as a thinking person.

And Adrienne Harris, without whom psychoanalysis would never have enticed me. Her deep intelligence, mentorship, and friendship have allowed this book to be. Adrienne Harris and Muriel Dimen were my first analytic supervisors, guides, and companions, offering me entry and delight. Adrienne saw something in me, something I could not quite see in myself, and that forward imagining of me was powerful. Just as consequentially, she and Muriel led me into a community of like-minded colleagues: Francisco González, Orna Guralnik, Stephen Hartman, Julie Leavitt, and Eyal Rozmarin, my bicoastal queer writing and playing group where we create charged, intimate spaces in which learning, relationality, and love are inextricably linked. Telephone wires (before we had telehealth) buzzed. Welcomed into the minds, and living rooms, of this circle of theorists, I discovered a level of intellectual and political kinship I hadn't expected in psychoanalysis. I made home.

Closer in, I am grateful for those in Boston I have been in intellectual community with, including Al Praeger and Peter Wohlauer, beautiful men who taught me to translate the unconscious. And to Mal Slavin, who taught me how to get close to a patient without fear. And for Stephen Cooper, who invited me to write my first psychoanalytic article, believing I could. And for my analyst, who is good, so very good. And also very bad.

Most especially I thank my colleagues and friends at Massachusetts Institute for Psychoanalysis, where I cut my analytic teeth, flourished, learned to teach, became a leader, helped foment change, struggled, disavowed, and loved some more and will always love some more. Thank you. In particular, thank you to my candidates, students, and supervisees for always captivating me and keeping it fresh. And thanks to Larry Chud and Deb Dowd for being my buddies through much MIP blah blah all those years. And Ginger, for her recognition. And to the anti-racism task force, where over a few intense years, I have spent much time with colleagues who have helped steady me in the face of so much pushback and downright hostility: Elizabeth Bernstein, Elizabeth Corpt, Carter Carter, Deb Dowd, Linda Gelda, Selina Guerra, Lynne Layton, Linda Luz-Alterman, Jen Neuwalder, Dina Pasalis, and Barbara Pizer. And of course, to Sarah, who I travel through so much of life with. Thank you for coming to MIP to keep me company.

I also want to thank my various study groups, which have been homes for my thinking: Kaethe Weingarten and her Feminist Supervision group; the Relational Group with so many beloved colleagues; the Bion group with Jack Beinashowitz, Stephen Cooper, Larry Chud, Richard Frankel, Jane Kite, and Humphrey Morris; my intergenerational Study Group on Race with Ann Holder, Gina Lee, Jesse McGleughlin, and John white. And especially my supervision group with David Raniere and Richard Frankel, each a creative and powerful thinker with whom to feel the incredible anguish of our work. I also want to thank Humphrey Morris for his brilliant intellectual offerings and curation of works of beauty for his Psychoanalytic Reading Group on the intersection of art, philosophy, and psychoanalysis. This group is where I first read Barthes and Benjamin and became inspired to paint. And to the journal *Psychoanalytic Dialogues*, which allows me to edit cutting-edge work all the while making community with the most intelligent people. These have all been crucial spaces of intellectual growth and pleasure.

The papers in this book go so far back it is hard to know who *not* to thank for their contribution. Certainly, I deeply appreciate my writing group and also Jack Foehl, Miriam Kahn, Lynne Layton, Julia Matthews, Humphrey Morris, Avgi Saketopoulou, and Stephen Seligman, who read now or long ago—they all read with such intelligence. And I have received lively thinking and extraordinary editorial help from Laurie Abraham, Adrienne Harris, Christine Maksimowicz, and Suzi Naiburg; they have also put up with the very irascible me. I want to give a special shout-out to Stephen Hartman, who always helps when no one else has time, though he doesn't either, and to beloved friend Barbara McQueen, who appeared from nowhere to rekindle a lovely friendship from college. Barbara and Dina Pasalis bravely read the whole book, making it richer and more heartfelt. Muah, muah. And thank you, Georgina Clutterbuck and Kate Hawes, for your patience and skill bringing this book forward.

Last, it is not nothing to write from and about breach, mine and my patients. Also, not nothing to write a book about what didn't work so well, or only worked later. And to risk my patients' vulnerability and psychic pain and to show my own. To my beloved accompaniers: I am lucky to be in intimate relationships with you and to have your generosity turned towards me in so many ways, including your letting me tell my story through and with you. "I knew you, you knew me. We looked at each other, shining on each other. Shining-on sun. Sailing-on moon" (Minnie Bruce Pratt, 2022).

The author gratefully acknowledges permission to republish the following material:

"The Analyst's Necessary Vertigo," Jade McGleughlin, *Psychoanalytic Dialogues*, vol. 21, no. 5, 2011, Taylor & Francis Ltd, reprinted by permission of the publisher (Taylor & Francis Ltd, http://www.tandfonline.com).

"Do We Find or Lose Ourselves in the Negative?" Jade McGleughlin, *Psychoanalytic Dialogues*, vol. 25, no. 2, 2015, Taylor & Francis Ltd, reprinted by permission of the publisher (Taylor & Francis Ltd, http://www.tandfonline.com).

"Answering Gestures," Jade McGleughlin, *Psychoanalytic Dialogues*, vol. 25, no. 2, 2015, Taylor & Francis Ltd, reprinted by permission of the publisher (Taylor & Francis Ltd, http://www.tandfonline.com).

"The Impossibility of Meaning: Joining and Rejoining: Reply to Cooney, Ferro, and Stern," Jade McGleughlin, *Psychoanalytic Dialogues*, vol. 30, no. 2, 2020, Taylor & Francis Ltd, reprinted by permission of the publisher (Taylor & Francis Ltd, http://www.tandfonline.com).

"The Analyst's Necessary Nonsovereignty and the Generative Power of the Negative," Jade McGleughlin, *Psychoanalytic Dialogues*, vol. 30, no. 2, 2020, Taylor & Francis Ltd, reprinted by permission of the publisher (Taylor & Francis Ltd, http://www.tandfonline.com).

"Rethinking Oedipus or Not," Jade McGleughlin, *Psychoanalytic Dialogues*, vol. 31, no. 3, 2021, Taylor & Francis Ltd, reprinted by permission of the publisher (Taylor & Francis Ltd, http://www.tandfonline.com).

"Translation," Jade McGleughlin, *Studies in Gender and Sexuality*, vol. 21, no. 1, 53–57, 2020, Taylor & Francis Ltd, reprinted by permission of the publisher (Taylor & Francis Ltd, http://www.tandfonline.com).

The lines from "Phantasia for Elvira Shatayev," from *The Dream of a Common Language: Poems 1974–1977* by Adrienne Rich. Copyright © 1978 by W. W. Norton & Company, Inc. Used by permission of W. W. Norton & Company, Inc.

The lines from "Diving into the Wreck," from *Diving into the Wreck: Poems 1971–1972* by Adrienne Rich. Copyright © 1973 by W. W. Norton & Company, Inc. Used by permission of W. W. Norton & Company, Inc.

An Excerpt from *The Gates* by Muriel Rukeyser. Copyright © Muriel Rukeyser, 1976. Reprinted by permission of the Estate of Muriel Rukeyser.

An Extract from "The Love Song of J. Alfred Prufrock," *The Complete Poems and Plays of T.S. Eliot* by T.S. Eliot. Reprinted by permission of the publisher, Faber and Faber Ltd.

"For the Stranger" © 1978 by Carolyn Forché

An excerpt from *Proxies* © 2016 by Brian Blanchfield.

An excerpt from "The Condition of Black Life is One of Mourning" by Claudia Rankine. From *The New York Times*. © 2015 The New York Times Company. All rights reserved. Used under license.

An excerpt from "Not Waving but Drowning," *Collected Poems and Drawings of Stevie Smith* by Stevie Smith. Reprinted by permission of the publisher, Faber and Faber Ltd.

An excerpt from "Not Waving but Drowning," by Stevie Smith, from *All the Poems*, copyright © 1937, 1938, 1942, 1950, 1957, 1962, 1966, 1971, 1972 by Stevie Smith. Copyright © 2016 by the Estate of James MacGibbon. Copyright © 2015 by Will May. Reprinted by permission of New Directions Publishing Corp.

An excerpt of "The Dead Lecturer" by LeRoi Jones, permission by Chris Calhoun Agency, © Estate of Amiri Baraka

Three lines from "Blue Moon," Minnie Bruce Pratt, *Magnified*, copyright 2021 Minnie Bruce Pratt. Published by Wesleyan University Press. Used by permission.

"Modersohn-Becker," copyright © 1991 by Anne Michaels; from *Poems* by Anne Michaels. Used by permission of Alfred A. Knopf, an imprint of the Knopf Doubleday Publishing Group, a division of Penguin Random House LLC. All rights reserved.

Extracts from *Fugitive Pieces* by Anne Michaels and extracts from *The Weight of Oranges/Miner's Pond* by Anne Michaels. *Fugitive Pieces*, copyright © 1996, Anne Michaels, used by permission of The Wylie Agency (UK) Limited. *The*

Weight of Oranges/Miner's Pond, copyright © 1997, Anne Michaels, used by permission of The Wylie Agency (UK) Limited.

"Modersohn-Becker" from *The Weight of Oranges/Miner's Pond*: Poems by Anne Michaels, Copyright © 1986, 1991, 1997 Anne Michaels. Reprinted by permission of McClelland & Stewart, a division of Penguin Random House Canada Limited. All rights reserved.

"The Space Heater" from *One Secret Thing* by Sharon Olds, copyright © 2008 by Sharon Olds. Used by permission of Alfred A. Knopf, an imprint of the Knopf Doubleday Publishing Group, a division of Penguin Random House LLC. All rights reserved.

From *One Secret Thing* by Sharon Olds published by Jonathan Cape. Copyright © Sharon Olds 2009. Reprinted by permission of Penguin Books Limited.

Hiroshima mon amour directed by Alain Resnais © 1959 Argos Films. Thanks to: Sabine Azéma, Camille Bordes-Resnais and Argos Films.

Preface

I want to welcome you into a deep and expansive experience, reading this book of collected papers by Jade McGleughlin. I have been reading Jade's work for a number of years, and our conversations and explorations of clinical work are long-standing. Despite the familiarity of our connection, the experience of reading this book opens a depth and power of engagement that was both expectable, familiar, and profoundly transformative.

We are used to analytic writing in which we're guided into an increasingly layered comprehension of how the analyst sees and understands the patient. While this book unquestionably does that, its commitment is fundamentally much deeper and more complex. This book is a commitment to demonstrate in exquisite detail that the patient/analysand's changes are contingent on the profound and unexpected changes in the analyst. I say this and immediately want to notice that while writing about countertransference is widely practiced, this set of papers takes the presence of countertransference to a new level. So much so that I question the rightness or sufficiency of the term "countertransference" to capture the way Jade works and writes.

Many of the clinical chapters are an account of treatment in which the transformations in the analyst must and often do precede and provoke the moments of growth and change in the analysand. And this requires the analyst's nonsovereignty and entanglement—a perspective that describes two-person treatment in a whole different key. Reading this book, I found myself thinking that a lot of people probably go through quite similar transformative steps in the arcs and routines of the work, but we do not write ourselves into the clinical story or narrate the shifting internal states of the analyst in the way and to the degree McGleughlin has. It is a crucial contribution. Neither analyst nor patient can truly know herself and even less tell the other's story, necessitating a fundamental rethinking of theory and technique.

The work in this book is not only, I am saying, a radical expansion of what a two-person analytic system can be and do; it is also a movement through the study of clinical treatments, biography and autobiography, the analysis of film and texts. Throughout it all, the character and experience of the writer is vividly and profoundly educative. But there is yet another pre-occupation and focus in this book that is significant. McGleughlin applies the idea of intersectionality: the interpenetration of race, class, and gender in social formation, including psychoanalytic treatment. In doing so, she makes an exquisite and determined case for imagining and understanding that our work arises, is shaped, and invaded by social and political, as well as interpersonal, interlocking systems.

These transactional systems lead to transformation, and change, but also can contribute to or enforce stalemates and terminations. Varying aspects of voice and presence are given authority in this work in ways that engage the clinician as analyst and patient, as supervisor and supervisee. What is unusual and precious in this book is McGleughlin's voice. Moving among many distinct aspects of clinical and theoretical work, across distinct models of mind and of treatment, professional and personal spaces, McGleughlin writes in a style and a voice that is uniquely personal and engaged.

Adrienne Harris

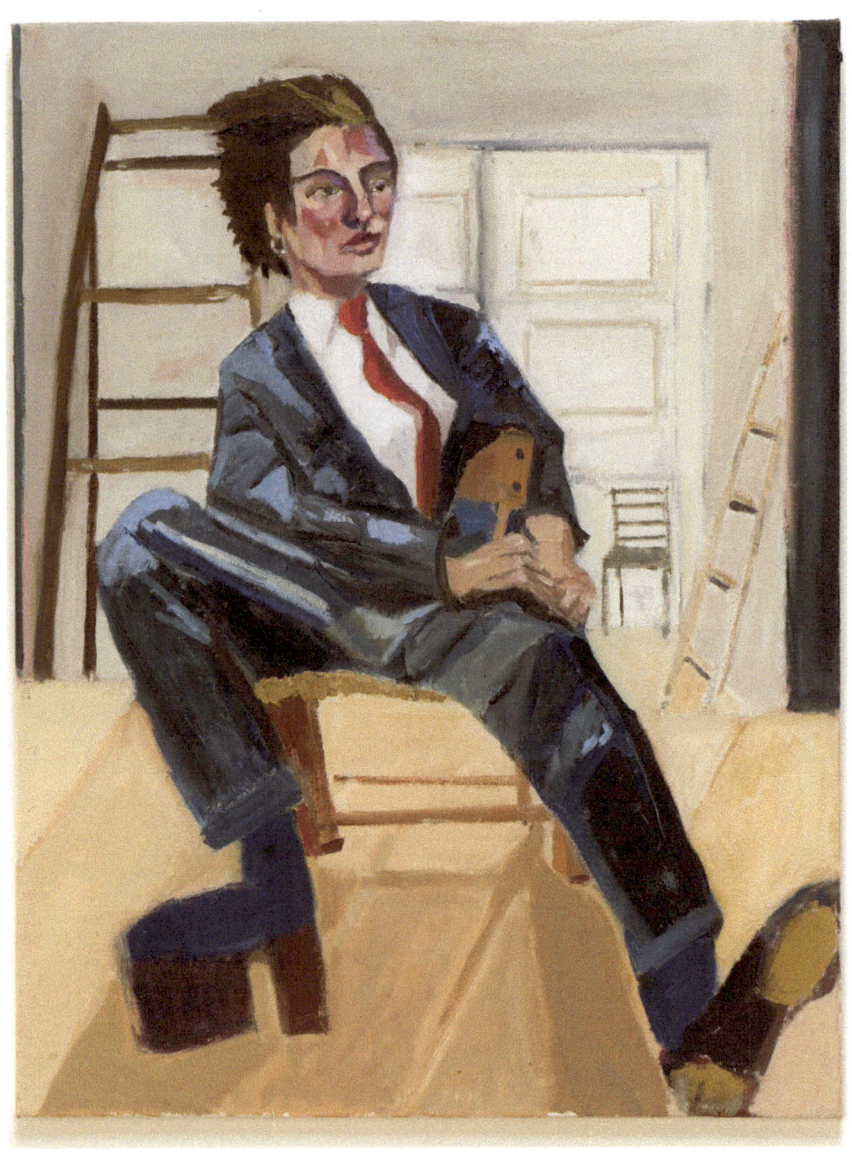

Figure 0.1 After Winnicott. Oil on canvas. 28x22. McGleughlin

Introduction

On being a bricoleur

Beginnings

In my first job out of college, in 1982, I worked in residential treatment with teenage girls. A white girl, I'll call her Marie, frequently snuck out. One night I caught her on the dangerously rickety outdoor fire escape. When I asked her to come inside, she quipped, "I am not on the fire escape." Certainly, she was, or so it seemed to my 21-one-year-old self, the snow swirling around her, the cold air raising goosebumps on my skin. Soon police, firefighters, social workers, and senior clinicians would arrive, lights flashing, whistles blowing. The other girls were watching me. Marie had to come in. She was breaking the rules. And I was responsible.

> Our interaction went like this:
> "Please come in from the fire escape."
> "I am not on the fire escape."
> "Please come inside."
> "I am inside."
> "You are not inside."
> "I am too."
> I wait, then tear up. Wait.
> Finally, I say, "Your inside is very cold for me. . . I wonder if you might visit mine."
> She comes in.

This interaction became a powerful guiding tale for me about not knowing and the need to crawl inside a story and look out with my patient. In fact, it was my inauguration into the ontological in clinical work, where thinking is decentered and being together takes center stage.

DOI: 10.4324/9781032670348-1

Marie taught me more. Asked to account for herself, she would always tell her story by laying out all the pieces, stringing disparate events together, utterly confusing us. If we interrupted, she'd start all over again, from *her* beginning. She could not do it any other way or eliminate a single bit. It was as if she were gathering and hoarding every tiny scrap.

Of course, my colleagues and I thought she was manipulating us or trying to keep track of her lies. We suspected a kind of sociopathy—not least because when we finally arrived where she took us, "the end" was hard to believe or nonsensical. Instead, Marie taught me about letting a narrative emerge as it does in a flip-book. She was *constructing* a self, piece by piece, in her own way, out of thin air. If she skipped a beat or reversed something, I wasn't with her, she didn't exist to herself. I didn't know how trauma disrupts time and storylines, or that we were probably in a transitional space, in which "inner reality and external life both contribute . . . a respite from the perpetual human task of keeping inner and outer reality separate yet interrelated" (Winnicott 1971a, 2).

Only later when I read Barthes's (1980) *Camera Lucida* did I realize that Marie, and other patients who turn the tables on us, offer us an experience of punctum, that which *disturbs* and "creates the pressure of the unspeakable that wants to be spoken" (Barthes 1980, 19) (Chapter 2). Marie was not a psychotherapy patient of mine—I did milieu work—but she required a lot of me. She was special, perplexing, piercing, the first in a long line of patients with whom I encountered a sustained way of experiencing beyond what I knew, somewhere between perception and language. Sometimes I was experientially undone. Certain of our patients, sometimes just one across a whole clinical career, sometimes many, or sometimes just an utterance or glance in a treatment, call forth our own primordial states. What happens when our usual therapeutic scaffolding does not hold us or our patients in the face of great affective disruption? And what can be reorienting? The clinical chapters in this book are about what a few of those patients taught me.

The ontological

I want to set the story of Marie and me in the context of what Ogden (2019) identified as a radical shift "in emphasis" (p. 662) in psychoanalysis over the last 70 years from an epistemological sensibility to an ontological one. Noting Winnicott's profound move from the symbolic *meaning* of play to the *experience* of playing and Bion's from the symbolic meaning of dreams to the experience of dreaming, Ogden establishes an ontological tradition with these two analysts as the principal contributors.[1] In this framework, knowledge or insight the analyst and patient acquire are no longer paramount; the therapeutic action is to facilitate the patient's "creatively discovering meaning for himself, and in that state of being, becoming more fully alive" (Ogden 2019, 661).

With Marie, I am intuitively creating a space in which we can live something new together, not thinking new thoughts but entering "states of being" [that] come to life in the . . . relationship that were previously unimaginable by the patient" (Ogden 2019, 667). From an ontological viewpoint, it didn't matter what stand-in I might have been in the transference, what old or new object I might become. What mattered was how together *in the moment* we got out of a "closed loop that repeats itself endlessly" of "experiencing the present as if it were the past" (Ogden 2019, 664). In our case, the loop of "Please come in from the fire escape"/"I am not on the fire escape" was interrupted when something shifted in me as we faced each other.

What allowed that to happen? I like to think that I had the presence of mind to pause and imagine, that I immersed myself in Marie's image of how she was not standing there. Maybe in a flash of unconscious connection, I located *my own* not being there, my runaway self. Maybe I wanted to dream with her about how we really were somewhere else, not on that fire escape at all, standing there/not standing there, but practicing going-on-being (Winnicott 1949). I like to think I might have matched something in my style, rhythm, and wondering to hers. And that in the time/gravity/ space continuum, we were together, simultaneously inside and out, on ground and in the air, then and now, apart and together.

Still, it was more capricious than that—and certainly desperate.

However I managed to talk from within Marie's story—matching her language and perception, "Your inside is very cold for me. I wonder if you might visit mine"—I now see that in that Winnicottian way, Marie and I entered that "overlap of two areas of playing, . . . and that unable to play before, we were brought into a state of being able to play" (Winnicott 1971b, 38). It was not the content of my words that facilitated movement; it was "working in and with the state of being involved in playing" that Ogden (2019) so clearly places in an ontological tradition.

With 15-year-old Marie perched on the fire escape with only marginal scaffolding and iced out of everyday living, my job is to bring her in. I will need to impose limits, boundaries, and borders, joining the infamous line of authorities designed "to help." Her alienation and mine, her identification and mine, are in play. My authority is clear, though so is my identification: Marie needs to feel my likeness, my kinship. My possible betrayal hangs in the balance between us but so too a thin thread, skin to skin, mind to mind, body to body. Snow to snow. In the bright winter light, I am/we are alive to what is happening between us in a force field that runs through us. We are, each and together, with her/our inside/outside Möbius strip and a whole lot of chutzpah, outsiders needing just then to go somewhere else.

While I locate myself squarely in Ogden's (2019) retrospective gathering of theorists and clinicians who lean toward the ontological, my exchanges with Marie were informed by aspects of the sensibility that are less clearly articulated and not as easily mapped in Ogden: the place of the social and the relational. To enter Marie's reality, I showed my vulnerability, found my own place of homelessness, and spoke from that place, making a bridge for us to cross together. These are ideas that I'll expand on in the following chapters.

Not coincidentally, Marie is a queer child, a perpetual outsider, not really invited in; she "unbelongs" (Leavitt 2022) to the group. As such, she exists "in a liminal refraction that is always moving to the outer reaches: internal experiences of self, cast against . . . the social milieu, social groups, social norms, social messaging" (Leavitt 2021). I am queer too, and though Marie doesn't "know" this, she also does. Marie intuits and I sense that we might belong to the same tribe of outsiders, that we might share "a notion of an unconscious that is *not within* subjects but *between* them: a collective queer unconscious" (Rozmarin 2019). She feels something with me but doesn't know what it is or its use. In that felt invisible bond, something else akin to being and being with each other may become possible.

Origin stories: thinking with others

Another formative ontological story stands out. It's 1980. I'm in a college class of an equal number of Black women and white women. In the middle of the room is one of my favorite professors Gloria Joseph. "Good intentions pave the road to hell," she booms to the white girls. It is an incantation. She is addressing our tendency to "know a lot" but do less. She is coaxing us away from our books. *Knowing* is of limited use, Joseph makes clear, unless we can develop from people who *read about* white supremacy to people who practice *being* anti-racists.

The class changed me (and us) irrevocably. It was not just what Joseph and coprofessor Jill Lewis said (1981), though their knowledge was formidable, but it was the process of our group living an experience together; being more than knowing. The affective currents that circulated among us changed us in ways not easily captured in language but registered as perpetual and perpetuating zingers. In the fishbowl of the classroom, we each became more fully alive. We absorbed, painfully, how power was unequally distributed according to race, culture, and sexuality, and that those distinctions shaped our shifting and fractal identities and our capacity to make personal/political change (Crenshaw 1991). What each of us could risk towards liberatory struggles—the forums we could enter or demonstrations we could stage or cites of power we could challenge (rage is a privilege)—laid bare our individual differences, as well as social, structural ones. An identity politic was not a fixed category but a way of seeing the world that takes account of who accumulates power and who is left behind.

This experience introduced me to intersectionality (Combahee 1983), and the idea that categories of race inalterably change categories of gender. At the time we applied the concept to a critique of white feminism, but it's since been more broadly applied as a means of thinking about sameness and difference and their relation to power. As the Combahee River Collective taught, categories are fluid, always permeated by other categories, "always in the process of creating and being created by dynamics of power" (Cho, Crenshaw, and McCall 2013, 795). The emphasis, in other words, is on what intersectionality *does* rather than what it is. Action was meaningful, knowing was deepening, and living through these radical encounters with difference was life-changing.

Psychoanalytic ideas entered my consciousness in 1983 when, just after I graduated from college, another favorite professor Margaret Cerullo gave me the unfinished manuscript for what would become Benjamin's (1988) *Bonds of Love*. Thinking through women's sexual subjectivity and agency added depth to my analysis of radical political movements (I had studied archival Black, Women, and Gay liberation newspapers from the late 1950s through the 1970s for my thesis), including the effect on the real-world relationships of desire that transformed the participants in the early Women's Liberation movement. Putting the projects together in graduate school allowed me to challenge the family as the exclusive site of the development of sexuality (as we were being taught) and augment that thinking with an awareness of how political movements could also be powerful venues for the development of intersubjectivity (Chapter 14). For me theories were more than just theories. Embodied, I used them to form my own adult relationships, endeavoring to hold autonomy and connection in tension and metabolize how recognition from a powerful other could augur sexual agency (Chapter 13). Psychoanalysis, a profession previously dusty in my mind, lit up. Desire was in the fore.

Feminism, anti-racism, and queer liberation were crucial influences as I entered psychoanalytic work. Harris and other feminist psychoanalysts had loosened the gender binary so firmly planted in psychoanalytic thought, introducing nonlinear systems theory and offering a view of the irreducible and determining influence of the social in the psychic (Dimen 2011). They challenged the centrality of heterosexuality, making room for the future work of queer and trans clinicians (Corbett, Hansbury, Saketopoulou). And they shined the spotlight on the power relations embedded in authority, putting the lie to the claim that theory was innocent, objective, neutral. Without this revolution in thought, I doubt I would have ever been enticed to enter psychoanalysis.

As with my formative classes in college, my psychoanalytic training was rigorous and rich. But the intellectual communities I became part of were charged, intimate spaces where learning and relationality were inextricably linked.

Who is left out

Reading through the lens of those who accumulate power and those who are left out, I was alerted to the question of who Ogden (2019) included as his immediate ancestors. I was particularly struck by the omission of Sandor Ferenczi and Edgar Levenson. Ferenczi focused on the heart of the analytic situation—the relationship between patient and analyst—conceptualizing it as an intersubjective exchange: a dialogue of the unconsciousness of two separate persons, each subject and object to the other (Aron and Harris 1993). He paved the way for a psychoanalysis in which clinical process trumps clinical knowing and being is constituted through relationship. This, in turn, anticipated much of the current focus on the role of the analyst's subjectivity and vulnerability, which I explore in this book as relevant to a more ontological psychoanalysis. Ferenczi's disagreements with Freud set the agenda for the contemporary debates between the ontological and epistemological perspectives: technique/metapsychology, experience/

insight, subjectivity/theory, empathy/interpretation, two-person/one-person psychology).

As for Levenson, he brought the Interpersonalist tradition to psychoanalysis in the 1970s, picking up the thread of Sullivan in the '50s. Levenson's work was part of a multidisciplinary paradigm shift that put "perspectivism and phenomenology, or connectedness and contextualization over certainty and hierarchical knowing" (Foehl 2008, 1234)—a course-change that has only widened and deepened over the last 50 years. He explicitly moved away from prioritizing the intrapsychic; critiqued the abstraction of metapsychology; questioned techniques hewing to abstract theory; challenged the primacy of interpretations of unconscious fantasy and transference; and eschewed objectivist understandings.

Certainty and uncertainty, analytic authority, and the myth of the separate self

Although Levenson was not one of my formative influences, he laid out several other principles that seem integral to an ontological sensibility and that undergird my project. These include the questioning of analytic certainty and the assumption that the analyst can understand and interpret clinical process for either her patient or herself, with the challenge to analytic authority that necessarily follows. The crumbling of the edifice of analytic knowing presaged the move toward the examination of clinical process and away from the search for (unknowable) causes for why things are the way they are for a person—a switch evident in Ogden's (2019) privileging the process of becoming more fully alive over focus on unconscious internal fantasy or object relations.[2]

Of course, Ogden may have innumerable reasons for leaving Levenson off his list, including aesthetic preference. Levenson's (1983) infamous question, "What's going on around here?" has a very different flavor from Ogden's (2019) "What do you want to be when you grow up?" Both of them put process before content and regard therapeutic action as "beyond understanding" (Foehl 2008, 1233). But Levenson stresses what is happening *between* the analyst and analysand because he rejects the Cartesian notion that there is a "self" separate from the interpersonal context. His interest in field phenomena, negative capacity, and "the flow of consciousness that underlies the therapeutic process" (Foehl 2017, 2) are also ideas I engage as essential to the ontological cast of my perspective.

By contrast, Ogden's (2019) question assumes the importance of the private, discrete nature of the self. He deeply appreciates Winnicott's extraordinary conceptualization of psychic growth as "weave[ing] other-than-me objects (people, poems, experiences) into the personal pattern" (Chapter 3). But, again, the pattern is "personal." In concordance with Winnicott (and Levenson 1983), Ogden does note the bidirectionality of psychic growth. The mother/analyst needs to have a mind that responds to the mind of the baby/patient, but he ultimately swerves away from the logical extension of his theorizing: the inevitable and continuous interpenetrating mix-up that is a main theme of the chapters that follow.

To see how the differences in theorizing manifest, consider Ogden's (2019) discussion of the possibility that growth might stall if either analyst or analysand struggles to enter a state of playing. If the analyst identifies himself as the source of the trouble, "the situation would likely require that the analyst return to analysis (p. 666). But that implies that the analyst can "know" where the problem lies and that an individual, historical cause can be uncovered (in the person of the psychoanalyst), which flips us back into the realm of one-person theories and epistemology: a "problem" is knowable, fixable, and produced outside of its context.

By suggesting an individual solution to the problem, Ogden moves from the radical implications of the shift from knowing to being. Imagining certainty is understandably seductive, because without it, analysts confront a thorny technical problem: How can we be part of a field that includes the unknowable and the negative *and* be its interpreter? How can we be full participants in the field while also acknowledging that our role as psychoanalysts sets up an asymmetry of responsibilities?

The view that therapeutic action involves providing an interpersonal context in which "previously unimaginable" forms of experiencing emerge (Ogden 2019) points, in my estimation, to the field as both the point of study and the location of resolution in the search for the play that's gone missing.

I think Ogden (2019) is getting close to an obliteration of some borders when he introduces Bion's (1967) idea that being

> supplant[s] understanding; the analyst does not come to know or understand or comprehend or apprehend the reality of what is happening in the session, he 'intuits' it, he becomes 'at one' with it, he is fully present in experiencing the present moment.
>
> (p. 670)

This is the radical potential of Ogden's ontological framing: creating a different kind of horizontal encounter with the other. Of course, knowing—however we might come to it, including unconscious communication—is imbricated in being. The epistemological and ontological are inseparable and exist in a dialectical relationship, as Ogden (2019) underscores. But I want to go further to suggest that the *being* I find most clinically expansive is a *being with* such that the subjectivities of analyst and patient are less distinct and can't be disentangled.

Developmentally speaking, experiencing aliveness, Ogden tells us, happens with the real mother, who is not a person distinct from the baby (Winnicott 1971a). While a mother has capacities her baby does not, her baby's subjectivity is a *process* inseparable from the mother and the surround. And, if we proceed from that premise, how do we reconceive the analytic frame and stance when psyche, Ogden reminds us, is not a *thing* to be built but a process, an experiencing of "imaginative aliveness" (Ogden 2023, 9)? In fact, the ontological turn suggests psyche and soma (and by inference subjectivity) are not nouns at all, but verbs (Winnicott 1949).

The emotional truth of a situation, to use Bion's language, will be found between us, not inside us. For me, rooting our work in perspectivism and phenomenology, connectedness and contextualization, precludes a certain kind of personal sovereignty, analytic authority, and belief in the separateness of selves. When the analyst's inability to know herself isn't fully acknowledged or embodied, the ontological approach is denuded.

Nonsovereignty

While the idea of nonsovereignty isn't new, its far-reaching clinical implications need elaboration. In place of the familiar psychoanalytic concept of subjectivity, I use the words *sovereignty* and *nonsovereignty* as employed by literary and cultural theorists Berlant and Edelman (2014) (Edelman is also a psychoanalyst) because their language minimizes the primacy of analytic self-knowledge, authority, and self-control. What is foregrounded instead is our fundamental misrecognition of ourselves—and it's not just our unconscious selves that elude our grasp. Aspects of being that exist outside the realm of representation (Chapter 15) have been only barely formulated by psychoanalysts.

Relinquishing the expectation of a reified, self-contained, sovereign subject suggests we are shaped not only through our personal history and intergenerational inheritance but also through the affects that pass between us in the present, making us open and vulnerable to each other and to experiences that cannot always be represented (Chapter 16). Adopting an ontological clinical paradigm thus requires a complete revision of our thinking about individual history, symptoms, relationships, and the psychoanalytic encounter. And it emphasizes the interdependent ways we are connected as humans to all living creatures and to earth itself (Levenson 1972, 220). This is the work the Intersubjectivists like Stolorow, Atwood, and Orange began decades ago (Stolorow and Atwood 1992; Stolorow, Atwood, and Orange 2002).

Gone missing

I raise Ogden's (2019) exclusion of Ferenczi and Levenson not to say that they got there first and go unacknowledged, nor to express my wish for theorists to talk to one another across separate, siloed schools of thought and practice, though I want that fiercely. Rather I raise it as a window into the larger issue of how we tell our stories, whether historical or clinical, and what and who doesn't make the cut. Historically, Interpersonal and Relational theorists were the banished stepchildren of psychoanalysis; they were believed to focus too little on the unconscious and too much on process. That changed somewhat when Object Relational and Bionian analysts came to write about analysis as an intersubjective process and to value the way the unconscious lives in the field and within the flow in the room. But Interpersonal and Relational schools still go unacknowledged despite the gravitation toward the principles they've long articulated.

While Ogden (2019) writes that his paper is "an account of the movement in my own thinking" (p. 663), it is inevitably more. He is one of our most widely read and admired contemporary psychoanalysts, and his inimitable voice necessarily and deservedly holds authority. He has put his finger on the pulse of the current moment and given it a new name—at least new in psychoanalysis (often decades behind other disciplines). Illustrated with close clinical process, his article is already defining for the profession, and for me too. Wittingly or not, Ogden has also established a history of who counts as our great original ontological thinkers. In fact, his 2019 paper will likely become the article-of-record for characterizing the sea-change underway in how we conceptualize and do clinical work, because Ogden wrote it and because he centers Bion's and Winnicott's contributions.

When our most renowned thinkers cite only our most renowned thinkers, other ideas are foreclosed or, at least, not developed (Ahmed 2017). Never reading or engaging—or worse, subtracting or erasing—voices that have been ignored by mainstream psychoanalysis—has ethical consequences. It echoes early displacements of thinkers deemed too politically risky, like Ferenczi, who is perhaps our earliest ontological psychoanalyst. Historically, such ostracism has had a deleterious effect on the expansion of psychoanalytic ideas. I hope for a contemporary psychoanalysis that disassembles its siloed schools and intradisciplinary purity.

Another way to tell this story

If I were to tell the story of the development of an ontological psychoanalysis, I might base it in feminist and queer theory, for which being is a fundamental mode of knowing (Chapter 4). I'd start by borrowing from feminist scientist Haraway's (1991) "diffractive" methodology, through which we locate ourselves in our entanglement with the other, a theme amplified throughout this book (and which I've already begun to do in my tangle and untangle with Ogden, a beloved thinker to me). Following Haraway's lead, we'd look closely at psychoanalysis' heterogeneous history, show how each branch of our field changes, contributes, and detracts from what we are calling an ontological sensibility.

The school that probably most manifests this comparative and braided methodology is the Relational. Relationalists have directly employed Haraway's diffractive methodology, and though they've sought unifying themes, they've at least begun an examination of a "history of interaction, interference, reinforcement, difference" among these bodies of thought (Dolphijn and van der Tuin 2012, 51).[3] An analysis of systemic racism in psychoanalysis that draws on critical race theory and social criticism is broadening the canon further. Barad, using Haraway, writes, "Diffractions do not displace the same elsewhere, in more or less distorted form, thereby giving rise to industries of [story-making about origins and truths]. Rather, diffraction can be a metaphor for another kind of critical consciousness" (Dolphin and van der Tuin 2012, 51). I love this idea. The implication is that differences are engaged for how they might sharpen one's own thought and encourage new ways of seeing and being with the other—my own thinking always emerges in dialogue with others. Cooper (2007, 2014) captures this in his notion of a pluralistic third and use of bridge theory to compare concepts across schools. Thinking in a diffractive mode brings in perspectives that have been excluded—a principle gaining in importance as psychoanalysts finally acknowledge that social oppressions are interpellated in the unconscious.

In this moment of racial reckoning—where we are learning much about who writes history (usually history's "victors") and how a story is told—I want us to be prodigious with our citations. Casting a wide net in our efforts to re-vision what has been a narrow psychoanalysis potentially creates a much bigger "we." Of course, some voices cannot be gathered up at all, because our field has drawn such a rigid boundary around who gets to be a psychoanalyst. With nonwhite communities consistently omitted from our understanding of the universal, there are sites of erasure and silence that must be part of our collective work of translation (Chapter 10). While the last ten years have seen more writing from Black psychoanalysts such as Holmes, Jones, Lewis, Pogue Whyte, Powell, Stephens, and Stoute, to name some, the century before suffered from the whiteness and exclusivity of the profession.

Importantly, and ironically, the very use of the word ontology as a philosophical perspective has been heavily criticized for its failure to take up the problem of Blackness and being. Black thinkers have been arguing that the term "human" can't encompass Blackness in an anti-Black world and have described the terror of living outside "the precincts of humanity and humanism" (Warren 2018, 4). Wilderson (2020) notes that Black people inhabit a metaphysical "nothing," against which white people define themselves, and that humanism is thus based on investing Blacks with nonbeing (Wilderson 2020). Blackness remains co-determinate with slavery, as Afropessimists such as Wilderson (2020) and Hartman (1997) explicate. This may offer one answer as to why, for example, the violence directed toward Black life can't be eliminated even after it is exposed; Black people fail to register as beings who can be hurt.

> In other words, the mind would have to see a person with a heritage of rights and claims, whose rights and claims are being violated. This is not the way Slaves, Blacks, function in the collective unconscious. Who ever heard of an injured plow?
>
> (Wilderson 2020, 225)

Within psychoanalysis, the term ontology is relatively new and will be deeply suspect if we do not interrogate its exclusion of Blackness.

The idea that we psychoanalysts might speak not just from what we know but from what we don't has become almost a cliché (it was not when I began my project in 2000). I'm hoping that a growing profession will help make "not knowing" less an ideal and more part of clinical practice, as I try to show in my own work in the following chapters. Embracing this principle, we expand not just our theory but the process of being with each other in diverse communities of thinkers (Chapter 10). Engaging absences and discarded presences gets at a key idea of this book: speaking from the register of not knowing allows creative transformations to occur, sometimes in ways that disrupt order, time, and stability. Or not. Perhaps this ontology is what Foucault names as an "untamed ontology," an ontology that lies "on the other side of all things that are" and "even beyond those that can be" (Halberstam 2020, 12) (Chapter 14). The ontological psychoanalysis I imagine includes "the space rendered by the absence of meaning and direction" (Halberstam 2020, 14).

Ontological clinical work or what I learned from what I couldn't accomplish

Each of the major clinical papers in the book—and specifically *how* they are written—tries to imagine a way of analytic being and writing that honor what is enigmatic and beyond our grasp. Centering analytic vulnerability, vertigo, and nonsovereignty, the clinical chapters can be understood as an effort to see what I have learned from what I *couldn't* create with another. The clinical illustrations are engagements with patients whose anguish is communicated not through *what* is said but how it is said, "its force or the emotional music, the para-verbal qualities of rhythm, pitch, force, volume . . ." (Levine 2023). In early chapters, my observations about analytic participation, what it actually entails, were based on hunches emerging from the vertigo of the clinical work. The later chapters benefit from the increased *theorizing* about enactments arising out of deficits in representational capacity. Howard Levine, who has helped elucidate unrepresented states that leave patients awash in affect storms and prone to impulsive actions and somatic discharge (Levine 2013, 2022), believes that representation requires binding, containment, and transformation of these primal energies. In cases where the difficulties lie beyond neurosis, the analyst's task is to lend her alpha function to patients to help them build their psychic structures. The end product of that work, Levine argues (2022), is expected to take the form of representations that become the building blocks of potentially communicable thoughts and ideas.

Yet if we are working from a more ontological slant and think of psyche not as a reified thing to be built but as a process inseparable from us, do we need a new way of thinking, playing, and writing? The analyst must be capable of being disturbed enough to *feel with* the patient and at the same time sane enough to think with or for her, until her own ability to think becomes established. Yes that, but also the analyst is the patient, too.

In fact, there is a growing sense among analysts that their own strain and burden are in some ways necessary to the treatment of poorly symbolized states. But the pain of the work is rarely described. We have focused on managing the countertransference, but often only as an instrument for the accurate and detailed observation of the other. While attending to the affective states that register inside of us may indeed be enormously useful to gather information about patients, countertransferential considerations alone are inadequate to understand the analyst's experience. For me, the concept is both too "one person" and too "two person" to really address a clinical situation characterized by an always moving, bidirectional unconscious field (see Chapter 2). Of course, I am not the only one who believes that. Field theorists both Bionian and Relational have all substantially moved toward thinking about the bidirectional nature of the analytic process.

But even the notion of the field relies on an analyst's reading or narrating or servicing it (Chapter 15), as if we can stand apart from the interpenetrating mix-up of self and other, a more unidirectional form of therapeutic action. In field theory we only hear of turbulence that begins with the patient and flows to the analyst—obscuring what can't be represented and ignoring the clinician's inability to know herself, even as the theory acknowledges that. This implicit sovereignty not only shrouds the unconscious symmetry between patient and analyst but also strengthens the hard-to-shake belief in a knowing self, separate from other selves. And it downplays the creativity born of destruction: breaking up old meanings to allow reconfiguring.

I argue that when the analyst primarily demonstrates competence and does not reveal the dissolution of the links of her own mind, or her negative capability, possibilities that emerge from *living together*, each unbearably alone, in a shared, contained entropy are foreclosed. I came to view the analyst's extraordinary efforts to reach her patient as requiring her to work from places of unknowing, to engage the "breach" of her own trauma, sometimes from its unsymbolized realm (Chapters 2, 7, 9). As you will hear in the cases I present, there is an evolution from patient and analyst *relating* to their *living together* within a cocreated process neither could have imagined by themselves.

Unrepresented states, which always exist in dialectical tension with symbolization, concentrate our attention on the power of what is unmarked (Phelan 1994). Keeping the negative alive as a concept helps us value sensing and perceiving, and alerts us to something not there, to be felt, whatever that might be. More and more, I attend to the energy that thrums between and around us, unbounded in space and time and beyond our perceptual range, creating chaos and excess but also potential and creativity. This energy makes manifests the enigmatic and interrupts the fixity of identity (Berlant and Edelman 2014). Encountering the negative, we disrupt our sovereignty (Chapter 15). This book is one effort to think through what a deeply entwined self, other, and world might mean for the analyst's therapeutic method, action, ethics, and, finally, writing.

Ontological writing and art and painting in particular

If we believe in the ontological slant's intrinsic value that for transformative work to happen we need to be "at one with" our patients in a shared *unknown* psychic reality that has not come into being (Bion 1967; McGleughlin 2015a; Ogden 2016), our writing has not kept pace. Clinical stories are expressions of our own theories, experience, modes of understanding, and interpreting—clinical data constituted rather than encountered (Schafer 1980). They're, in fact, fictions, but presented as both historical and narrative truth (Spence 1984), and they retain a sharp divide between subject and object and convey our unquestioned authority. There is little room for the analyst's *nonsovereignty*; we are invested in our belief that we know ourselves and tell it like it is (McGleughlin 2015a). Yet knowing that a clinical story is a shared experience of patient and analyst, how do we speak without othering, surveying from the outside? Our writing is influenced by a "network of constraints and censorship" (Johnson 1998, 168) through which we edit out multiplicity, sensation, and incoherence. In the name of clarity, we privilege the objectivity and linearity that can be anathema to the work. As soon as I start to tell you about a case, I stand outside it and assume an interpretative authority that robs you of being in an experience in which you might come more fully alive.

Instead of this kind of writing, I want to invite you into that Winnicottian (1971b) overlap of two people playing, such that reader and writer who were "unable to play before . . . [are] brought into a state of being able to play" (p. 38). But how?

The collected essays span 2000–2021 and elaborate on the central problem of how to engage patients and ourselves when verbal representation fails. How to enter that scene of breach with our patients and then how to involve the reader/listener? Using film, visual art, and a range of theory, you will see that themes of how we tell a clinical story, how we bring the reader affectively into that story (enacted writing), the necessary vertigo and the necessary nonsovereignty of the analyst, and the creative and generative potential of the negative each take the stage as we think about the place the analyst reaches from.

This is also a book about how we tell the clinical story of the other. How we tell these stories matters a great deal. To these ends, I offer a series of overlapping clinical and at times personal stories to help us think about new ways of being with our patients—what we might have once called technique—through different ways of being with you, my readers. Rather than employ writing that "impress(es) itself upon a wiggling world like a snap-grid of shape-setting interpretability" (Gregg and Seigworth 2010, 4) or leading with my authority, my intention is to trouble the analyst's sovereignty as theoretician, clinician, and writer. Experimental writing that evokes our own vulnerability may be one way to engage our own nonsovereignty.

While I attempt a different kind of assemblage and decentering weighted toward the reader's involvement with the text, it is hard to write in experimental forms. I had hoped to create a shared sensory experience that manifests the limits of representation and highlights *perceiving* characteristic of the work and writing of someone like Agnes Martin (Chapter 15 and 16), but we will have to count on her for that! Still, rather than reading forward toward putative ends, I urge a more process-oriented experience.

The way I've put this book together creates its own kind of narrative, a personal one, that allows you to trace the development of my thinking about clinical storytelling and experience it in action—as it opens up. As you will see, my thinking begins with the idea of the difficult-to-reach patient but quickly develops to think about the difficult-to-reach analyst. Yet a focus on the subjectivity of either patient or analyst ultimately falls short, and I invite you to move with me across genres, disciplines, and modes of writing as I consider the multiplicity of forces and engagements of the analytic field. The *process of joining me* through the book as I lay out the evolution in my thinking and practice may be as useful as the content of any one chapter itself.

Yet my book can also be entered anywhere. At the beginning of each major section, I detail its core themes and introduce individual chapters. You will find some inevitable repetition as I make different efforts to capture complex ideas. But in truth, like Marie, I want to bring you everywhere I've been in the hopes that if you live it with me, you can come to see it as I do. I want you to know how I got from here to there. I *don't* want to metabolize everything first and feed it back to you. I hold a powerful fantasy that if I drag you along with me, you can be where I am.

Still, you have your own mind, internal objects, ways of anticipating, and this is necessarily so. In writing, we are always staging an encounter with an other. Every telling is a kind of performance (McGleughlin 2015b). Whether or not we are self-disclosing, we are showing more than we know, telling a story about ourselves as if it were only about the other.

When we acknowledge the performativity of our writing, we upend our telling of the other's story as if it were theirs. Instead, experience is lived in and through the subjectivity of the reader/observer, disrupting traditional notions of who is viewed and who is viewer: we invest the image with "the ability to look at us in return" Benjamin (1935/2008). Movement is less through the trajectory of time and more though reflective, interactive seeing/experiencing, moving/being moved states, writer to reader, reader to writer. The instability of form that never claims to represent the real and is always changing reflects the instability and timelessness of subjectivity. Artist Marlene Dumas says it this way: "When involved in an exchange with a person or a thing, even just a line, you are not only an 'I' but also a 'Me.'" What *me* do we then see in such an exchange? Forms of art and artistic forms of writing can privilege what we don't know and allow for emergent possibility between writer and reader and within readers. This is psychoanalytic telling as art; it gives "the gift of implication" (Smith 2013).

If psychoanalytic writing is its own kind of landscape, there exists a history, a geography with which we must contend. As Swartz (2019) writes in reference to removing racist monuments on her South African university campus, landscapes

> are alive with meaning and ferociously signal not only their history but also their claims to future time. They become the setting for resisting change to historical narratives; for this reason, they also represent barriers to change in the search for new perspectives on both histories and future possibilities.
>
> (p. 169)

I think of analytic writing as such a landscape or monument: it has been a taken-for-granted, solid background for the development of theory. And yet "it is neither solid nor continuous [nor, I would add, scientific] and is always enmeshed with the phantastic and phantomic" (p. 168). The demolishing of a monument "ruptures [and] shakes the solidity of an imaginary" (p. 168).

To sever analytic writing from its ghosts requires a change in the symbolic. This might happen when alternative narratives supplant traditional theorizing in our social unconscious (González 2009). And we imagine new ways of living and loving and telling our stories. New narratives require new thinking, often born from disruption as opposed to assimilation, a rather queer way of seeing (Ahmed 2019). I hope for a vitalized psychoanalytic storytelling tradition that reflects the growth of the field and that challenges existing power relationships between the see-er and the person who is being seen.

Painting

One last story.

I am a (very) novice painter.

"I started again; where everything starts: the body". (Anne Michaels (2001, 87)).

The source of light is the painter's body," writes the poet Anne Michaels (2001, 83).

Right. OK. We are the source of light, but it is no small task to be that light. Objects turn out not to be hats or life jackets or noses or parallel lines or the color red. They are triangles and missing spaces, light and shadow. Every mark changes every other. Each line you paint rearranges the one before and must be reworked in relation to the next. Mark, erase, mark, repeat. Repetition is our effort to get it right, closer to the thing, to sense its values, shapes, tone, and affective moment. It is harrowing.

And humbling. The teacher tells me, "Jade, a box is made up of straight lines." I say, "That is my straight line," and we circle.

I was in my fifties that I began to paint for the first time. After participating in an interdisciplinary group studying psychoanalysis and the visual image, I wanted to try my hand. Never an artist, representational oil painting seemed like a stretch. I couldn't even doodle, much less draw. Yet my work as a psychoanalyst had propelled me to want to play visually with what can't quite be captured in language. And being a psychoanalyst actually prepared me to paint. It wasn't just the long hours of observation of people but also being immersed in an experience of the enigmatic message of the other living in each of us. Then, too, my own long psychoanalysis, and the process of the work included in this book, had given me a different sense of being alive. Early messages that I couldn't cut or paste or color in the lines gave way to news of difference. Seeing my paintings emerge was the first time I didn't feel counterfeit. Here they were, and they had to be mine. Something showed up across the body of my work, in every painting. I had a style, undeniably visible and yet outside my conscious mind. It seemed it wasn't just performative or recycled (of course it was) but the accumulation of something in me, over there but always changing.

Tracing my own movement across time, I can see the way I have become and am becoming.

And the way I am undone. Some paintings will accompany us as the book unfolds.

Notes

1 In a footnote, Ogden explains that he can't comment on all analysts who have influenced this orientation but includes a list of twenty. He contrasts them with those who represent the epistemological tradition, principally Freud and Klein, who privilege knowing and understanding.
2 Bromberg (1998, 2002, 2006) wrote significantly from these perspectives as well, brokering new ways to think about the unconscious and centering a way of working that relies on object relations but also clinically shifts therapeutic action from the importance of knowing to the importance of being, especially of sensing.
3 Some psychoanalysts criticize Greenberg and Mitchell (1983) for who they left out and for underemphasizing Winnicott's crucial contribution to notions of relationality (Cooper 2021).

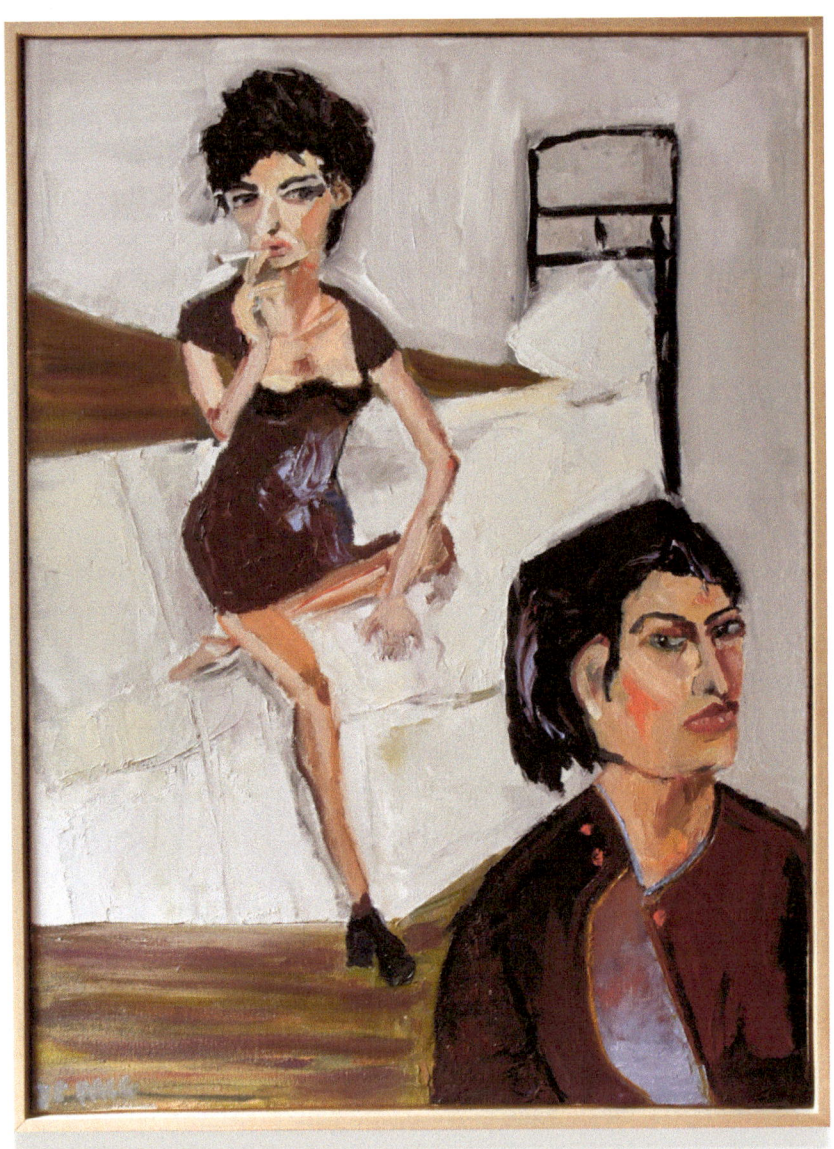

Figure Pl.1 Dust Ruffle. Oil on canvas. 20x 24. McGleughlin

Part 1

The analyst's necessary vertigo (2011)

Introduction

In the spring of 2000, I began an extraordinary analysis with a patient I call Sarah. Much of the treatment did not exist in the register of language. I learned through a powerful symbiotic drama what Sarah could not yet know, feel, or remember in words. The two of us co-created that drama, and most intensely experienced it when Sarah stopped speaking during our sessions—for months at a time, five days a week. Time became psychotic time. There were no facts, no history, no grounding narrative to hold onto. The treatment was the most tumultuous of my career, in part because of what the sustained and agitated silence did to me. Almost every paper I write connects in some way to that baffling, shaping experience, in which I felt I came as close to an objectless existence—the void at the center—as humanly possible (for me).

Now I think the juxtaposition between the slow, still, sometimes utterly silent work and the cacophony of sounds it gave rise to within me attuned me to "a state of things which, contrary to appearances, continues to exist even when the sense cannot perceive it, not only in the external world, but in the internal world consciousness" (Green 1999, 16). That radical shift into silence allowed a concentration on absence in a form and frequency I had never known: waves, rhythms, cycles of feeling vibrating in a liminal zone suspended out of time and space. In the years following the treatment, I've come to wonder if the kinds of waves and vibrations I sensed in the presence of Sarah may be resonances of perceptions from our earliest infancy before perceptions are located and/or locatable. We do not remember them, as they are not stored in our verbal or narrative memory. Rather, they live in our bodies.

DOI: 10.4324/9781032670348-2

What happened to me with Sarah might resemble what Shaw (2006) calls the post-modern sublime. He describes it as a state in which we are defeated in our ability "to apprehend, know or express a thought or sensation" (p. 3), and in which "experience slips out of conventional understanding . . . such that words fail . . . points of comparison disappear" (p. 2). We are thrown into "the absolutely unknowable void, upon whose brink we finite beings must dizzily hover" (Milbank 2004, quoted in Shaw 2006, 3). In that defeat, forces overtake us, and something beyond representation—but largely defined by the limits of representation—captures and transports us beyond the confines of our own consciousness. I have struggled to make positive use of the ineffable experience of this work.

I refer to this experience of being buffeted by powerful, unknowable forces as contacting "the negative." What does this look and feel like in treatment? How does it impact the ways in which we respond to our patients when there is not yet a patient-self to whom we can relate? I further elaborate this idea of the negative in Part 4.

The first paper in Part 1, "The Analyst's Necessary Vertigo," written in 2008, attempts to address my shift from an idea of the difficult-to-reach patient to the difficult-to-reach analyst. I argue that to reach/build some patients' sense of self (and eventually of the other) may require clinicians to "reach" toward a place of corresponding deficit in themselves, to sink into the foundations of their own (non)being. While some theorists might consider such a move a product of the analyst's own pathology or self-protective omnipotence, I argue that extraordinary efforts may be necessary to meet some patients' needs.

If "The Analyst's Necessary Vertigo" can be understood structurally as the "bones" of Part 1, Chapter 2, "Love letter to a patient or the raw story" may be its thrumming heart. It conveys my own free-form inner dialogue, parsed with excerpts from the novel *The Passion* (1989), by Jeanette Winterson, and fragments of poetry—all meant to convey an experience I could not narrate in more conventional form; that is to say, the feeling of drowning, inchoate sensation, and whirling vertigo that sometimes accompanied Sarah's treatment. This was my graduation paper from psychoanalytic training, and though I have presented it and tinkered with it countless times for over 22 years, I come back to the original here without a lot of the theory. Perhaps this is what it is to attempt to write about the experience of "the negative" with a patient, where time is no time at all.

Both "Vertigo" and "The Raw Story" are early efforts to metabolize this difficult treatment by writing outside of a strictly "objective" form of psychoanalytic writing. I wrote "Vertigo" (2008/2011) after "The Raw Story" (2001), but here the later paper appears first. It may seem odd to hear reflections on a case before reading it. I ordered the chapters this way to offer ballast to you, the reader, because "The Raw Story" is so filled with my own unsteadiness. Likely I want to shore up your sense of me as a robust and reliable analyst/writer.

When I wrote "The Raw Story" in 2001, I wasn't consciously trying to draw the reader into the affective states I suffered, but to steady myself against the lonely vertigo of the work. Later, presenting the piece, I inadvertently learned that reading my unmetabolized "telling" could in fact *enact* the feeling of drowning in the chaos of the case. In 2001, a visiting British analyst called "Raw Story" "performance art," registering his protest against reading the work as psychoanalysis. That felt wrong, but I couldn't quite defend myself.

While ideas about the necessity of undergoing the situation with our patients in live, enacted experience, and/or "the field contracting the patient's illness" (Ferro and Civitarese 2013), were less formulated then, 20 years later it is clear that in cases of very archaic trauma, creating/recreating and living in more sensory and sometimes enacted states with our patients may be necessary when their experience is outside symbolic representation. Elements of early trauma show themselves in action where intolerable affects may shift back and forth, shareable and unshareable, toxic and mutative, like the queen of spades in a game of Old Maid (Davies 2004).

Today, I am more confident that draining the tumultuous vertigo of the case from the writing would not convey the case's clinical imperatives, and that, in fact, performative writing might be an important addition to our psychoanalytic canon (see Chapter 4). Still, on any given day, I can veer from worry about allowing you, the reader, into such an intimate, vulnerable experience with that 2001 me, to shame about wanting to drag you along in the melodrama of the writing, to reinvigorated belief in the importance of the analyst sharing her world. And I hope that for my patients this raw, unprocessed material in their analyst will not cause vertigo of its own.

In the next two pieces of Part 1, "Afterword(s) on writing: we always tell it slant" and "Afterword(s) on technique: the necessary reach," I move us out of this dreaming space into a waking one—from "punctum" to "studium" (as defined and elaborated in "Vertigo"). How can we think about experimental writing and the fiction of our supposedly more objective case reports? Is there more to understand about the narration of this treatment now that you, too, have experienced something of this work in "the negative" with Sarah? I am interested in the pedagogical insights to be gathered in the case's wreckage, and also its pleasures.

In "Afterword(s) on writing," I explain why I'm telling you Sarah's story in multiple registers: the more "objective" (yet for psychoanalytic writing, still relatively loose) approach of the "Vertigo"; the feeling-laden, wide-ranging "Raw Story," which is something like a journal kept to hold onto myself during the intensely difficult and bewildering treatment; and, finally, the "Afterword(s) on technique," which steps back to consider how I did what I did and the theoretical underpinnings that guided me and, sometimes, left me wanting. There I draw on two relational supervisions to tease out more about analytic stance, formulation, and clinical approach. I compare a self-psychological-relational approach and a more object-relational approach, highlighting tensions between techniques in greater depth than in "The Analyst's Necessary Vertigo."

My goal is not to bombard you with repetitive information but to demonstrate that *how* we tell a story determines the reader's understanding of the characters and meanings. This, in turn, leads to a major theme of this book, that our writing does not so much describe the truths of a case but creates them. This is not *Rashomon*—you only have my take, at times informed by "experts"—and that's also the point, to emphasize the analyst's power as narrator, the possibilities and dangers.

Finally, in Chapter 5, "Two Case Vignettes: How Sarah Helped Me Help Troy and Christina," I apply some of the generative learning from my work with Sarah.

As you will see, in all five of these early chapters, my theoretical focus is on the patient's psyche, transference, projections, and intrapsychic conflict. I unpack my own countertransference and use of self as I confront the difficulties of understanding this case through the framework of intersubjective relating and relationality. But when I wrote all these pieces, I had not yet begun to conceive of patient and analyst as part of a *bidirectional field*, within which all the significant phenomena must be considered in their bipersonal dimension. (see Part 2.) Moreover, while these chapters contain building blocks for a therapeutic stance and style that privileges *being* over *knowing* and the analyst's nonsovereignty, I had not yet consciously developed my thinking about more ontological styles of working, where inner and outer, self and other, are more entangled. I *felt* that entanglement, but I still felt shame about it. As difficult and sometimes heartbreaking the work with Sarah was, it has shaped my way of thinking, perceiving, and feeling, and my capacity to be in relation.

Chapter 1

The analyst's necessary vertigo (2008/2011)

I want help with something heavy, and I turn to my 16-year-old son. He says without rancor, "I refuse to help you, but I project my most helpful thoughts towards you." I'm startled. Where did he get this idea? Is this unconscious identification with what it means to be an analyst? Have I engendered this cheekiness?

At first irritated, I am soon delighted by his wry remark, his deadpan delivery, his adolescent assertion, and I feel much better as I make my way down several flights of stairs to haul up the wood. I am smiling, contained, accompanied, chuckling, set free from my own demands, my nagging mother voice. He has done a lot lately. But on my way back up, my elbows tug. I can feel my months of physical therapy give way, tendons pulled again, too far. Snap. My arms give, the wood drops. I can't do it. I need his help. Real help.

Max's comments briefly held open a space of play, of boundaried self and separate other, a different kind of mother/son relation. But this position grows more complicated with each upward step, breaks down in my old body, in the impossibility of the task, in my genuine helplessness.

What does it mean to help our most difficult-to-reach patients? What does "difficult to reach" mean? Does this language convey a broad attitude toward a patient? Are we drawing attention to a group of patients who are challenging? Is this not-so-ordinary analytic language of "difficult to reach" descriptive? Evasive? Does it aim to skirt pathologizing language, or does it subtly re-pathologize the patient, locating the problem in the individual? Is it one-person psychology? Or is it a comment on the analyst's suffering? Does this shift in language, euphemistic as it is, suggest inadequacy in our method? Are we suggesting that something different is required of us? A different kind of reach? Reach means to extend as far as; to come to; to pass or give something; to make movement toward; to arrive at or get to; to

DOI: 10.4324/9781032670348-3

strive or yearn; to stretch. It is an act of going toward. What does it mean for the analyst to reach? And how far? Who among us wants to claim reach as our therapeutic action?

Take my patient John. He only knows I am really in it with him if I jump far outside my way. He wants me to feel the danger of what it is like to be him, the precarious way he keeps on going from the wreckage of mayhem and disaster to something off-balance, tilted, but generative. He wants to feel me open to this demand to live here with him, at the brutal pace of falling, in the tender intimacy of the catch. He wants me to feel the invitation of his desire to be alive; the way a hundred nerve endings sing electric when the arm is twisted. He wants the bruise, needs the resolve of my ministrations. Likes this pitch. When he eats cake, he prefers the cherry (Aeroplane 2010). He likes the deepness of penetration, the tangled-up nature of limbs and psyches. Is this memory? Wish? Enactment? Is this me who calls this out? As Friedman (2005) noted, "When you are dealing with emotional memory (procedural memory, non-declarative memory) you are not just dealing with the pattern of behavior, or even the form of wishes; you are dealing with the form of the you" (p. 422). Friedman means, I think, that the psychoanalytic discovery of transference throws into question which me John wants and which me I am.

In this liminal space, I try to "take the transference," try to live in John's need of this certain me that causes me to stretch past my safety. How much, Friedman asked, can we be what a patient wants us to be and still impel him to change? (p. 422). I do this, allow myself to be in this mix-up with awareness of risk and the possibility—the inevitability of enactment and, I hope, reflection.

And if I dare to speak his way? Freud tells us, according to Phillips (2006), that to speak is to articulate one's wants, to make known to oneself what is absent . . . and the performance of wanting, in mood, in language, in action puts one's life in danger. There is the danger of punishment . . . (castration) and the danger of acknowledged dependence, and the potential for loss (p. 18).

This seems like a lot to do as the analyst. I live off-balance. I live in fear of the excess in this reach.

John lives in the other side of my fear. He fears what Barthes (1980), in discussing a certain group of well-composed photographs, called *studium*: a visual concept, a way of seeing the image that evokes commitment or interest without acuity; unconcerned desire on the order of liking, not loving;

an interest that comes from one's training or culture; a kind of education that allows one to discover the picture taker, the intentions that motivate or animate his practice, but as spectator. John wants to make me exist not as someone on the outside, but as participant. He fears he is someone I take analytic interest in, compassion for, studium. He wants to be what Barthes called *punctum*: in photographs, the visual detail that stands out, the thing that disturbs the image.

Barthes wrote about seeing and being seen prior to, or outside of language: studium and punctum are ways of looking and being looked at. They hold the tension between language and image. And, indeed, John wants more than my speech. Like Barthes, John wants to evoke a different kind of mood. My words are not communications except of this: they are conveyors of my way of seeing him.

John wants me to see him his way. He wants to be someone who stirs internal agitation, who creates "the pressure of the unspeakable that wants to be spoken" (Barthes 1980, 19). He wants to penetrate, animate my unspeakable in speech with him. He wants to be the punctum, the thing that disturbs, the piercing.

Certainly, all patients have the potential to pierce us. Perhaps it is even our job to look for and to be open to the way each patient has the ability to move us, touch us, whether or not they ever do (H. Morris, personal communication, March 3, 2011). And in many treatments, there is oscillation between a background of good, solid analytic work (studium) and arresting moments described in a variety of different analytic languages (punctum). Or within a lot of studium, there is always the potential for punctum. These concepts live in dialectical tension. Still, sometimes, whole treatments are characterized less by movement between studium and punctum, and more by the analyst's vertigo. By wound. John and a few other of my patients' analyses are dominated by punctum; the reach requires something from me that feels dangerous, moving, painful, deeply involving. Does this deeply affected me do better work? Does punctum help or hurt? Dialectic abounds and confounds.

About ten years ago, I began presenting my most difficult-to-reach patient to every consultant I could think of. My patient was brilliant. She had a quiet, contained, humble intelligence that permeated her being and moved me deeply. I desperately wanted to help her through her pain, and yet I couldn't. There was a tormenting dread and fragile beauty that permeated the atmosphere and lived in me in a vise grip of punctum.

My strong sense of her goodness and integrity were lost on her because she could not locate herself, her thoughts, her feelings, and I could not "find her." I was often reaching to her, and offering my mind and my feelings as a bridge to her mind. Sometimes I felt I was registering her affective states as they came to be known in me, and other times I was just looking for a point of entry. The work was grueling. I had never encountered such pain, loneliness, inaccessibility, and inability. And I had never felt so deregulated. My tremendous effort and willingness to offer, yield, wait, risk, endure, and reach were not experienced as such. She said she felt nothing from me and that I did not register in her mind. She told me, "You hide. What you risk is what you value." I was shocked by this reversal, given how much of the treatment took place in the playing ground of my mind and how vulnerable and overexposed I felt.

Episodes of connection occasionally led to a deepening of the treatment, but just as often they led to her violent self-attacks that I did not learn about until later. So I would feel exquisite pleasure in our rare moments of meeting, but she would feel nauseous and sick. It was disorienting to discover that my pleasure was her pain.

Her inability at times to put even the most rudimentary words to her experience meant that the work that took place in our individual psyches only became known through the roller-coaster action between us at these disastrous disjunctures. She would tell me I was a dementor sucking the life force from her, that she could not breathe in the air I breathed out. She often withdrew, and the longer her silence, sometimes five days a week for months, the more I felt erased, even annihilated. Yet she told me I didn't exist enough for her silences to be communications to me, much less aggression. Consumed and overtaken by our work, I could not truly believe her report of my nonexistence because her focus on my misattunement felt quite powerful and agentic. The room overflowed with affect. Our wildly disparate experiences caused a kind of vertigo. There was no consensual reality.

Perhaps if I had thought of my patient as operating from the psychotic part of her mind, I would have been guided toward different treatment decisions. Her radically uneven mix of self-states—the highest level of education and intellectual acumen side-by-side with profound difficulty in thinking and relating—confused me. I understood our trouble as a negative therapeutic reaction and continued to try to unlock the impasse by understanding the transference/countertransference dilemmas. Her prolonged silences and her attacks on me appeared to be reactions to therapeutic injury. Led by this awareness to a model of trauma and repair, I tried to pursue what was happening in the space between us as if that conversation was possible. And because my relational orientation led me to search for my own contribution to our impasse, I became involved in my own badness. I blamed myself for the treatment ruptures, rather than truly understanding what my patient was trying to communicate: I was sitting with a woman who did not have an "I." Enactment followed enactment.

Hard as I tried, I couldn't seem to help her. Eventually, neither of us could take it anymore. She told me before she left, "You always disappear, you shift, you're not whole." I thought of the healer in Toni Cade Bambara's *The Salt Eaters* (1980) who says, "Wholeness is no trifling matter," and agreed. I didn't really believe in wholeness as a possibility or goal. I thought more about shifting self-states and Bromberg's idea (1998) that maybe the goal was to stand in the spaces. But my patient's words weren't untrue. There was something I couldn't contain, and I was bruised from my effort to reach her, shamed by it, by what it took from me, how much I had to want the treatment, and her.

Indeed, I spent the next ten years writing and giving talks about the complexity of the analyst's psyche and its contribution to impasse. Certainly, I knew these same affects of grief, shame, and badness lived in me in unintegrated ways. She had run into something inside of me that I couldn't rework; some way I couldn't see I would falter. I am the difficult-to-reach analyst, and she is the aggrieved but patient healer. She wonders if I can be cured. Beneath a lot of openness, vulnerability, and self-reflection, a raw, slippery, elusive me moves off in the face of hurt. Most patients don't run up against this part of me. Still, now I am thinking, Were those treatments dominated by studium? Patients whom I liked, even loved, but didn't feel wounded by and therefore didn't damage with my love or trauma à la Fairbairn and Guntrip? Punctum, Barthes (1980) told us, is an addition, whether or not it is triggered. In his language it is what we add to the picture and what is nevertheless already there (p. 55): "The punctum, then, is a kind of subtle beyond—as if the image launched desire beyond what it permits us to see" (p. 59). My unconscious is not hidden. It is out in the open. My own history haunts.

I retained my problematic certainty that I must be the major source of the problem. My own lack, my own fault lines, were too much like hers. The problem was punctum, the prick. She and I colluded in a powerful idea that if only I were more attuned, she could be helped.

Caper (1999) might say we were in a folie à deux. The patient provokes a state of mind in the analyst that corresponds to what the patient is projecting into her in fantasy or projective counteridentification. In other words, a patient's fantasy meets up with a corresponding fantasy of the analyst. In this case we shared the powerful idea that the problem of nonintegration was mine. We could both have more hope.

Caper (1999) asked why the analyst goes along with a folie à deux and accepts the patient's fantasy. He pulls out the part of Freud that argues that the analyst's need to cure is a defense against his own sadism. For Caper, the analyst has only one real function—to bring the patient into fresh contact with himself. The analyst does this, Caper insisted, by helping the patient to become aware of repressed or split-off parts of the personality, not by trying to resolve or integrate the conflict. This is difficult for most of us to do, he suggested, because it leaves the analysis hostage to the *patient's* ability to resolve the conflict. Our own failure to come to terms with our destructive impulses means we can't let the outcome of our work rest on the patient's shoulders. Caper told us that if the analyst can recognize his need to relieve the patient's suffering as a by-product of his own unconscious conflict, he will be free of his need to heal the patient (pp. 21–22). Through this lens, the need to cure arises from the analyst's unintegrated psyche.

We are offered a different but similar story in relational literature. Harris (2009), in her beautiful paper on the analyst's contribution to impasse, "You Must Remember This," cited Davies's work on a failed case in which Harris extrapolated the idea that early in training, junior analysts may become overly involved with haunting tragic patients for whom we go beyond all limits, precisely because the effort to heal the patient represents an attempt on the analyst's part to repair or heal an internal object she has yet to fully grieve. Harris traced the kinds of developmentally based attachment difficulties likely to be found in many analysts that lead to an omnipotence that keeps them overreaching. I am both persuaded and provoked by this line of thinking. I can see clearly how my own failures to mourn have led to a tendency to want to breathe life into states of psychic deadness, and a refusal to accept certain limits that keep me suffering and are of limited use to the patient. And I join Harris (2009) and others in noting the profound and overdue insight that impasse may loosen when the analyst has access to unbearable affects and is able to metabolize, shift, grieve, change, and speak from this slightly altered state. Still, I came to question that my problem was overreach. What really allows change is indeterminable. Capricious. It is a different kind of omnipotence to imagine otherwise.

As Phillips (2006) pointed out, the psychoanalyst has two aims more at odds with each other than Freud would acknowledge. On the one hand, he aims to cure, to relieve suffering, to help make life more worth living, but on the other hand, he aims for what is technically called "maximum symbolization." He wants to respond only in ways that will facilitate the expression of unconscious desire. He wants to let the unconscious speak (p. 17).

For many contemporary theorists, uncovering the unconscious is no longer considered the major form of therapeutic action. Nonetheless, it remains a highly contemporary question: Does articulation of wants give people the life they prefer? Can we change wishes? Should I have helped John alter his desire?

Freud (1937) knew, as he made clear in *Analysis Terminable and Interminable*, how unchanging people are. As Friedman (2005) described, the analytic setup is designed to disrupt business as usual between two intimates in order to overcome the intentions of both. The conditions for psychoanalysis after all, he reminded us, were aimed at creating conditions disruptive enough to overcome the difficulty of change. The historic tension remains about which will best accomplish that.

This question is highlighted with patients for whom the issue of their very existence takes center stage. What does the work of maximal symbolization look like when patients do not have the developmental capacity to access the mind, the experience of a self, much less a self that houses intrapsychic conflict? In this context, what do we mean by a patient's wish or desire? For many people, enactment takes the place of remembering, but when patients have major deficits arising from early pre-symbolized trauma, it may be the primary form of communication. In relational language we speak of enactment, but the concept no longer conveys much about the qualities of an enacting "mind." I have come to believe that something is lost in not articulating clearly enough, as some of the one-person literature does, what may be required for patients to have stable psychic structure (as it was once called). Self/other differentiation, intrapsychic conflict—these are features that make possible more relational treatment.

Several authors (Lombardi, Robbins, Searles), have emphasized long periods of time in which destructive reenactments and undifferentiated and unintegrated forms of mentation are not only routine; they are required before higher-order symbolic thought and communication is possible.

Unlike Caper or Harris, those who study unrepresented states do not believe treatment in which the analyst must take responsibility for the care of the patient (and the analysis) are unanalytic, or a product of the clinician's omnipotence. Instead, great activity on the part of the analyst is seen as essential to establishing a broad reflective perspective and a capacity for intrapsychic conflict (Robbins 1996, 768).

Stories from several one-person theorists about the internal worlds of their patients, and the kind of tormenting reversals and transferences they suffered as analysts, gave me grounding. Green (1972), for instance, wrote that when a patient has internalized a psychically dead parent as a way to nurture and cure that parent so the parent is not totally lost to them, the transference contains a reversal. According to Green, I had to breathe life back into my patient by imbuing her with my aliveness. She had to feel she had succeeded in garnering my special attention, that I was narcissistically invested in her. Under these conditions, Green thought a patient could begin to bear the confrontation with the dead mother entombed inside her.

Steiner (1993) also described long silences in which the patient is projecting the desire to make contact onto the analyst and the analyst must hold all the desire for the treatment replete with the humiliation of always having to be the pursuer, the holder of the want. Like Green, he challenged the idea of withdrawal as actual disengagement and instead named this an intense sadomasochistic interaction designed "to avoid psychic reality."

I was grateful for these theories because they normalized my experience and released me from my preoccupation with my badness through a focus on what the patient might be activating in me from her own childhood experience. As long as the crazy was in her, I could feel empathy again for my patient, held hostage to her inner world of complicated gangs neutralizing, binding, and controlling anxiety, keeping pain and destructiveness at bay through her withdrawal. My wild affective self-states were really her feelings as they came to rest in me. My masochism was not my own. Here reach became merely technique.

Yet as important a corrective as these theories were to my misplaced attention on my own subjectivity and contribution to the impasse, they had several problems. Both were wedded to a conflict model. Steiner and Green speak of the unintegrated mental organization of very disturbed patients, and yet, like many contemporary theorists, they conceptualize these people's minds as possessing many attributes of a so-called more mature, neurotic mind, thus seeming to bypass what may be real deficits in self-development. These theories implicitly suggest that because the analyst feels something visceral, it follows that the patient has produced that feeling. So my patient was to blame for my affective disruption, something I desperately wanted to believe.

Robbins (1996) noted reliance on concepts like projective identification, which require "an unconscious intent to not only evacuate bad feeling defensively but place it in the mind of the other, implies the operation of developed representations of self, other, and the intended affective communication between" (p. 756). With a patient like mine, this kind of formulation seems problematic because it potentially skirts the developmental deficit being enacted. Patients at this level are not able to "differentiate a primitive albeit unrealistic (all-good) self from a projectively identified (all-bad) object, and to maintain an integrative linkage with that object (p. 755).

For my patient, it is likely that massive early neglect and misattunement had *precluded* the integration that enables the experience of intrapsychic conflict. Aspects of her personality, and traumatic history, never took form as experience, implicit or explicit, because there was no intersubjective system in which they could emerge (Orange, Atwood, and Stolorow 1997). Put in other language, she had, in this self-state, no experience of herself, her mind, or her feelings. There was no subjectivity with which to answer questions or reflect. She rarely knew what a feeling was or how it felt.

Rather than think about her mind as fragmenting defensively, trauma had left gaps, areas that had not come into being. Robbins (1996) noted that in these situations it would be more apt to talk about the presence and influence of affective and cognitive deficits that were required to survive, and which now characterize the transference, rather than about the defense. In other words, the capacity for intrapsychic conflict as well as the constructive, growth-promoting aspect of it, are no longer natural, as is the case with neurotic patients; they "must be developed from the somatic anlage that have kept the patient physically alive" (p. 767).

Both Robbins (1996) and Lombardi (2005, 2010) noted that in cases of difficulty in sustaining affect representations, if the analyst insists the patient is projecting anger and the patient has no corresponding internal representation, then he can only experience the interpretation as an attribution or an attack. Before other work proceeds, it may be necessary to translate and symbolize bodily states into affective experience (Lombardi 2005, 2010). Indeed, when I interpreted my patient's attempts to evacuate feelings, this was confusing to her. A conflict model and the techniques

I associated with it were not helpful. I was contained by the theory, but my patient felt alienated.

The theory that best described my patient's experience was the work of Stolorow, Atwood, and Orange (2002). Their phenomenological view of nonbeing felt closer to her experience—both its formlessness and its terrors—than most theories. They capture something unique about the suffering of patients who feel they do not exist in ordinary terms—and advocate a profound de-centering from one's own world to become deeply immersed in that of the other. Yet the wild feelings this case (and others) have evoked in me made this more traditional self-psychological "selfless" stance unachievable. My feelings of erasure made such a stance feel like an annihilation of my being. I came to feel their ideas did not help *me* with the enormous, wrenching complexity of what a human de-centering process actually entails, not in empathic/technical terms but in relational terms (i.e., real, human love and hate). The work required a deeper opening to myself, to bear my patient's annihilatory absence. While they imply the necessity of the analyst's struggle, this aspect goes largely undescribed.

For my patient, though, neither was a relational approach entirely helpful. Relational theory helped me craft an intersubjective story in which both of our damaged internal worlds were in intense unconscious communication and contributed to the difficulty in the work.

But the technique that followed, conceptualizing the treatment as a two-person field in which both analyst and patient are available to use each other's competing subjectivities to understand the patient—a seminal relational idea—was impossible prior to my patient's capacity to reflect on the experience of herself or recognition of me. Though often underemphasized in clinical reports, the capacity to work intersubjectively in Benjamin's (1995) terms is an achievement.

What then is relational work when a patient's experiential world and yours cannot coexist within a shared experience? When both patient and analyst are unable to see themselves through the eyes of the other and so there is a "collision of realities" that precludes using the other to reshape the "truth" that exists in each of our minds (Bromberg 2006)? Bromberg offered, "When disassociation has significantly organized the development of mental structure, not only has the capacity to bear internal conflict suffered, but also the capacity for intersubjectivity is foreclosed" (p. 7/8). When this is the case, experience cannot be told; it must get reopened and reexperienced in a new context. What does this look like? How do we begin to lay the foundation to shift dissociative structures? This work requires extraordinary effort that may resemble overreaching, based on our own omnipotence and failure to mourn rather than a response to a patient's developmental need.

That our omnipotence protects us from our own shame and grief by keeping us reaching rather than mourning is suspect. I have come to think of omnipotence, like enactment, as ubiquitous and inevitable. My own grandiose "deal with the devil" never protected me from grief; I reached and reached and, in reaching, felt a terrible shame for having to be, one more time, the pursuer. These feelings were reactivated with my patient. I was and am that small child following my mother from room to room trying to get her attention. And also I believe pursuing can be the price of the treatment. I straddle these contradictions.

Whether we believe in the explicit prohibition of cure in Caper's story, or the implicit warning of omnipotence in Harris's version, both target a kind of excess on the part of the analyst—an intrapsychic need to serve ourselves rather than our patients. We have become The Analyst Who Loves (and Hates) Too Much. Our wound is unhealed. Punctum made us do it.

Of course punctum made us do it. Whether we have managed our sadism or mourned our losses, all of us reach (or don't) from particular places that animate our practices. The question is, what is the analyst's own relationship with that place from which they reach? What differentiates the kind of reaching that ends up being generative, connective, cohering, meaningful from that which doesn't? I think Harris would want us to find a way to talk more openly about the sources of our particular ways of reaching without reducing them to the analyst's pathology or presuming that these aspects of our subjectivity can be well symbolized (by the analyst) or brought into a two-person way of relating to the patient in the room.

Do I reach toward that "raw, slippery elusive me that moves off in the face of hurt"? That part of me that "disappears, shifts"? As analysts, we talk about how to reach those wordless parts in our patients, but how are we living with the corresponding or complementary parts in ourselves that compel us to reach in the ways we do? Perhaps this is the space where our models are most impoverished: they do not represent a way (procedurally) of being in relationship with those parts of ourselves.

We are left with a one-person literature that is vivid in its depiction of the internal world of patients whose minds are not structured within a linguistic frame, and yet the concepts and language of those studying unintegrated states can also be alienating. One-person theories capture the affective disruption a patient will engender, but they emphasize our separateness and difference from our patients. This work succeeds by us pulling ourselves out of the pool; differentiating our presumably more neurotic minds from their more primitive ones, leaving us with our health intact and authority unchecked—something relational theory has taught us to question.

So why return to what feel like antiquated notions of a mind separate from the relationship in which it emerges? Why recall a unitary (stable) self when we believe we are a mix-up of more and less developed states, all of them necessary (Ogden 1989)? Why venture back to Cartesian notions when we have more sophisticated ideas about self as process, not structure? Clearer understanding of archaic states might have led to different treatment parameters and better technique for my patient. If I had really understood her states of nonbeing and had been less intimidated by her sharp mind—more ready to believe in her concomitant inability to think, reflect, and communicate—I would have pushed less on the "us." If I had thought of her as not like me, I would have suffered less vertigo and perhaps been more attuned. Yet neither one-person objectivist thinking nor relational negotiation was right. I needed a model that made explicit what was required in working with the psychotic part of a personality within a relational frame.

This would require a keen focus on what was happening in the singular mind of my patient whose world was solitary and not yet primarily object related, but a focus that came from my solidly relational self. I that knew I helped produce and shaped some of what I saw, and either facilitated or interfered with her developmental processes. Relational training invites us to use our subjectivity and ourselves deeply, and it is this willingness with which we must travel back to ourselves to find the separate other.

So how do we gain access to a person's state of noncoherence? Most of us would not choose to live in this terrifying place of human suffering, and yet when experience is enacted, that is exactly how we may come to know it. In Searles's (1965, 631–632) language, to gain access to that "amorphous sensory amalgam of undifferentiated experience" that patients enact, we must be inducted into a symbiotic experience: somatic, unbearable, unthinkable, unrememberable elements live between patient and analyst (Robbins 1996, 772).

Becoming mixed up with the other, what Paul Russell (1983) has called "the crunch" is relevant to some extent to all analytic pairs, but I am describing something unique about work with patients who struggle with very early relational trauma. In some way, compellingly and impossibly, chaos has to take place with these patients because they have to be able to compel the analyst to move down to the foundations of their own being with them. As Lombardi (2005) offered,

> The fact that the analyst . . . is able to hear the profound resonances arising from primordial aspects of the analyst's own corporality in its connection with primitive instincts (Freud 1915a; Winnicott 1949) . . . seems to be, in these clinical contexts, decisive for the patient's develop-ment. The analyst, delving deeply into a relationship with him- or her-self, offers, in the intersubjective exchange of the analytic relationship, a critical catalytic element that enables the patient to approach his or her own internal level, benefiting from the organizing role of the boundaries of the body and the relationship with the other, leading ultimately to the patient's ability to construct appropriate ego boundaries.
>
> (p. 1095)

My patient and others like her require us to access the most profound expe-rience of our own aloneness. The work requires a return to our own basic fault lines as a way to feel into their experiential world. I came to see that if I could find some way to bear my own helplessness and despair, and convey that to her, this shifted the atmosphere between us. The subtlety of moving from trying to find her to finding her by accepting something in me was not yet apparent.

I agree with Slavin (2011) and Lombardi (2005) that there is some-thing potentially generative and powerful when a patient can involve us in a primal way in our own places of deepest pain. When we are willing to return to the place of corresponding deficit within ourselves, to heal our own internal splits in our effort to reach the other, a channel toward change and transformation can open. When the analyst's pathology or failure to grieve are read only as sources of interference, something in the paradox is diluted. Perhaps I am implying the inverse of Caper's view; namely, that we have to help our patients in those places we can't yet help ourselves (Raniere, personal communication, 2011). There is something for us to manage internally about this paradox that goes beyond the work of what we usually refer to as grieving. This is always an ongoing task.

This willingness and capacity to be provoked and live again in symbiotic mix-up with our patients offers a form of hope and love and vision of the other that uniquely puts the analyst in touch with both the suffering and the potential of the people we treat. Countertransference, like transference, is both distortion and a vitally accurate reading of the other. It is not our pathology or the patient's that is determinant, but what is experienced separately and together, including the struggle to make meaning in the face of meaninglessness. It is here perhaps that punctum has value. Does accompaniment, our own involvement with the struggle, which can often require extraordinary reach, alter the existential landscape, the mortal fear we all confront? The analyst wrestles over and over in life with these issues. The love lies in the willingness to wrestle with it, grieve it, never fully together (Slavin and Kriegman 1998).

My patient is back again after an eight-year absence. She never had any interest in cure. Attempts to "treat" her felt like either a bypassing of who she was or an attempt to cure her of herself. It wasn't "better" she wanted to be exactly. And she didn't want to learn to be intelligible either. She didn't want to speak at all. She wanted to stay alive in the room, and later, in the room with me.

Now time is passing by, and when she realizes that, she cries out. She does not know much more about herself, has almost no relationships in the world, and is tormented by internal demons. She has repeated the failures of the treatment elsewhere, but the one thing she knows now that she didn't then is that the failure of the treatment had something to do with her. The knowledge relieves me, but it doesn't help her. There is no I within her, and without my reach we are nowhere. She comes again, still, because she wonders, Am I any better?

Am I any better? As Harris prophesizes, there is something I have given up, something in my own imagination about my ability to "do better" or "work harder" that I have let go of, and in this I suffer less. But I fear the equanimity of my state in me means that we're just not quite back in it yet. Barthes (1980) said, "Not surprising, then, that despite its clarity, punctum should be revealed only after the fact, when the photograph is no longer in front of me and I think back on it" (p. 53). Like the displaced temporality of psychoanalysis, clarity is sharpened later.

Whatever outdated ideas I had that change meant she should start a session, or articulate a want, or have something to say, might be the same old misunderstandings I always had. When I ask, "How are you?" and there is no "you" to answer, a lot is required of me. Overfunctioning, in analytic language, with the difficult-to-reach patient, is the parameter. I will project my most helpful thoughts, I will contain her most toxic parts, but certainly I will carry desire, hate, terrible annihilation anxiety, time, money, identification, structure, process, punctum, pleasure. And I will be my mother's daughter.

Now I spend a lot of time thinking how quickly I will have to empty my mother's rent- controlled apartment when she dies. She isn't sick, but I am haunted by the speed in which I know she will be gone, by the lack of time I will have. I will not linger with her things. If she dies at the end of a month, it could be just a day or two I have. There won't be much to take. She culls, or simply rids herself of things, certainly paper, people, sentiment. I can't imagine what I'll throw away. Nothing. I already know I'll hoard her. She will in death, like in life, be elusive, ephemeral; this is the her who lives in me—too raw to touch, too slippery to hold. I will need real help carrying when she goes.

Who am I to love
so deeply? As against
a dark heavy darkness, pressed against my eyes. Wetting
my face, a constant trembling rain.
    Along life, to you. My friend.
I tell that to myself, slowly, sucking my lip. A silence of motives/
empties
the day of meaning
    What is intimate
enough? What is
beautiful?
    It is slow unto meaning for
any life. If I am an animal, there
is proof of my living. The fawns
and calves
of my age. But it is steel that falls
As a thin mist into my consciousness. As a fine
ugly spray. I have made
some futile ethic
with.

"Changed my life?" As the dead man
pacing at the edge of the sea. As
the lips, closed
for so long, at the sight
of motionless
birds.

There is no one to entrust with
meaning. (These sails go by, these small
deadly animals.)

And meaning? These words?
Were there some blue expanse
of world. Some other
flesh, resting
at the proof
of the world . . .

You could say of me
that I was truly
simpleminded.

> —LeRoi Jones, from *The Dead*
> *Lecturer*, p. 42

Chapter 2

Love letter to a patient or the raw story (2001)

"Do I move toward form, / do I use all my fears?"
—Muriel Rukeyser, from "Double Ode," in *The Gates* (1976)

Version 1, September—the undoing of a psychoanalyst

My patient Sarah and I have just reached the other side of a terrible impasse that has threatened to destroy the analysis. Spring and summer have been marked by profound silence, unendurable pain, and constant chaos. Sarah has felt that it is too painful to come to sessions, sometimes too painful to speak by phone. Each day threatens to be the last day. The analysis is under constant assault.

My summer vacation brings some reprieve—needed space for both of us. Still, we speak once a week by phone, and each conversation slowly restores some equanimity. A chance encounter during my vacation reminds Sarah of the pleasure of my company. She comes back into the office in September after months of physical absence, or psychic retreat, and we are both giddy.

I feel a small window open; I am standing with her in that frame.

> There is only this train
> Slipping through pastures of snow,
> A sleigh reaching down
> To touch its buried runners.
> We meet on the shaking platform,
> The wind's broken teeth sinking into us . . .
> Telegraph posts chop the winter fields
> Into white blocks, in each window . . .

DOI: 10.4324/9781032670348-4

There are few clues as to where
We are: the baled wheat scattered
Everywhere like missing coffins.
> ("The Stranger,"
> Forché 1981, 46)

My giddiness feels about the pleasure of *being on the same train together, meeting,* for this rare moment; the way this small window frames something we can both see, even death. It is an unexpected vista we share on an otherwise snow-blanketed world.

"Burning together in the snow / We will not live / to settle for less/ We have dreamed of this / all of our lives" ("Phantasia for Elvira Shatayev", Rich 1978, 6).

But this new feeling makes her ill—literally sick and tense—a pain between her ribs stabbing her in the back. She can't breathe when she has it. When she leaves my office, she gets sick; explosive expulsion. She calls her sickness a "bifurcation." She cannot reconcile the pleasure of being with me and the absolute "inefficacy" of our relationship—so she is ill.

In this brief interlude—when she can tell me how she leaves a shell or husk in the room with me while she removes her body to privately absorb the feelings between us—we are living in the world of words together. Not words enough so that she might not be sick, but words enough that when I note her absence in the room, she can tell me she and her body are elsewhere working hard. Soon she will be depleted by her effort to let me be with her. She feels she must talk for me, and she resents it. More, it exhausts her. She can't.

I think of Freud's Dora and what cannot be spoken—or even known—between us. Our desire. Our destruction. No way to tolerate the feelings between us in a linguistic or affective register. Thus, a conversion. The emergence of a hysterical symptom.

When, in the following weeks, Sarah comes to feel my admiration for her integrity and my genuine delight in her, her pain dissolves. (I would like you to know how good she is—how decent, ethical, honest; generous and faithful; disciplined, resolute, square behind her words).

I finally see that my internal fear of over-involvement with her has led to a lack of verbal generosity on my part. There is a split inside of me between how I hold her in my mind, my reverie about her, and what I share with her.

Each time she has rejected me, I have offered her less of myself. We had mutually regulated ourselves right into a cold, contactless existence.

Now she feels the gleam, and I sense her relief, buoyancy even. She can't believe I hold her in my mind, much less hold her there with pleasure. Because she destroys me at each separation, she has imagined her own gruesome death inside me. She believes only in her own invisibility, her failure to affect the other. Now she can hear something new, something else.

There is an opening.

Why haven't I been able to give this to her sooner? Why hasn't she been able to see?

And who am I in this moment for her? There is so much I can't know. And who is she for me that this moment of her return feels so alive and vital? I think about my pleasure in being let in, or rather, not being shut out. Some ancient dread lifted. And how that dread has kept me from really being with her.

My own failure to mourn is what I am up against in myself. And then there is my omnipotence—the curative fantasy. This dogged, misplaced persistence—is it what has allowed the work to go on, or what stops it?

I can make her better. Heroic rescue, some might say. I am not so sure. I think of the conditions for loving.

I spin tops, I shoot marbles, I slay dragons, I steer boats clear of lobster pots. For a brief moment, we have lived in perfect pitch. In wonderment, our senses opened, the world pulsing with life.

Whoosh.

The orange ball glides through the hoop.

And then it's over. Thud.

Oh, I know how to stop on roller skates, to be at the bottom of hills, the end of movies, the line between where I take off and the close of your eyelid, the slowing of your grin.

The more she allows herself to love me, the more threat she is under. Every time we connect, a terrible violence follows. She dreams:

There's this apocalypse coming. I know it's coming. At first, I think everybody else knows, but they either don't know or they won't take it seriously. I can't convince them. It has to do with the sea. There is a storm coming, but they think it is just a storm. The waves are getting whiter and wilder. And they're dismissing it like it doesn't matter. No, no. . . . I've seen this before, I tell them. I've seen this storm. Once before I saw the sea like this. The sea is screaming at me. It's mass destruction.

Then everybody is assembled, like on the deck of a ship, but it wasn't a deck. But they're all nice and neatly rowed and dutiful. I don't know if I said it, or if I was thinking it, but I thought if this is the end, this is not where I want to be. With them. I am not waiting here with them.

I wander off. I could see this wave, not a regular crashing wave. I could see the sea scream. It was not an ocean. I know I am going to die.

This wildness we have whipped up, this affective storm of loving, is surely death. I am contained, dutiful at best. Sarah has been here before, and she is not waiting for the end with me. She has wandered off.

There is a violence to her splitting. She must have felt (without feeling), I love you so much I have to kill you.

The dream heralds the shift away. A day later we have a familiar miss. I have said the wrong thing, used the wrong tone, failed to notice something. We are instantly catapulted back into wordlessness. There is only aloneness, a place of persecution and complementarity. There is no third. Now my interpretations, queries, and silence chase her away.

Each of us stops ourselves from risking more. Sarah cannot come into her sessions. She cannot endure them. The fall begins to feel like the previous spring—a cancelled session, then a missed session, no call, a question about the next time we will meet.

I have done this to her. Made her disappear. I am her unremembered parent. Murderer by misattuned love. I cannot bear this feeling of having done again something so injurious, so deadly.

And there is what she is doing to me when she leaves. I am her unremembered child self, abandoned and alone. Punished. I don't mind living in this place of deep feeling for her, but I do mind when living with her means living without her.

When I live so intensely with you, your sudden disappearances catapult me into relation with my own entombed "dead mother." I am agitated. This is too much feeling here with you, my patient.

To live in this raw exposed part of myself requires her. She has awakened me but won't engage with me. I know I will be left on the deck to die dutifully, like a soldier without her, I must have felt.

When I wonder out loud with her about her disappearances, she is incredulous. She hasn't a clue as to what I am talking about. I play no part. There is nothing happening here, she insists. It's as though she is saying, You don't register. You're not even on the screen. She feels only a familiar deadening. Blankness. Psychic retreat.

Still, it is hard to live exclusively within her story. To fully align myself within her subjective world because her only way of allowing me into that world is through her silent disappearances that last for months. There is no symbolic register. There is only the elaboration of her feeling as it comes to reside in me at the moment of her psychic departures. I feel Sarah's feeling palpably in my body: and it feels like there has been a catastrophe. And I have caused it. The atmosphere in the room that I perceive is thick; angry, defeated, stony. I cannot be an emotionally uninvolved interpreter. It is the denial *of anything happening* in that space that causes my vertigo.

I have erased her, annihilated her. She erases me, annihilates me. Yet they are not the same. The transference is diffuse. The boundaries permeable. We have between us the undifferentiated, unintegrated elements of our minds.

I hear Freud warning, this is a transgressive transference.

I hear Forché: There is no train. The landscape blurs. White.

My analyst self (I am just developing and trying so hard to lose) whispers to me, Remember your Klein. *Your efforts to show her how she uses her absence, her silence, not just to protect herself but to punish you are not wrong—just years away. Of course, she has aggression.* And yet, is it aggression? I give her unconscious motivation, agency, conflict. Yet when I ask her, "How are you?" there exists no "you" to answer.

She requests my deep involvement, but she cannot let us think about it. When we do, we have moved out of being. That move is violent for her. She must tear herself from herself to "think" in this way (Bion 1959).

The you who can be with me in a reflective mode has already abandoned the you who needs me most. I ask you to abandon her in favor of this talking you. You know it is an abandonment. And so you leave again and again.

I will have to find a way to use my own feeling of having been done in, to keep putting in words that which is being enacted. I think of Paul Russell's (1998) work on affective competency. How we must do this over and over until the capacity to feel becomes a possibility. And while I am supplying stable patterns of reflective thought, fantasy, and feeling, there is this excruciating encounter with myself.

Each time she breaks contact with me, I must reach for her. In each reaching I feel diminished and ashamed. My own desperate longings, my masochism, my failure to mourn. These will have to be revisited. Without her, in order to begin to exist for her. *Yet if I let the treatment drift off again, we live in your neglect.*

When I mark a limit or a boundary that I need, when I assert the frame, that she come, that she leave, that she pay me, I assault her with my words, my needs. It is me wanting, needing. She is cool, aloof, untouched. I am the ill parent.

Green (1972) offers language to understand the reversal:

> "The patient spends his life nourishing his dead, as though he alone has charge of it". . .

> He keeps the dead mother prisoner, and she remains his personal property". . . ."The mother has become the infant of the child. It is for him to repair her narcissistic wound". . . ."Dead and present but present none the less. The subject [patient] can take care of her, attempt to awaken her, to cure her. But in return, if cured, she awakens and is animate and lives, the subject loses her again, for she abandons him to go about her own affairs . . . the subject is caught between two losses.

> (pp. 163–64).

Sarah keeps me locked inside of her. She will cure me, she will make me stay. I must suffer these fates as she suffered: uncertain, vulnerable, raw, exposed, needing her. But I want to reflect on her need of me to be in those states. I don't want to be in these states. I want to be the psychoanalyst. I don't want to be her. She thinks of this as my authenticity. I think of it as my undoing.[1]

But this is who I get to be for now. If I awaken, and am alive and well, she will lose me. My competencies, my attunement, my best analytic self— these are too dangerous. These qualities imply my separateness which she cannot conceive of or bear. I cannot bargain enough space to exist as separate enough to help.

This is how she lives with me. In lieu of verbal interchange between our separate selves, I am inducted into a symbiotic experience: somatic, unbearable, unthinkable, unrememberable elements live between us (Searles 1965).

I want my alterity. I need at least to theorize her aggression to manage all my own deaths. This steadies me. I read Steiner's *Psychic Retreats* (1993) like a lifeline. He describes patients who present formidable technical problems including long periods of silence in which the patient is project-ing the desire to make contact onto the analyst. Steiner's descriptions saved me. My dance with Sarah, so urgent and disrupting, this version of sado-masochism, was being danced all over town. Hallelujah.

Tempered hallelujah.

Steiner knows, this *is* about the patient. He seems steady, sure. I am less sure. Because I am less sure or because she needs me less sure?

All the theoretical frames that hold me during this work—ideas of projective identification, of evacuation, of sadomasochism, of psychic retreat—these fail her. I want to say to her, *And I know that if I inter-vene from this knowledge base, one that holds you up as subject and actor, these are word bombs that I deliver. They are not means of com-munication. They are actions. Acts of hate. They blow things up. For you. For now.*

Even when I merely hold these ideas in my mind, she knows that I have left her. At first, I think this is because they make me steadier, surer in my gaze. A psychoanalyst. It takes me longer to see that there is neither the internal structure nor not the mutual recognition to support this work.

But even when I hold the theory, I feel better. I can locate myself again. Find my footing. But you are gone. To find myself, I lose you. One or the other. This is the tension. There is no both and. No dialectical tension. And yet, we move somewhere new.

Version 2

How is it that one day life's orderly and you are content, a little cynical perhaps but on the whole just so, and then without warning you find the solid floor is a trapdoor and you are now in another place whose geog-raphy is uncertain and whose customs are strange?

(Winterson 1989, 68)

I first met Sarah inside my living room on my couch. She came into the wrong part of my house. My office occupies my first floor and my house the second and third. I gave the usual directions. Many years. No mistakes. Deep-blue door on the right. Door's open. Enter right into the waiting room. Sit down. I'll come get you.

And I leave the other door unlocked. The one that leads up a flight of stairs, deep colored, into a cathedral-ceilinged living room. I wait the long ten long minutes of my previous patient hour with her in my house. I think to myself, Move slowly, as I tumble up my stair from my office. I was always waiting for her, to reach her, to tell her, she was in the wrong place.

When I find her, she sits across the room under the sharp-eyed stare of my two Berman kitty cats facing her down across the living room. Imperious, suspicious, sumptuous, beautiful. Inviting and refusing closeness and touch.

She is sitting very still. Sweat pouring from her. Overwhelmed shocked. She tells me right off, "I am a stranger in a strange land. "

> *Travelers at least have a choice. Those who set sail know that things will not be the same as at home. Explorers are prepared. But for us, who travel along the blood vessels, who come to cities of the interior by chance, there is no preparation.*
>
> (Winterson 1989, 68)

My heart is pounding. I sweep my eyes over what she is seeing. Intimate photos of my partner and me, the children, our family and friends line mantel and shelves. Toys are strewn about—and books. Paintings cover almost every inch of walls. Beauty. Chaos. Some order. Lots of life. I try to imagine how she will see it. And I feel her terror enter me. Later I will feel that I invaded her, took her over, shocked her into frozen wordless dread.

Curiously, I did not feel intruded on. But I know the meaning of a house. I've read Freud. She is in me.

Passion is not so much an emotion as a destiny (Winterson, p. 68).

She has no memory of the room. I do not live inside her, she says.

My person trapped here on the page, in my house, in my transference, in the tone of this story. It's my story. She demanded it be my story. It was that reversal I suffered.

Maybe I could stop right here. The first five minutes of the first hour contains the whole story.

Had I invited her or had she stolen into my house? I feel I have done something wrong, entered her forcefully. And in my panic in having done this, like in my childhood, all that matters is to find her, to bring her back. I *cannot* have her disappear. This immediately sets up an overreaching on my part. I will be pursuing her throughout the treatment. I will hold the movement, affect, love, hate, life. And I will fear the toxicity of these feeling states. I will feel I have made her disappear with my love. I will be her child self, left and alone. You can hear my concordant identification (Racker 1968).

And Sarah? By walking into my house, Sarah establishes herself as a person who enters, who possesses motility, proceeds without permission. But she cannot be that with me and remain true to her internal objects. She has formed her sense of self in relation to parents who could tolerate no agency, hardly presence. She can barely exist. Wanting is forbidden, even curiosity. An agentic self would be profoundly disloyal to the intimate self she has created/been allowed. In order to remain safe, she disappears, dissociates. Goes missing.

So much of the time I was looking for her. So much was about lost and found, hide and seek. Mine and hers. Does that mean we were two?

Neither of us wants to believe in her activity. Only mine. The pull up, into my body, through the terracotta of my stairwell to the rose and rust inside. This is a defining symbol. For me. How she came into me. It's true. She was inside of me from the start. Happily. And not just happily. Terror too—hers and mine. Pleasure and unpleasure. Green's co-excitation. Tensional intensity. The requisition of fused sensations (Green 1972).

She tells me, "English is a second language."

We who are fluent find life is a foreign language. Somewhere between the swamp and the mountains. Somewhere between fear and sex. Somewhere between God and the Devil passion is and the way there is sudden and the way back is worse.

(Winterson, p. 68)

I wanted to be in this with her. But I wanted asymmetry. I wanted that too.

Passion out of passion's obstacles. And me? Every game threatens a wild card. The unpredictable, the out of control. Even with a steady hand and a crystal ball we couldn't rule the world the way we wanted it. There are storms at sea and there are storms inland. Only the convent windows look serenely out to both.

(Winterson p. 71)

My house was no convent, and she did not go home. Will you stay, I ask? Come down this way, back in, through the other door, it's calmer. Not so much to see. Muted sunbaked sand, a little olive and gold. Opaque.

All the questions here from the very beginning.

Come dwell here, where I choose, where I can have you, patient, guest, interloper, lover, thief, player.

All the nouns have action. All the metaphors are geographic.

The treatment is a kind of ongoing hysteria. Not just Sarah's, mine. But I think a kind of madness is required.

****

Sarah wears no watch. She requests I move my clocks. The loud sound of the passage of time distresses her. She asks for so little.

In the military, she was taken captive in another country. Her identity mistook. Four days. Four desperate nights. Little water or food, sweltering heat, no human contact. Near death. Then immersed in water.

I dream I am swimming. Strong elegant strokes cut through the water. Four strokes for the whole lap. This was her fourth time so close to death.

I start in water. She on dry land. But it isn't so. We are both submerged, yet she is still, arid, whereas I am messy, wet, spilling.

Have we fallen down a looking glass though neither of us is any Alice? Could there be two mad hatters? Certainly, there is a mirror.

On brief leave, when she went missing, no one looked for her. No one noticed she was gone. Eventually diplomats intervened. A book deal was offered. Mistaken identity. Espionage. Murder. That—murder—has always been with us. To render this devastation into a drama of the devastation is nothing less than an annihilation of sorts.

And Sarah doesn't want to tell the story of the wreck. She's quite under-stated. Panic the first night. After that, no feeling, no fear—only strategy. How to avoid the heat of the day and the cold of the night in the outside cell. A rescue that misfires. Hope surfaces, but the liberators think she is someone else, and she is left again. She cannot draw attention. The real insult, she says, was her parents' nonresponse after the rescue. No visit to the hospital. Nothing. Her realization that all she has in her life is her own self-loathing.

Later she told me during the ten years death inhabited her every wak-ing thought before the trauma, and before she decided to live, if she had been able to conceive of dying in captivity, she would be dead. In such a death you needn't have been. No acknowledgment that you lived by killing yourself. Instead, you were disappeared. No body. Just gone as if you never were because you weren't. It met all the requirements.

She told me she gave up fantasies of dying because at some point she knew she wouldn't kill herself and there was too much pleasure in the fantasies. She couldn't allow herself the indulgence. Yet, in the first month of treatment she told me the following two dreams dreamt years before the trauma, before she met me. The only dreams she'd had in ten years, she said.

I am in my house with other people. Someone came in. Broke in. There was a violent episode. The person mowed everybody down including me. It was very bloody. Slaughtered us. And yet I was still there. The person who had killed all five of us was sitting at the table and I had to serve them food and water, which I did. Then I woke.

She can't be killed because she doesn't live. She's not enough alive to live. Only alive enough to keep serving others. It's haunting. It is a haunting.

A prisoner was missing. I went to look for him. I didn't find him. I went to bed in my dream. I felt someone on me. There was a person in bed next to me bludgeoned to death with a brick. It was the prisoner. There was blood all over me. I was wearing pieces of his skull.

We wear each other tight against the chests, seeping into each other, in pieces broken up in one, then the other. This is what it felt like. Yet she insists on our separateness. Pieces and parts. She and me. Her missing. My mess.

There has always been murder here. Mine and hers. And murderers. Sub-jugation and surrender. . .

> If we go on we might stop
> in the street in the very place
> where someone disappeared
> and the words Come with us! we might
> hear them. If that happened, we would
> lead our lives with our hands
> tied together. That is why we feel
> It is enough to listen
> to the wind jostling lemons . . . the cries of those who vanish
> might take years to get here (Forché, in "San Onofre, California, in *The Country Between Us*, 1981, 9)

I was so impatient. My hands bound. I wanted to hear the scent of lemon. That's this story. How I followed the disappeared. Did I lead? I have my own "dead mother."

Followed found entered—became that split-off part of the self that desperately needs understanding but which is not available because she has/I have located it in the other, and it is years before she will/I will get here (Joseph 1975)?

****

Although wherever you are going is always in front of you, there is no such thing as straight ahead. No as the crow flies short cut will help you reach the café just over the water. The short cuts are where the cats go, through the gaps, round the corners that seem to take you the opposite way.

(Winterson 1989, 49)

Every day I am in the room with her, following the cats, round the corners, and she is travelling away from me into a treatment without words. Yet in the beginning, she talked. One month three times a week. This is what I learned. Haltingly:

Her grandparents raised her. A grand/mother who is cold and distant, critical. And doesn't like crying. A grand/father who was warmer but tormented, intermittently violent. How she watched herself from the bottom of the stairs when she was 7 fall down them after her grand/father slapped her and she tumbled unconscious to wake in another room, ears ringing, her grand/mother saying her father was sorry. It's the time, one of two, she can remember her mother ever acknowledging the violence. And the adolescent remembrance where he ripped her shirt off of her when she tried to leave, holding her to him, with her mother on her knees begging him to let her go. She remembers both stories by the fact of her mother's interventions. She doesn't bother to tell any others. How her father would come and go at night on "house calls." She thought he was a burglar stealing in the night.

The telling undoes her.

Sarah begins to recede. I become blurry to her, as do the questions I ask. I wonder aloud about the important people in her life. *I don't understand.* I ask in a different way. *I don't know what you mean.*

Soon direct questions simply go unanswered.

You are opaque.

Her parents forget to include her in a family reunion being planned.

I don't know who you are.

She can't locate me. I am unintelligible, imprecise, sloppy, clumsy. She stops talking. Every day she comes. And doesn't talk. For 50 minutes.

The more silence, the more despair. She is really gone. No thoughts or feelings, no fantasy. These moments are about primary object loss. I *have* disappeared. There is a massive decathexis of me and, of course, her mother before me. She has "psychical holes." She is blank, in blank/blanc mourning (Green 1972, 46).

I think of Searles (1965) and his description of psychological sensory deprivation. The way a certain kind of blankness reveals an immersion in a chaotically dedifferentiated amalgam of experience in which memories, fantasies, somatic sensations, and perceptions of the outer world are not separable from one another. Later I come to realize that I do not really exist for her.

There is no difference between inside and outside. There is no other. Almost a kind of autism. I am in her autism. Empathically experiencing her state of isolation. Her absence of another.

In the suffocation of that silence, I *recognize that she needs to know me.* I offer a poem:

I wanted the doctor to turn it off
But I couldn't seem to ask, . . .

But he said, "of course" as if I had asked,
And he stood and approached the heater, and then
Stood on one foot, and threw himself
Toward the wall with one hand, and with the other hand
Reached down, behind the couch, to pull
The plug out. I looked away,
I had not known he would have to bend
Like that. And I was so moved, that he

> Would act undignified, to help me,
> That I cried, not trying to stop, but as if
> The moans made sentences, which bore

Some human message. (Sharon Olds, "The Space Heater," in *The New Yorker*, 2001)

It seems that in this unconscious acknowledgement of her need and my vulnerability, a space opens between us. A sliver of light. The next day, she brings this.

Psalm 23

The Lord is my Shepherd

I shall not want   .

He maketh me to lie down in green pastures . . . he restoreth my soul (King James Bible, 1611)

I am stunned by the hope.

But here, in this mercurial city, it is required you do awake your faith. With faith, all things are possible (Winterson, p. 49).

I need more faith.

In that small opening, she notices the church across the street. Disconcerting how she has to look at a cross and the words the Blessed Sacrament. Later she would say she was getting converted by me.

How as a small child she had, over and over, driven by the church of the sacred heart and read the scared heart.

Then she falls silent again. She has said too much.

> *The astute gambler always keeps something back, something to play with another time: a pocket watch, a hunting dog. But the devil's gambler keeps back something precious, something to gamble with only once in a lifetime. Behind the secret panel he keeps it, the valuable, fabulous thing that no one suspects he has.*
>
> (Winterson, p. 90)

You can't risk anything with me here, she says. *You hide. What you risk reveals what you value* (p. 90). These were the terms.

I am hiding how alive she is for me. At times I grope near but can't see her. Like the helicopter overhead, hovering, raising hope but ultimately blind.

But when I find her, find her dead mother, it is worse. "Behind the blank mourning one catches a glimpse of the mad passion the mother is . . ." *(Green 1972*, 162*)*. He writes,

> When the analyst succeeds in touching an important part of the nuclear complex of the dead mother, for a brief instant, the patient feels himself to be empty, blank, as though he were deprived of a stop-gap, and a guard against madness.
>
> (Green 1972, 46)

She tells me about the pleasure in the deep softness of my voice.

Then how that admission cost her. *We cannot live in pleasure.* Green (1972) suggests that to feel the pleasure of the analyst's narcissistic investment provokes profound anxiety.

Her silence overflows with self-contempt.

I offer another poem. Mary Oliver (1986). One in which Oliver writes about not having to be good or having to repent. All that is required is to love what you love.

Sarah begins to speak again.

Sarah has an I. She thinks of herself as a person thinking thoughts. She makes meaning. Takes responsibility for her own actions. She remembers me. A new experience gets added to something from before. We have a past. I can exist as separate. She could lose me, hurt me. *Is this anxiety?* she asks.

And then I fail again. By not taking heed of my own gift of the poem. I am not showing her my delight. I wouldn't let myself love her out loud. Loving your thinking?

The past is recast. I am not the same person I have been. I am the person she always knew would destroy her. We have no history. Everything is arbitrary, erratic. She is buffeted about by thoughts, feelings as if by external forces. Everything we see is what is. There is only the real. We live inside it.

Would it help to theorize it? To give these shifts a name? A Melanie Klein name (Klein 1948)? Positions?

And there is silence.

If she speaks, she will lose her endangered sense of being barely alive. She is trying to maintain herself. I do not properly attend to this key need.

Sarah can only hold onto herself by sacrificing our relatedness.

She thinks I do not understand how ill she is, how fragile. She is trying to spare me, spare us, the sure disaster that will follow her loving and hating me.

She dreams: .

I'm on a beach. In the water, there are seals everywhere. At first they are beautiful. Then I realize they are dead, and they are not natural deaths, but rather the effect of waste. There are tubes in their mouths. Small, bristled vacuum cleaner attachments the size of fists. They can't breathe. They're also tied in ropes I realize as I move closer. They haven't died from this but from something really catastrophic. Some systemic disaster has happened.

There's a woman walking down—talking to another woman or maybe someone in the house. I feel bad for her. She doesn't yet know what really happened, why the seals are dying.

She bound and gagged. The trauma of our attachment. The catastrophe that looms. But Sarah doesn't care much about the symbol, the sucking tube, what gags her.

She keeps dreaming these dreams. The terror is what stays with her.

How can I talk about the place of deep identification, especially given my knowledge of own flagging analysis in the background? The bad patient who can't be helped, the bad analyst who cannot help. Stolorow and Atwood's intersubjective conjunction (1992). I know this "crunch" (Russell 2006) and offer her my Paul Russell (my first analyst who died) and his idea. But the work is so new, and we, so quick to this impasse, and I, so discouraged.

Someone more senior can help her, someone farther along, finished in his or her analysis. Someone who loves her less and whose identifications aren't so close. I suggest a consultation.

Her despair grew at its mention. That helps me. (I kept needing her help.) I remember, something is holding in the process. How can I have been so easily fooled? Over and over I pay attention to defense. That is my first leave taking (that I count).

To shift these organizing principles (Stolorow and Atwood 1992) is such hard work.

There is the day she asks me what I am thinking. "About 'The Love Song of J. Alfred Prufrock'" (Eliot 1915), I say. She looks up, genuinely interested. *Really?* she asks. "Yes," I say.

Why are you thinking of it? she queries. I reply:

I do not think that they will sing to me . . . .
We have lingered in the chambers of the sea
By sea-girls wreathed with seaweed red and brown
Till human voices wake us, and we drown.

(Eliot 1915)

What's that last line? she asks. "The end of the poem," I say. What is happening here, in the room. *No,* she says. *I recited the poem my whole way here, you see. I don't think that's how the poem ends.* But it does, I think.

That seems to make things worse. Makes her queasy. The way our minds might drift to a place we share, the synchronicity we can't quite translate. We need other people's words.

After that, she tells me she can't come in the room with me. She knows that the breath I breathe out, she will breathe in. Who am I, this stranger looming so close?

Like when I wonder if she knows Carolyn Forché. She is startled. She has been thinking of Forché just as I ask her. "Is there a specific poem?" I ask. She can't say. Later she tells me it was "The Stranger." The poem I began this paper with. More silence.

And I am reading and thinking of Adrienne Rich's poem "Diving into the Wreck":

The thing I came for:
The wreck and not the story of the wreck.

(Rich 1973, 197)

I keep diving into the wreck.

At the end of July, some relief comes. She asks me to hold a letter. Unopened. Too toxic for her to have at hand, too painful to read, too valuable to throw away. The letter is from someone who broke her heart and disappeared. We call them "the person-who-left-town." Their name is unspeakable.

I feel I have been given a valuable gift. A sign or symbol I can hold onto. And I do.

It is after that we have our first psychoanalytic moment of free association. She is thinking of an old woman on a bus with a beautiful face, alive in conversation. And into her mind comes thoughts of a serial killer she read about. A little later she is thinking of the person-who left-town's tender kiss and how into her mind comes the memory of her father beating her.

We live in these moments of free association one day and then the next I am off base.

I am so fast she tells me. Rushing from one thing to the next. Imagining I might start making love just where I stopped the day before. No prelude. Just a barbaric reentry.

I am always off. *Like a fifth-grade boy having sex*, she says. *Some template of how it goes. First to first, then second, then third. Fixed erotic zones, frenzied pressure.* Clumsy, awkward, impatient, dumb. I believed her. But fifth-grade boy? Fifth grade? A small 10-year-old?

Then I leave for three weeks. It's September.

She's always unadorned except for one small amethyst ring.

I have begun to wear a small ring of my daughter's. I think because I am needing to remember to get it sized for her. My own mother (who has given me little) has given it to my daughter from her mother (who likewise gave my mother little; my mother steals the ring at her death). Stunning in its constant change of color, deep blue like the sea, then violet, still later turquoise. All vacation I turn it on my finger.

Sarah does not look at me. She looks at the ring. I wonder out loud with her. Perhaps I am trying to hold her, too, in the absence. She feels queasy. She looks up.

You're revolted by me, she says. She can feel it from me in waves. "Hate," I query? "Oh no. I have not heard. Hate is voluntary. Revulsion is involuntary." *You can't help yourself*, she tells me.

I am stunned. Can she not feel my love?

While I've been away, she has returned to the town where the person-whose-name-we dare not speak disappeared to. She does not like to talk to me about the story. She feels (and she is right) that I do not fully believe her. I don't think the person just mysteriously left. I think she had a part to play in the terrible misunderstanding.

I am the person who left town. We are one. I cannot hold them fully responsible.

It is my second major leaving. I've begun to count.

She's seen her old therapist while there. Perhaps, he says, you cannot talk to her (me) because you "have a crush." *Have a crush?* she said, incredulous.

Later she thinks it's true. She has an aesthetic and visceral response to me. That's why she stays, but it can't help her—quite the opposite.

Red-faced and worried, she also tells me she's seen a new therapist. She's guilty. She doesn't want to hurt me. If we'd met another way, she thinks perhaps a conversation would be possible.

Later she tells me how I flinched when she told me. For several weeks, she sees the new therapist. She doesn't want to tell me how sure, how smart, how steady she is. She can't compare, it's not a fair comparison. I want the world for her. I am pleased. I know I am failing . . . If she can find help with her. . . . The next time I ask Sarah about the therapy, she doesn't want to speak of it, and the next time it's over, she says. I think it's been three, maybe four times. A year later an analyst I admire in the city has room for me. I have waited patiently on her waiting list. She is much sought after. "Let me tell you about my Sarah," I say.

But we can't talk. The analyst knows her, saw her, this most enigmatic woman, for the entirety of the fall the previous year. The woman was having trouble with her analyst. Each week the analyst had been certain that Sarah would leave her current analyst and begin analysis with her. They had connected, the analyst tells me, but then Sarah had stopped talking, paying, coming. And faded away.

Relief. Release. *It really isn't just me.*

I remember transference.

Had I known it was that consultant? If I had, it would not have been my first dissociation.

Yom Kippur. Time to atone in my book. To see if we have missed the mark.

There is a christening in her family. Her parents ignore her. She hasn't really spoken to them since she was jailed. She attends the service, but they don't see her. I feel her invisibility and how it will cost us. I can't get her attention. Nothing interests her. She is emptied hollow.

Something holds me with her. It is not my failure this time. I am with her. I am not afraid. I hold steady. Some hope comes from this steadiness. I have a basket filled with food. Just a bit, I say to myself. One sweet drop at a time.

She tells me she is drinking me in on a body level, my soft warm voice inviting her to muse with me. And then the dizzying punishment, she cannot cross to receive my offering. And the concurrent reality of being bludgeoned by this assaulting softness. My invitation as attack. I am unsteadied by the back and forth of this rhythm (Reed 2001).

She went to therapy with her parents in her twenties. She tried to talk with them about being a battered child. Her grand/father neither confirmed nor denied the abuse. He had a kind of blankness about him, she said.

There is a leaden feeling between us. No wiggle room.

She shares some things. The agony of fully having given herself to the person who left town, the not knowing how, the shame and humiliation at her underdeveloped self.

The next day she can't be in the room. It's a huge physical force. I am a dementor. I suck the life force from her. She is made weak, limp, melancholy (the danger of merging).

She says I am a riptide. "Yes," I say. "If I stand on the shore and call to you a way out, I am too far, if I come into the water with you, we will both drown."

Blankness comes. Sarah arranges to meet her grand/parents for dinner, but in lieu of choosing a restaurant ahead of time, it is decided they will meet on a street corner. It is costing her a lot to go. In dread. She is leaving a crucial meeting at work for them. She doesn't tell them. She is pressed, working hard for this as she traverses the city to come to them nowhere specific but far away from her. She is on public transportation. She tells them she will be a little late.

They don't wait. She is crushed. She calls me. *Is it the only time ever?* We don't say much, but the call matters. At first.

Being gotten through to feels like being penetrated and beaten. Soon she feels nothing. Soon I am nothing. Soon I will hurt her. With each bludgeoning, it is like leaving a scene of the crime. I have no idea how much damage I've done to her insides.

We add a fourth session. She dreams her first dream about therapy.

I had a dream. My only thought about it is that you will be thrilled.

"Thrilled?"

I'll be giving up something of myself.

I think of Ghent (1990). Surrender? Submission? I will try not to want it.

I've never seen her more animated as she tells the dream. It's like a Venn diagram. A place where all things come together. She gestures. She reenacts. I think, I've never seen her move before. I hardly see her breathe.

We are in your office. I don't know where I am. You're really excited, animated about something. You're telling me a story about this woman. She's your patient. I think, though, Why are you telling me about her session if she is your patient? Anyway, there's been a renowned woman in your office.

An expert. I must say you're impressed by her, this pain expert, and you're reenacting the session and telling me about the connection she's discovered between the brain and the arm. You come over to the couch and sit here (where she now is). You're reenacting what the expert says.

Who's the expert on pain? What roles are being reversed? Only later do I think of dreams of supervision (Blechner 2001).

She tells me I will learn from her. I think so too, my expert. She does not remember this part of what I said.

Sarah tells me at the end of this session, *I know you've been very generous with yourself.* On the day she gives me her dream.

A year later she will remind me of how when she told me I had a lot to learn from her, I had turned that into generic relational learning. And when she had commented on my generosity, I had disowned it as personal, made it the price of doing business, and how these rejections silenced her for a year. . . . I couldn't let her heal me.

The next day I don't open the office door.

This is what I was thinking. How she looked up for the first time in five long months and noticed the room. How she took in my flowers, which sit behind my head. I decide to change the water for them, for her, to keep them fresh. I leave my room, fill the vase from my outside hose. I keep my eye on the sidewalk. I watch for her, but it is early still and I go back and wait. She doesn't come. I don't fill the hour with any of the things I might. I sit quietly at my desk, first anticipating her, then missing her. First a little, then with some aching. Forty minutes pass, and suddenly I know that she is with me. I open my waiting room door. She is there. "When did you come?" I almost shout. She looks dead.

I've been here the whole time.

"Why didn't you knock?"

I didn't hear you.

Nor had I. She hadn't made a sound. Not a cough, not a turning of a magazine, not a breath. I hear everything from there to here.

No words. Again, for weeks.

Later she said she read, she went to the bathroom, was no stealth patient. I cannot, do not believe it. It was the first day she wanted to come, she said. To talk of the dream. Later she says at her moments of surrender I don't open the door. At the moment she exists, she tells me I will disappear. It's getting hard not to believe her. I think I am enacting her dread of being disappeared. We are living in annihilation anxiety.

Now she exists again by not being found. She is so withdrawn. Not a muscle moves. You couldn't move her like a mountain.

Her withdrawal allows her own motility. Her dead mother tucked inside. Nothing can enter this space, nothing can emerge from it. There is room for nothing else (Green 1972).

I need to be there. *Reliably*, she says when she finally speaks again.

We have come to an arrangement. I will leave her a message on Sundays.

I am away at a yoga retreat. On the first Sunday, I leave her a message about being glad to share a corner of the earth with her, alluding to the Oliver poem I brought to the treatment. Then I become frightened of having revealed too much.

The next day I am taken by a guide through magnificent woods. We walk and walk. I want to bring a friend back later but worry that I will get lost. The guide assures me I will be fine. That she will give me a map.

My friend and I embark later that afternoon, map in hand, at first unused as we follow the clearly marked trail. Soon things are more confusing. And the map is of another forest. For many hours we are lost, darkness falls, and while at first we are sure we will be found, we increasingly become less sure, then not sure at all? Eventually we are rescued by a large search party of men in trucks with dogs almost as scary as being lost. Should I reveal that we were within 100 feet in several different directions to exit the woods but could not be located?

Should I have told her?

I think of Benjamin (1998) and the problem of constructing the analyst/other who already speaks and the patient/other who does not yet speak for herself. This suffering other requires recognition by the subject who does speak, but this recognition will be effective only if it incorporates a moment of identification, and so disrupts the closed identity of the subject. Likewise, the other's attainment of speech can proceed only by her identification with the speaking subject, by which she is in danger of losing her own identity as other. If the patient must become the analyst, the analyst must also become the patient.

Surely this isn't quite what Benjamin had in mind?

When I see her on Monday, she is chatty, pleasant. I had not existed at all, but she tells me I came alive for her when I call on Sunday. Thoughts of me play in her mind, though she can't catch them. I am rising from the dead. It is the first time I have registered with her. It has cost me a lot, my weekend suffering alone and out with my desire, but it seems worth it. Is it mine?

I have the old maid now. The queen of spades (Davies 2004), it's mine. I am swirling, twirling, hurling. She lives inside me. Take it back, I think.

On Wednesday she tells me her heart is fractured. I say your heart is broken, and we miss again.

And then another holiday. They are always bad. Thanksgiving. I give her a window I will call in. I am 20 minutes late.

She doesn't notice I am calling on Thanksgiving. Only that I am late.

I cannot believe that I am late. I have watched the clock.

She comes Friday but won't speak. She cancels Monday and Tuesday. She comes Wednesday but won't speak.

The absence between us feels complex, nuanced. Seizes hold of us again, shadows us, threatens to propel us toward oblivion. But Green says absence is a necessary condition for a vital life—an intermediary situation between presence (intrusion) and loss (annihilation).

She tells me we have no tonal resonance. We do not both start at C.

She cancels all appointments in December. Each day I leave a message. Each night she calls back as if she might come the next day. Later I learn her sister has been critically ill. She might die. She is managing the crisis. She never says.

When she returns, she dreams.

I had a dream last week. I was very badly injured. I couldn't get in to see whom I need. I have to force myself in, literally, but I am badly injured, bleeding. I don't know how I know, but I have a gruesome scar under my right eye.[2]

I am in the emergency room—they keep saying other people are in front of me, but I don't see them. Finally I convince them to let me in, it's my turn, and the person, I guess it's the doctor, opens their arms. I am furious all they have is open arms.

She tells me there is a scar in my *Eye*. It's gruesome. All I have is open arms.

In January she says she came to know she might actually keep me faint, indistinct. Her old therapist's comments about my presence, her attraction, something about all this needs to be kept at bay. She says it's not just me.

Again, she tells me the story of her love who left. She uses all the language, literally the words, she uses to describe our relation. The lover had a deep ambivalence about her; there was something not integrated about them; they would say they loved her and would justify their nonloving behavior by throwing theories around. The lover's love was self-contained; they didn't need Sarah for it. It was dangerous relationship, she said, and I refused to see it, encouraging it through my neutrality.

Does she hear the similarities? *Yes*, she says. But she doesn't question my capacity, just my commitment. But isn't it the other way around?

I do better. I am empathic. I feel with her the devastation of this relationship, her anguish of having allowed herself to trust, the betrayal and deadly grief. I know what we are up against.

You have to risk everything, she tells me.

Later in the month she is travelling and has to call me for our sessions. The conversations are different, deeper, more involved. In them Sarah talks. When she comes back she acts as if they'd never happened. She has my failure on her lips. She tells me she talks of knitting while I talk of weaving. She is *phonetic*, and I am *whole language*.

But something new becomes possible.

She realizes I am just a person, not so scary. If she and her lover were yin and yang, she and I are positive and negative. She is Goofus to my Gallant. We are back to *Highlights*, her childhood. Why do you have to be bad to my good? I wonder. But I know, I think.

Late fall becomes winter, becomes spring. A step forward, four back. Each contact precipitates closeness and catastrophe. There is nothing small.

I have seen a line from "Hymn," a poem of Ammons (1986) used as a quote by Ogden. I tell her the line. Sarah brings me the poem. Later I buy his book.

> I know if I find you I will have to leave earth
> And go on out . . . And if I find you I must go out deep into your
> Far resolutions
> And if I find you I must stay here with the separate leaves.
>
> (p.9)

And she answers me with Stevie Smith's "Not Waving but Drowning" (1983):

> Nobody heard him, the dead man,
> But still he lay moaning:

I was much further out then you thought
And not waving but drowning . . .

(p. 301)

We circle around.

She denies pleasure as a discipline. She tells me she is like a good spy. When she is captured, she knows nothing. I see her laugh for the first time. Throw her wild mane of Black hair back and laugh. She tells me I will learn something from her about a fruit ripening and that there is a time for everything under the sun.

Sarah dreams more and more. Annihilation and murder—but this, like the treatment, begins to shift as well.

There is a wholescale terrorist attack. There are no lights. It is completely dark and I cannot get my car out of the parking lot. Something is wrong with the trains and I have to drive. I am driving to get somewhere safe, out to the woods.

There is a fork in the road. I go down one path, but it is completely dark. Desolate. Then I hear a voice. It is a great voice like a radio announcer's voice. Soft and deep. I think I should go toward that voice, that must be the right fork.

It is hard for me to stop here or anywhere. I want to tell you all her dreams and how they transform. And the other poems and associations. But there isn't an end in sight.

It is almost spring. Sarah's birthday has just passed, and we share something lovely about what we are building together. It is a moment of uncertainty, fragility, hope.

Notes

1 Judy Teicholz (2000) describes the "authentic" analyst as the one who reflects back to a patient how the patient's behavior affects the analyst, so that the patient might see how others react to her. The "empathic" analyst addresses how her own behavior has affected the patient and how much sense the patient's behavior makes in light of the analyst's thoughts and feelings.

2 (Should I tell you how in that same time my son is run over by a cyclist, has a gruesome cut now scar under his right eye. How trapped on a bridge we couldn't get him to the hospital at first, the ambulance missing us, how we carried him and couldn't get him help?)

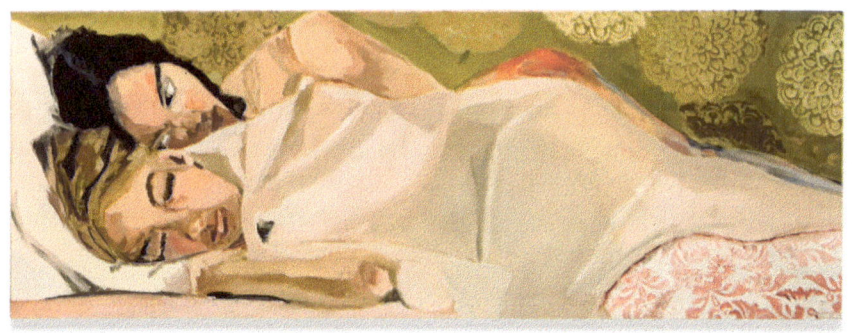

Figure 2.1 Waiting. Oil on canvas. 36x12. McGleughlin

Chapter 3

Afterword(s) on writing

We always tell it slant—clinical stories create truths, not describe them (2020)

I have included two distinct accounts of my work with Sarah here to demonstrate how differently we feel about a case and its subjects depending on how the story has been told. In the first version, "The Analyst's Necessary Vertigo," I want to show how an analyst's reach matters, but without reducing the analyst's efforts to pathology, or presuming that her subjectivity can be well symbolized (especially by the analyst herself) or brought into a two-person way of relating to the patient in the room. The different versions of the case muse on the same questions, but "Vertigo" is told at a steady clip with a forward-moving narrative. And while I want you to wonder in a theoretical way who's the patient here, who's the healer, I am clearly the analyst. I seem credible, reflective, able to offer ideas, like an analyst might. Drawn in by the playful tone of the chapter's opening or the theory I've employed, you might even feel good about me as a colleague, despite any disagreements with my thinking. You have no reason to doubt me, or the portrait of the patient I have painted.

In "The Raw Story," I do something else. It's less like humming along associatively and more like slogging through peanut butter. While I did not intentionally seek to recreate the feeling of the case when I first wrote it, I was trying to write in the chaos, give the feeling of being both flooded with and immersed in something and simultaneously shut out from the experience. I had hoped by evoking the tone of hysteria, the drama, and melodrama of the case I could write myself into conveying that something in the field came about between me and the patient, something powerful that cannot be described as a meaning. This prose/theory/poem was inadvertently my first experiment in enacted writing, (Naiburg 2015) where the reader may be inducted into the experience the writer creates.

DOI: 10.4324/9781032670348-5

In writing this way, I become a suspicious narrator. I leave my professional voice and wade into a version of my inner workings, my own difficult reactions, their connections to my own trauma. So, reading it, you might feel worried about me, or critical of me. Perhaps you're off balance, with vertigo of your own. (Or maybe by now the piece is edited so thoroughly that the felt angst is gone. You might feel bored by the cycles of the same story.) It is easy to think, *Perhaps there* is *something really wrong with this analyst. Maybe it's not the patient at all.* I have tilted the frame towards analyst as patient.

While the enacted writing happened unconsciously, I was quite conscious about my wish to disrupt the dualistic and hierarchical notion of the patient as the subject of inquiry and the analyst as a superior expert who does the inquiring and ultimately the recognizing. Who's the subject? Who's the object? How are we entwined? Ferenczi, Racker, Searles, Gill, Levenson, Russell, Benjamin, and Hoffman have all recognized the importance of the patient as teacher and healer of the analyst. Sarah believes, and I do, too, that she will need to heal something in me so that I can help her. I've sought to expose these bidirectional effects to underscore this dynamic.

I also hope that this piece might make you wonder if cordoning off our internal worlds from readers may limit our ever-evolving theory and practice, given the increasing agreement that analysis involves two subjects and that the analyst's subjectivity invariably influences the treatment.

We do write about our own subjectivities, of course, but usually only in reference to the countertransference. In many clinical accounts, we surveil the patient as if we were realistic, accurate reporters. Indeed, it is very hard to write outside this frame. Yet in Part 1, and as the book goes on, you will see I am interrogating whether the pretense of objectivity serves the people we treat: is our outside-in look necessary in our writing, or, as can be true in clinical work, can it sometimes be nontherapeutic and potentially subjugating? While most contemporary analysts believe we are shaping what we see, our writing has not reflected our deep and personal, not just countertransferential, involvement as originators of experience in the affective field.

Difficult treatments are also described in our literature, and sometimes they even include the suffering of the analyst, but we are less likely to find analytic accounts that incorporate our subjectivities in a moment-to-moment, experientially alive way. Why don't we allow the reader inside this way? One reason might be that by the time a case is written up, its author is often more senior, and more prone to theorize than to palpably revisit her own distress or trauma. Perhaps this is as it should be, though it's as much of a description of how things are as a comment on whether they need always be that way.

Another explanation is that such a presentation would too closely resemble the minds of our patients, potentially exposing us and worrying them. As one example of the similarity between patient and analyst, you might notice how in the "Raw Story" Sarah and I move toward and away from each other. This offers a rethinking of the traditional Kleinian notion that patients are continually advancing and retreating from making a live connection with the therapist's psyche, shifting back and forth between depressive and paranoid-schizoid positions (Likierman 2006). This vacillation is often thought to reflect the patient's unconscious object relationship (2006). Might it be useful to have a similar literature for the analyst's corresponding movement toward or away, and a means to describe what could never be defined as one or the other's object relationship?

There are a variety of patient-centered reasons we leave our psychic involvement out of many accounts, but it also allows us to remain healthy, credible, in control. We want to maintain our power. As a field, so much of our analytic writing shows allegiance to Euro-American, male-centric academic scholarship, which has tended to obscure its subjective inclinations and investments (Fournier 2021). Since Freud's own early writing, we have felt compelled to present our work as something akin to scientific and objective, despite the very clear autobiographical and personal elements in Freud's own theory-making and clinical work. Freud's need to legitimize his revolutionary thinking and method has a very long tail. More than a century on, we're obscuring just how much of the analyst's subjectivity—her interests, her concerns, her focus—is invariably embedded in a case.

When analytic writers have tried to interweave the personal with the theoretical, their neutrality has been doubted (See Chapter 12), as has the intellectual credibility of their work. Historically, incorporating personal experience in theoretical writing has made one vulnerable to being criticized for narcissism, for lacking sufficient critical distance, or for failing to show rigor—all of which mean that this style of writing is professionally risky (Fournier 2021). As literary critic Barbara Johnson observes, "Any body of work that includes personal experience has tended to be excluded from the discourse of knowledge. Worse, the realm of the personal itself has been coded as female and devalued for that reason" (Fournier, p 15).

It is not just the analyst's inner world that is omitted from clinical accounts but the patient's as well. How is the voice of the patient really conveyed? In the case of Sarah, there is little history, little tethering to ground you. You might have been thinking, *I can't get the* feel *of Sarah's Sarah*. I don't share our verbatim dialogue; she has no voice of her own except through my projections, as was sometimes true in the work. (Sarah's one place of narration was her dreams, so I include those, but they are very abbreviated.) Certainly, Sarah remains on the edge, outside, liminal, in some substantial measure because of her silence. But regardless of the writing of this one case, I would like for us to wonder if we don't *always* render our patients voiceless. As you will see in stories later in the book, like Lenù's narration of Lila in Ferrante's Neapolitan Quartet, I am raising questions about telling stories about people who cannot or do not speak for themselves.

In a body of work called *Autotheory*, Fournier (2021) attempts to question what constitutes theory and to what extent it can make apparent the personal within it. She defines autotheory as moving

> between theory and philosophy . . . [between] the master discourses with their status as intellectually rigorous . . . and the experiential and the embodied often written by people who have had less access to these modes of discourse like women, queer, poor and BIPOC folks.
>
> (p. 14)

I don't know if this raw chapter would fall under this genre, a "self-conscious way of engaging with theory, as a discourse, frame, or mode of thinking and practice alongside lived experience" (Fournier 2021, 7), but I think so. The skepticism or suspicion that comes with writing in less academic or objectivist ways is something I invite with "The Raw Story."

Yet though that piece is framed with a vulnerability that implies authenticity, it's not the "real story" any more than is the paper "Vertigo." Expostulating from what Poletti writes, following Butler, the *story itself constitutes the case through the act of writing it*, rather than the expression of it (Fournier 2021). By widening the aperture in "The Raw Story," narrowing it in Vertigo," and displaying the writing's theoretical underpinnings in the technical section, what I am hoping to show throughout this section is that we as analysts are never depicting a life or relationship that exists prior to the act of writing about it. It comes into being *through* our writing of it. Writer Maggie Nelson perhaps says best in one pithy sentence: "Let the writing perform that the memory is false" (cited in Fournier 2021, 16).

If we claim our writing functions as objective, we are employing seeing as a way of knowing, which is always mimetic of our own self-image, because we see only what we know (Phelan 1994). As Butler argues, "The real is positioned both before and after its representation; and representation becomes a moment of the consolidation of the real" (Phelan 1994, 2). What we represent is temporal, no more solid than what we eliminate. But because we, as a field, write in the way we do, psychoanalysis reproduces a specific logic of the real, and this logical real promotes its own representation as if it were true, limiting other possibilities.

What makes our portrait? What affects or drives our hand? And what is cut out? Invisible? As in any portrait, we do not document reality, no matter how much realism marks our canvas. And while each picture an artist/writer creates is singular—motivated by the views, needs, feelings, ideas they want to convey at a specific moment—there is a recognizable style that is uniquely ours (and not our patients'), indicative of what we can and cannot see, what we are willing or unwilling to show (Phelan 1994).

Chapter 4

Afterword(s) on technique
Necessary reach (2009)

Two ways in: can theory help?

In my work with Sarah, I thought we could craft an intersubjective story in which we used our competing subjectivities to understand her mind. I relied on other stock ideas like working with the transference/countertransference in the here and now, exploring negative therapeutic reaction, utilizing cycles of trauma and repair, and examining my own failure. But I was relying on a relational red herring, because Sarah had serious trouble with what we formerly called stable psychic structure, self/other differentiation, and intrapsychic conflict. Or, in better language, she struggled to reflect on her experience, recognize me as separate from her, or feel alive—the prerequisites for more language-based, relationally oriented treatment.

Most of this chapter was written in 2009, after years of questioning and reflecting, writing and talking about this treatment with colleagues. It remains for me among the most poignant, if challenging, clinical experiences I have ever had. I learned an enormous amount. Here is one more way to think about the case.

It is 1999. For several years, I am simultaneously but separately supervised by two highly regarded relational psychoanalysts. Occasionally the three of us meet, struggling individually and collectively to understand how I can make genuine emotional contact with Sarah, a woman who enacts trauma rather than remembers it, for whom trauma is not yet encoded in verbal forms. While both supervisors shared basic premises about relational psychoanalysis, their approaches to the case were significantly different.

The first offered:

> Set boundaries, carve out your separate self, stop seeing your similarities, know how different you are. Stand tall. Intersubjective space is

DOI: 10.4324/9781032670348-6

always filled with distinction, difference and otherness. Full identification is a fantasy.

The second recommended:

Imagine yourself into being without agency, resource, or capacity; enter her experience in a full way. At every single moment of, "I can't do this another second, I can't give up my life and my sanity," just do it anyway, hold on at all costs and see. This will be the means for her to establish her own subjectivity.

The tension between the two perspectives, theoretical and technical, offered a compelling opportunity to examine the inherently comparative nature of relational theory as it meets clinical practice. I want to underscore our need to treat Relational Psychoanalysis not as a unitary, overarching meta-theory but as a way of thinking that embraces multiplicity. I was also trying, again, to metabolize the work.

Embedded in this essay, written seven years after the treatment finished, is the idea that both my patient and I had an array of self-states that became activated in our specific relational configuration. While this was not yet a stock relational idea in 1999, a developmental model featuring multiplicity was already gaining ground through infant attachment theory, chaos systems theory, and the pioneering work of Bromberg. Benjamin's concepts of shared identifications and mirroring complementarities would come in 2004, but when I wrote my first lengthy paper on this treatment in 2001, illustrating the breakdown of recognition in Benjamin's terms and our failure to ever achieve a place of "thirdness," there was little written on the impact of our complementarities and their paralyzing effect, which I only knew experientially.

A relational object-relations perspective

In the first supervisory dyad, we try to understand Sarah's silence through her treatment as it comes to rest inside of me. We pay close attention to how my countertransference oscillates between feelings of love/desire and annihilation/erasure to understand the patient's feelings of the same. We understand this to be direct unconscious communication.

The case is filled with so much near-death experience, the raw annihilation anxiety generated in each of us (patient and analyst), that this supervisor and I draw mainly on European continental theories (Steiner, Joseph, Green) and the work done with very disturbed children and psychotic patients (Milner, Alvarez, Searles, Robbins). Yet we also recognize the one-person aspect of this literature, so counterbalance it with the relational notions of the mutual, unconscious impact Sarah and I are having on each other. We believe one relational configuration may be my inhabitation of her child self: alone, abandoned, filled with longing.

For a long period in the treatment, we theorize that I am the holder of all conscious desire in the relationship, which leads to acute feelings of masochism and shame on my part. We understand that 1) these feeling states already existed inside of me and are activated by the treatment, and 2) that they regulate my ability to be in contact with Sarah—both relational ideas. Nonetheless, our focus is on the patient's self-states as they come to be located in me.

Through an object-relations perspective, my supervisor and I register Sarah's intense involvement with me as sadomasochistic: interpreting her psychic retreats, her evacuation of large parts of herself, and her communications as acts of unconscious aggression. Steiner (1993) gives us a frame with his descriptions of the elaborate defensive systems such patients use to bind, neutralize, and control anxiety, pain, and primitive destructiveness. The patient is projecting the desire to make contact onto the analyst, and the analyst must hold all the desire for the treatment, replete with the need to be the pursuer, the keeper of the want. Like Green (1972), Steiner disputes the idea of withdrawal as *actual disengagement*, instead regarding it as a sadomasochistic interaction designed to avoid abandonment or destructiveness or absence.

Sarah's repeated withdrawals feel teeming with connection to me, and Steiner (1993) helps bring me back into contact with her by shifting the focus from my own masochistic feelings (engendered by her departures) to her inner world: the complicated gangs (object relations) keeping pain and destructiveness at bay (p. 4). He notes that these pathological forms of organization are equally an *expression* of the destructiveness as a defense against it.

Where I diverge from the British school is to eschew direct interpretation because receiving, containing, and metabolizing a projection from Sarah—and giving it back to her in a less toxic form—proves impossible. Instead, drawing upon a more relational model, I conceive of enactments as the primary therapeutic agent. But as one might expect, and as you saw in the "The Raw Story," negotiating rupture and repair dialogically is premature.

In this first supervision, we also use Green's idea (1972) about how I am incorporated into Sarah's unacknowledged fantasy with a reversal of subject and object. According to Green, when a patient has internalized a psychically dead parent so as to have and hold that parent, to nurture and cure that parent—so the parent is not totally lost to them—the transference contains a reversal. In Green's formulation (1972), I have to breathe life back into Sarah by imbuing her with my aliveness. Sarah has to feel she is garnering my special attention, that I am narcissistically invested in her, through my pursuit of her. These are the conditions in which a patient can begin to bear the confrontation with the internally entombed dead mother and gradually separate from her.

Green (1972) helps me contain me feelings of inadequacy in another way. Sometimes when I connect with Sarah and thus leave the session elated, she goes home and punishes herself, dissociates, and stops coming to treatment. "When the analyst succeeds in touching an important aspect of the nuclear complex of the dead mother, for a brief instant, the patient feels himself to be empty, blank, as though he were deprived of a stop-gap, and a guard against madness" (Green 1972, 62). If the connection is exposed, Green explains, the mad passion for the mother buried inside emerges, and the patient will be overcome by overwhelming vivifying emotion. When this happens, naked despair shows itself. Put another way, Green is saying what happens is what is supposed to happen. Sarah cannot let me see what I mean to her.

I am grateful for these theories because they give me a way to feel less shame about my love of Sarah. It is necessary. I am managing my affects through theory that focuses on the *patient's* needs. Comfortable, right? Psychoanalysis as we know it. Though I feel better keeping this in mind, I also feel slightly disingenuous. This is not a technique. Sarah *is* special. She has my keen, genuine interest. And while the object-relations literature contains me (and my attendant fears and anxieties that I am doing it wrong), when I carry this perspective—even just this feeling—into the treatment, I lose Sarah. She knows intuitively, and I do too, that an account like Steiner's does not take up the self-states of the analyst, his inner world, the bidirectional nature of the field. If I get fully on board with Steiner, I cannot believe my patient's story. This is the conflict.

This is in 2001, and no one is talking in descriptive terms about how the analyst's pathology shapes the treatment. While impasse has already been conceptualized as bidirectional—a problem potentially lodged in the analyst—and while we've made the turn toward the analyst's mind, we have yet not seen the way this looks in clinical writing (at least not since Ferenczi). Davies (2004) has not yet written *Whose Bad Objects Are We Anyway?* I suspect, however, that the problem is not really just Sarah, it is me. The shame of this, the unbearableness of my affective state—the way her withdrawals catapult me into relation with my own unpredictable, now entombed, "dead mother"—prompts me to seek additional guidance.

A relational self-psychological perspective

With my second supervisor, my work with Sarah is chiefly viewed through the lens of a thwarted developmental process, marked by a tremendous deficit. The Object Relational theory that suggests that because the analyst feels something visceral it follows that the patient has produced this feeling seemed limited and confusing. I doubt that Sarah has sufficient agentic capacities to be responsible for my affective disruption. Because of adaptation to early developmental failures (rather than defenses against intrapsychic conflict), words have no meaning and cannot yet be symbols. Long periods of destructive enactments are expectable because words are implements of "destruction, seduction and coercion" (Robbins 1996, 769). A focus on defense is misleading. This leads me to Stolorow, et al. (1998), who note that concepts like projective identification, which require an unconscious intent to evacuate bad feeling into the mind of the other, imply the operation of developed (though perhaps unconscious) representations of self and other, and affective communication between them. With a patient like Sarah, this capability is potentially not yet formed.

I find myself equating the dynamics of our relationship to the way an undifferentiated being like a baby takes hold of the internal regulatory system of the mother in an attempt to survive (Slavin 2011). What seems vital to point out is that while such a formulation retains the flavor of deep mix-up of self and other, it does not assume an intent, even unconscious, to transfer to the other to eliminate unbearable affects. Instead, patients involve us in symbiotic dramas in order for us to know about experience that had never taken form as experience, implicit or explicit, because there was no intersubjective system in which they could emerge (Orange 2008).

This shift in my thinking is influenced by the self-psychological approach of my second supervision.

This supervisor asks me to imagine myself into a feeling state without agency, resource, capacity—to step into Sarah's experience without attention to my own self states. He wants me to believe Sarah's story that I don't exist for her, and not take her silences as communications, much less aggression toward me. In this frame, I try to decenter from my own affective experience of her and her clamoring nonverbal messages to me. This means entering a reality that feels completely obliterating. My supervisor calls upon me to do it nevertheless. Let time unfold. Enter her world, enter it with abandon. This is empathy.

Given my extremely aroused affective state, existing within Sarah's idea that I did not register in her psychic world often felt psychotic. Yet I discover when I *can* work this way, it seems to allow my patient more room to exist: she feels held (while I feel dysregulated). I might be, in Green's sense, the dead mother who she can heal.

In time I recognize that, depending on the theoretical stance I adopt, one of us feels "done to" in Benjamin's terms (2004)—either she is unseen or annihilated or I am. In both supervisory dyads, my responsibility for my participation within the treatment is assumed, but in the first model, I try to own and repair my mistakes. Sarah, however, cannot recognize these relational moments. She is not interested in what I have done. Or her own participation. Her innocence about her hostility is, we theorize, a product of an unintegrated psyche in which affect is globalized rather than appropriate to mental content.

By contrast, the second model requires that I actively turn away from *my* experience, which includes any acknowledgement of my misses and failures. In a way, I need to unlearn a version of relational work that assumes two participants in the room. Because Sarah's world is solitary and undifferentiated, it is premature to home in on the way we impact each other, or affectively regulate each other. Our focus is on what has not yet developed psychically for the patient.

My stance here might be thought of as a return to the less visible, silent presence of the classical analyst, at least as (he's) often caricatured. Despite how excruciating, and often impossible, it is to sustain such a state of attentive nonexistence, I find myself thinking that, in fact, it may be necessary with such patients, as someone like Grossmark (2018) would come to illustrate so beautifully. The second supervision takes me in this direction. It is my subjectivity that is intrusive and troublesome for the patient. Winnicott might call it impingement (Winnicott 1949), and prior to offering my authenticity or subjectivity, my quiet, non-intrusive presence seems essential.

Still, sometimes Sarah experiences my quietude as empty; not attuned to her but absent. When I express something of my empathy, I suggest my separate subjectivity, and that will often be experienced by her as dangerous. Moments of empathic meeting seem to actually *cause* rupture, inviting a more object relational framing. But unlike with an objectivist outside/in lens, or fully self-psychological one of joining and mirroring, I learned I needed to immerse myself in *my* states of nonbeing, not reflect or change hers. It is a return to my own horrifying place of nonexistence that begins to allow Sarah to recognize and register feeling states within herself, to create something, to surface, to establish "going-on-being," in Winnicott's terms (1949). It will be some time, however, before she feels conflict, before she begins in her terms to exist. I think I had to feel Sarah's sense of existential anxiety with and for her and in myself. Overall, I came to believe that this kind of enactment, involving the mix-up of the insides of two people, is a necessary mode of therapeutic action and empathy. Then we could live together in a shared affective space outside of language where she could feel rather than hear me. These ideas have shaped my life work.

My first supervisor bristles against all the suffering I'm enduring. She doubts this new Sarah I cook up with the second supervisor, the one who requires my utter submission, complete surrender, new parameters of the frame, who is *only* solitary or victim and has no agency. This supervisor reminds me of the bigness of Sarah's job, her intellect, her aggressive self with regard to all things professional. She wants me to see Sarah's agency in the analysis, its detrimental effects on me *and* on her. She wants me to search for the transference-countertransference significance of this one self-state of Sarah's having totally taken over the treatment (Davies 2004). She pushes me to include these shadings as part of the picture of Sarah that I draw.

To this first supervisor, Sarah's projections are just that, and I am susceptible to accepting those attributions as true rather than as part of Sarah's mind. Importantly, she notes that it is impossible to ameliorate or answer to her charges, and that my method of trying harder to get it right will necessarily fail. Because I've become seduced by Sarah's suffering, I'm imagining that it's my task to ameliorate and equilibrate her behavioral and emotional states (Robbins 1996), a losing battle. Sarah's envy of my life, my marriage, my children may be part of what is so unarticulated and costly, this supervisor says. My willingness to talk with Sarah, even on weekends, to get her back into the office after missed sessions (there are many), to pursue her, could be making her worse. She wonders if Sarah is guilty about how much I do for her, the way she can take me over. Maybe Sarah is worried that she is wearing me out, making me sick. This supervisor thinks I need to protect myself a bit more. Wonders about my omnipotence in the case, the extent of what I am willing to do, willing to endure. She wonders about my heroic rescue.

Robbin's: the case for a qualitatively different mind

In the course of this case, a third theorist, Robbins, seemed to bridge aspects of a more object relational and self-psychological stance, though he, too, maintained a solidly one-person theory. Long periods of destructive enactments are expectable because words are implements of "destruction, seduction and coercion" (Robbins 1996, 769). Because of the trouble Sarah had in maintaining a representation of her experience of herself or of me (object constancy), her difficulty reflecting on her mind rather than enacting it interpersonally, and the ongoing confusion between what was her mind and what was mine, Robbins would categorize her as a "primitive" patient, a term I am replacing imperfectly with "unintegrated" because of the racist history of that word (Brickman 2017). The key point here was that Robbins argued that the minds of unintegrated patients are qualitatively different from more neurotic ones—and it's a mistake for the analyst to proceed as if her mind operates like the patient's. That error, he says, "naturally leads the analyst to believe that formal requirements or technical interventions that would be useful to him in understanding himself are equally comprehensible and useful to his patient" (Robbins 1996, 66).

Indeed, my identifications with Sarah did keep me attempting to intervene in ways that had been of use to me. Sarah and I both possessed internally entombed "dead mothers," certainly one source of our being trapped in a dyadic complementarity, leading to the now-familiar impasse of doer/done (Benjamin 2004). And in my own analysis, in less dramatic ways, I struggled to integrate previously split-off aspects of myself and bring them into better resonance, better dialogue. My identification with Sarah, as a patient who was "failed" in the course of her development and again in treatment, might have muddied the waters.

Robbins' technical advice is to suggest parameters to help the patient become a subject capable of bearing the intrapsychic conflict intrinsic to relational intersubjectively: 1) Make eye contact to mirror and contain, much like the mother does for the infant; 2) Understand that free association can be disorganizing rather than revealing because associations remain unlinked—instead, relevant content will be enacted; 3) Maladaptive beliefs and adaptations to a crazy familial environment must be noted and challenged if the patient is to become integrated enough to experience intrapsychic conflict which is not yet a primary motivator of experience; 4) Alternatives to the patient's ways of thinking and behaving should be offered to encourage analysis of the origins of self-destructive beliefs and actions, as well as to promote conflict and choice in the present; 5) Judicious clarification and interpretative sharing of the countertransference may be not only useful but essential.

In fact, Sarah taught me these parameters. Not just through her enactments and our necessary failures but also through her verbal instructions: in her refusal to lie down, in her fear of free associating, in her insistence on her alienation from words, in her puzzlement over my frequent questions about what motivated her behavior and about why she was angry or sad, aggressive, or withdrawn. She taught me by rejecting a frame that indicated she had a choice to speak.

Perhaps what was most useful in Robbins' account of the "qualitatively different mind" was his discussion of the failures of a trauma and repair model, as well as the complications he added to conceptions of empathy and confrontation. Both were things neither supervision had quite been able to articulate. I think Robbins might agree with the object-relations supervisor's tendency to think that the analyst is vulnerable to becoming seduced by the patient's suffering, and thus will (futilely) endeavor to "fix" the patient's behavioral and emotional states. Like her, Robbins is clear that the therapist becomes a projective screen for the unintegrated personality "and inevitably participates in a drama in which the patient seeks to coerce compensation from him" (p. 769).

But, like the *second* supervisor, Robbins doesn't believe this is a problem signaling the pathology or omnipotence of the particular analyst. Go there with the patient, Robbins says, though he doesn't share the second supervisor's belief that joining with or understanding is necessarily empathy or the best technical strategy in such situations. While Robbins notes that the analyst sensitively and imaginatively enters the patient's world in all good treatments, he believes the empathic method is "fraught with pitfalls when dealing with an unintegrated and undifferentiated person, especially if the empathic stance is viewed as a preferable alternative to objectification and at times confrontation" (Robbins 1996, 61). Unlike Kohut (1972), who noted the difficulty of empathy for mentally fragile patients and found them conventionally unanalyzable, Robbins argues that with consistent confrontation, the patient will, over time, feel a fuller sense of being understood.

Robbins writes,

> Because so much of their functioning is based on enactment of primary unconscious elements such as rage, and not linked to stable, dynamically unconscious mental representations, and because they tend toward projective-introjective oscillations, confrontation by the analyst with things that seem objectively apparent to the patient may be tantamount to showing him a rage which he may uncritically and compliantly introject into a self-attacking badness identity and use to invalidate his own perceptions.
>
> (Robbins 1996, 71)

This felt particularly felt so resonant: Whenever I'd float my perception of what was happening in the room, Sarah would locate hostility in me and feel attacked but would then turn the perceived hostility on herself in a vicious self-attack.

I offer so much of Robbin's theory because I think that as a beginning analyst—particularly a relational one, taught to avoid one-person thinking—his technical suggestions would have been game changing. Nonetheless, I continue to chafe at the totalizing and pathologizing separation of my mind from a patient's, even one with real difficulties in integration. As Robbins notes, the patients he describes may be extremely high functioning in professional spheres, as Sarah was. But it is not just her exceptional accomplishments or luminous mind that cause me to abandon his frame. It also fails to capture who else Sarah is and who she is with me. In other self-states, not articulated in this set of writings, I experienced her extraordinary presence, facility, integrity, and capacity for intimacy. These qualities, along with many others, exist in a mixed-up jumble with the rest of her. In other words, rather than having a qualitatively different kind of mind,

Sarah seems to combine more "mature" and more "unintegrated" levels of functioning. She was often my teacher, and I am grateful.

I also depart from Robbins in my belief that any understanding of Sarah must be predicated on the idea that what is generated in the analytic pair is always context-specific, dialogic, and relational in the profoundest sense of that word—in the sense that every aspect of the experience emerges from not just the clinician's participation in the patient's world but the intermingling of *both* our worlds. Is this intersubjective relating? Yes. But not *relational relating*. Sarah and I were deeply embedded in an intersubjective experience, even though there was no common language or reflective capacity to understand that relating. And part of our intersubjective engagement involved multiple uncanny identifications that made the work extremely powerful *and* extremely painful to negotiate.

I feel increasingly convinced that I had to revisit aspects of myself in a way that caused real suffering for me so that Sarah could know something about my authenticity (in part as it emerged through her attempts to heal my internal splits). For Sarah and others subjected to early severe trauma, this chaos *must* take place because the patient has to be able to compel the analyst to move with them down to the foundations of their own being. The patient yet to develop an integrated sense of self will only grow and develop when actively engaged with another person's version of what she is struggling with. This was the ground on which important shifts in the treatment began to occur.

Chapter 5

Two case vignettes

How Sarah helped me help Troy and (almost) Christina (2014)

While relational theorists often write from one or two of Stephen Mitchell's original three poles—self, other, and the space created by the analytic pair—fewer have written directly about patients who suffer with issues of their very existence, for whom psychic breach and unrepresented mental states dominate. In his initial theorizing, Mitchell recognized the interpenetration of intrapsychic and intersubjective surfaces, and the necessity for one- and two-person psychologies, but he found drive theory incompatible with a relational view (Aron and Star 2012). If the relational model holds that the operations of the mind are fundamentally dyadic and that experience emerges in the interactive field between people, what is the place of the individual psyche? Neither one-person objectivist thinking nor relational negotiation is right. The U.S. relational cannon has sometimes emphasized the "we-ness" of the analytic pair, fully acknowledging the role of the analyst's subjective participation and the asymmetrical process of mutual recognition. Yet work with certain patients necessarily involves our separateness, the unknowability of ourselves and the other.

Patients whose treatments call upon me to bear feelings of annihilation and dread require a deeper opening to myself than most analytic literatures describes. This requires a keen focus on what is happening in the singular mind of the patient whose world is solitary and not primarily object-related, as well as attending to my relational self, because I know I help produce and shape what I see.

Take Troy. He is a white adolescent, sprightly, bright-eyed, and remarkably cheerful, smart, resourceful. He is the top student at his university. And he is also alone. Really alone—not only in the city where we live, but in his mind. On a day that the temperature is below zero, he arrives in short sleeves, smiling broadly. He isn't cold. He has a body he has chosen, crafted—an act of incredible agency for someone who can feel at sea in

DOI: 10.4324/9781032670348-7

the world. Now that he has this body, he wants to know about feelings, he says. He can't offer much but looks expectant, beckoning me with his earnest smile. He is waiting for me to show him. It would be easy to read his smile as anxious, his body as numb, but the words wouldn't have much meaning to him. Endeavoring to structure the sessions, I ask a lot of questions. He tries to answer, but he doesn't know how. He is concrete but also vague. There are no nouns, no referents. Questions are impossible, because before the why, there has to be a who. Troy feels large parts of him are missing. Feelings float unanchored. Later he will tell me his smile is to cover blankness.

We are at a loss. I feel a powerful sleepiness that I have twice before experienced in the treatment room. I hate the drifting, the fight to stay awake. Despite how much I really like Troy—might already love him—I come to dread the emptiness of the sessions, which has less to do with the paucity of words exchanged and more to do with the anxiety I sense in my body: an intensely felt demand on me to carry the treatment forward psychically, linguistically, and with my desire. This is a tell-tale signal: my body can feel that Troy has not lived through moments of harmony and unison with anyone. I think about Butler's (2015) ideas about how tactile impressions made on a body are the basis for sentience, feeling, cognition, and the beginnings of agency itself.

> One does not experience a primary touch, but a primary touch inaugurates experience. In fact, touch, understood as neither simply touching nor as being touched, not only is the animating condition of sentience but continues as the actively animating principle of feeling and knowing.
>
> (Butler 2015, 9)

In Alvarez's (1992) language, psychic touch—my willingness to enliven, seek, and engage an "undrawn" patient like Troy—will be necessary to catalyze growth. To process his pain and anxiety, Troy will need to feel my deep involvement, my readiness to join him on the stage where the drama is reenacted. We will have to build self-experience that might facilitate the capacity to use symbolic thought. I know I will be scrambling to fill space, and that that is not overreach but a requirement of working with unrepresented states (McGleughlin 2011). But I can't stay awake.

I want to parse a paradox. I try to consider the level of disturbance, anxiety, object-development, and relatedness in the foreground. Only then can

I understand how we might establish the broad, reflective perspective and capacity for intrapsychic conflict that will allow Troy's subjectivity, wish, and desire to emerge (Robbins 1996) and be created. It is not, as I might have once believed, an immediately intersubjective process. Recognizing a more autistic level of development, in Ogden's (1989) sense, guides me to think along a vertical axis. I can neither comment on Troy's internal object world nor address what is happening between us. Both approaches are too other/object-focused when I still register as place, not person, when I do not read as a separate other. Some kind of living together side by side will have to occur before words are connected to personal affective meaning, not merely concrete external phenomena.

At the same time, if we return to notions of psychic structure not as metaphor but as thing—when we reify developmental level or pathology—we may fail to consider multiple and shifting self-states, and the unpredictability of change. Recently, Troy saw a colleague during my absence. She felt neither sleepy nor a sense of dread with him. Her metabolizing of his utter aloneness provoked something unusual in her too—a move to action—an enactment. But she did not experience the anxiety permeating our field.

Does that call into question my hypothesis that his unrepresented mental states and level of annihilation-anxiety indicate something about his psychic structure? I don't think so, but it does underline a theoretical point that I believe has important clinical implications and distinguishes classical and field approaches from relational ones: how analysts work with their own psyches. It is not just that the patient will dream different dreams with each of us, and that our own histories will resonate uniquely, but also that our unmentalized states may be activated in determining ways. My own experience of aloneness means I reach from a particular place, one that, for better or worse, may give me access to a different state in Troy. And it fills me with anxiety. I can't go back there, but I will have to.

I have learned that to enter into Troy's experience of objectless existence, a symbiotic experience will have to enter our field. Somatic, unthinkable, unrememberable elements will arise; indeed they already did, in our opening moments, when dread and anxiety occupied each of our bodies (Searles 1965; Lombardi 2005). From that alive state, sensation can be translated to affect representation, mentalization, and, ultimately, fantasy. It is here that I've been greatly influenced by Bionian field theories such as the importance of the field contracting the patient's illness (Ferro and Civitarese 2013), the utility in somatic resonance (Lombardi 2005), functional symbiosis, and other forms of containment (Peltz and Goldberg 2013). I will have to travel back to my aloneness and Troy's.

Somatic experience comes to me in my dreams. After many months of drowsiness and a fight to stay alive in the room, I begin to have nightmares that are highly unusual for me: in their horror, in their starkness, and singularity. They have no narrative and take place over two months. The first is an empty street; some post-apocalyptic wasteland unfamiliar to me except in previews to movies I decline to watch. In the dreams, that street returns to me again and again—always the same harshly lit, narrow space, but in different seasons: in summer, hot and pulsing with a smell like cabbage, or an electric stove, acrid and burning. Then in winter, frozen, desolate, a ghastly scene of twisted ice. In other dreams, a deserted baby appears on the edge of a bright-green foamy pond, a sinkhole, later a stray child without an arm. There were never two figures in any one dream, never any sound.

I don't tell Troy about these dreams, but I am certain they are also his. But it was grueling for me to feel an aloneness I had rarely felt. I sense Troy's terrible loneliness as pain in my body. Something palpably shifts in me as I can *feel* his helplessness and my own. Dread lifts. I begin to talk to Troy about my sleepiness. He begins to answer. He settles. I settle. We are awake.

While I am consolidating a long and heartfelt process, Troy slowly came to feel his utter deprivation and solitariness, and we could know it together. I have not been sleepy since our opening phase, and while anxiety can return to us as a pair, we share a robust and vital connection, as does Troy now with his lover and friends.

In the Bionian field model, the route towards transformation lies in the analyst's capacity for reverie, for sensing the "bipersonal unconscious fantasy" of the analytic couple, and for the often-silent internal working through of the patient's projections (Ferro and Civitarese 2013). Perhaps this is what happened with my dreams. This view of the analyst as metabolizer of the other's pain appreciates our alpha function. But it downplays how, for instance, vibrating to Troy's traumatic aloneness (a two-person phenomenon) will require me to try to understand an objectless, terrifying state inside me (a more vertical, one-person exploration), which I can then invoke in our two-person relating. To reach the unrelated parts of our patients, their areas of early and profound failures and catastrophic aloneness, we must be willing to access our own affective/somatic mind. When we can use the analytic relationship to know our own places of incapacity, we may help the patient build the competence to bear theirs.

Let me turn to Christina. We meet, and I am overwhelmed by a sense that I have encountered her before, maybe even known her. I can't place her, but her familiarity tugs at me. White, a bit older than me. She tells me she feels impoverished. Her inner world is lonely. Everyone turns to her, thinks she is solid, big, commanding, but she is devitalized, depleted, alienated from her husband, the children who love her. In analysis, she is pensive. She chronicles one of the worst trauma histories I have ever heard, and she does it thoughtfully, with affect. The story and her demeanor don't match. That kind of trauma, this kind of poise and elegance. I "know" about her aloneness but don't feel it. I'm on alert. Her language is art. Each word is crafted, sculpted, shaped—like a multifaceted gem, drawing my binocular attention, riveting me. It is not poetry. It's precision. Relentless, always on point, her mind is sharp and clear. It's hard to think of her without language or capacity for thought or agency, but I need to.

Within months of starting treatment, Christina tells me that she is stunned by her access to long-buried feelings, at how buoyantly they emerge between us. Crying for the first time in a decade, she says she has never allowed herself to feel before. She is suffering, but she can't believe she found me. She loves me. She doesn't want to be obsequious, inappropriate with her praise, but she wants me to know how unexpected and rare this grace is. My countertransference, too, is powerful. My room seems swathed in beige and taupe and lofty grey. The accents are crisp, clean lines. My words are simple and elegant, too. I am unusually still, and in that stillness, we move together loose with holiness. Idealization has never felt quite like this before.

Is Christina trying to create the necessary conditions for maternal preoccupation, the love affair with one's infant? Or is it more grown up? Is she evacuating her good and giving it to me? What kind of special object is she creating me to be? And what of her sexual abuse and the presence of Eros so quickly? In the office we *seem* to be in the world of words, but I note the flooding id and rapid transferences, the speed with which things unfold. Any talking to the "her" who can spin language will not work. I need the child whose history has torn her in two. But that Christina has never come into being.

We have a long break ahead. Upon parting, she tells me a story that can only be interpreted as a murder I will have to watch, one that she already has endured. I hear what the trip might cost us, the peril we will be in.

When we come back, she tells me the structure of therapy is not right for her. She will instead talk to friends—with whom she can cathart without the clock! She narrates the humiliation when sessions end, the degradation of having been awoken only to be left to drown. She understands the rules, why I must stop at an hour, but she can't choose that kind of unsafety and human betrayal. And she was surprised to realize she didn't miss me. She was relieved while we were apart. Really relieved. I feel vertigo, I start to spin. The shift is crazy, abrupt. She seems like someone else. I think of defense. I have looked forward to this return, but I try to remember what else I know. About the danger of psychic touch and the terror of proximity, about how for her, each breath I breathe out she breathes in. About what has not come into being such that beneath her poise and precise articulation is a feral child who has never been constituted and is in grave danger.

Green (1975) notes that decathexis is the psychotic defense most involved with failed representation. If I interpret Christina's decathexis, I assume greater internalization than may exist. I know that if I insist that a patient is defending herself who has no corresponding internal representation of such feelings, of internal conflict, she can only experience the interpretation as misattribution (Stolorow, Brandchaft, and Atwood 1987). If I observe that we have ushered in the trauma, murdered and murdering, it assumes too much self/other differentiation. If I use my subjectivity—express my puzzlement about her new indifference against my excitement—I assume more relatedness than is possible, at least yet. For now, Christina can't think. There is no goodness, pleasure, potential, conflict, absence, anxiety, anger, or terror—all feelings available to me. She knows only that she cannot be in this relationship.

What would it look like for Christina and me to go on being knowing that she cannot be in relationship? It was not easy to take her at her word, to believe she felt nothing between us and was willing to give up the affective aliveness of our connection. But to interpret or even hold in mind her need to defend herself against this "falling in love," though it may be what happened, would be to ignore the real danger that analysis can be for some patients. Christina brings to the fore a limit in the structure of psychotherapy/analysis, which is that it may replicate earlier parental failures to hold. The challenge is to grasp Christina's very authentic perception, not distortion or defense, of the threat she perceives. Genuine understanding of the constraints on the analytic situation might allow something to emerge from the unrealness of analysis. As I have written (McGleughlin 2015a), if trauma cannot be told and is recognized primarily by the psychic breach it causes, we would need to access that breach in this encounter. And so, after a time, we did. That work required coming to know, for the first time, the loss of really loving and losing.

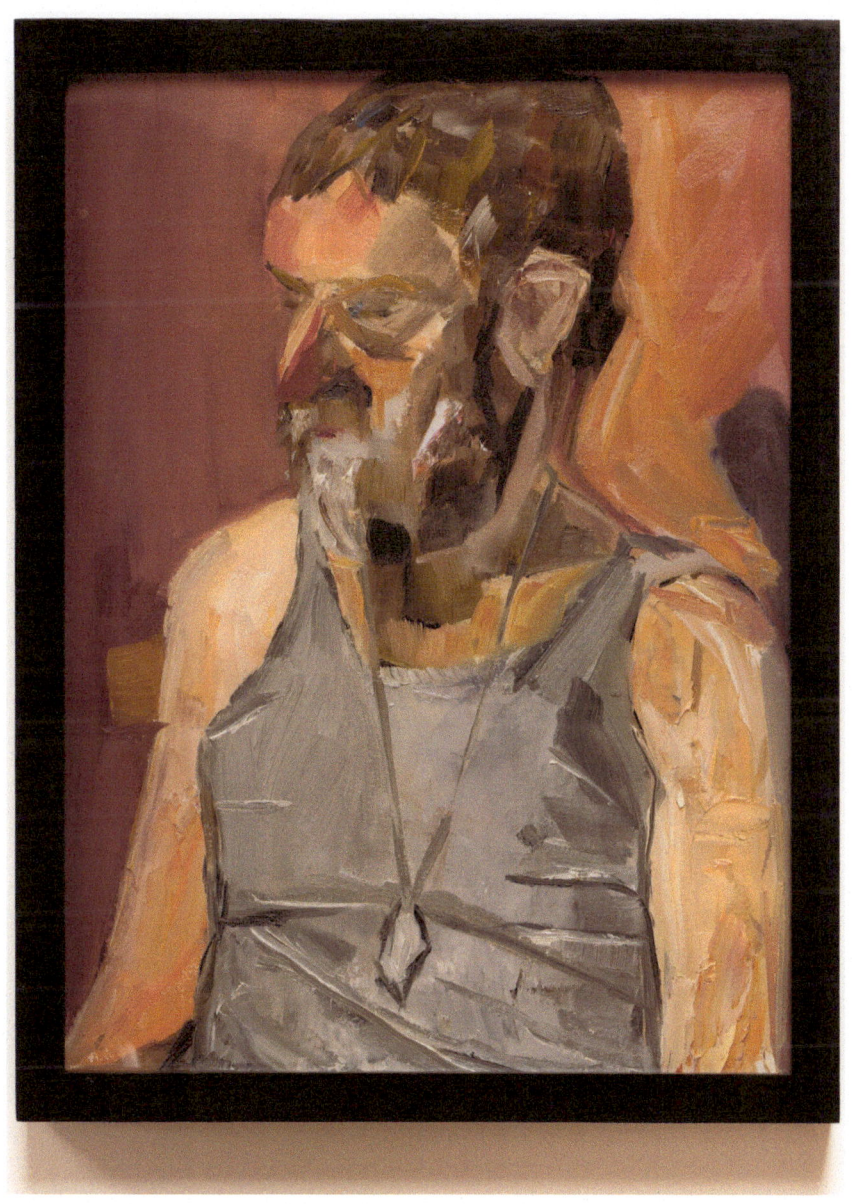

Figure 5.1 Lost. 12x16. Oil on paper. McGleughlin

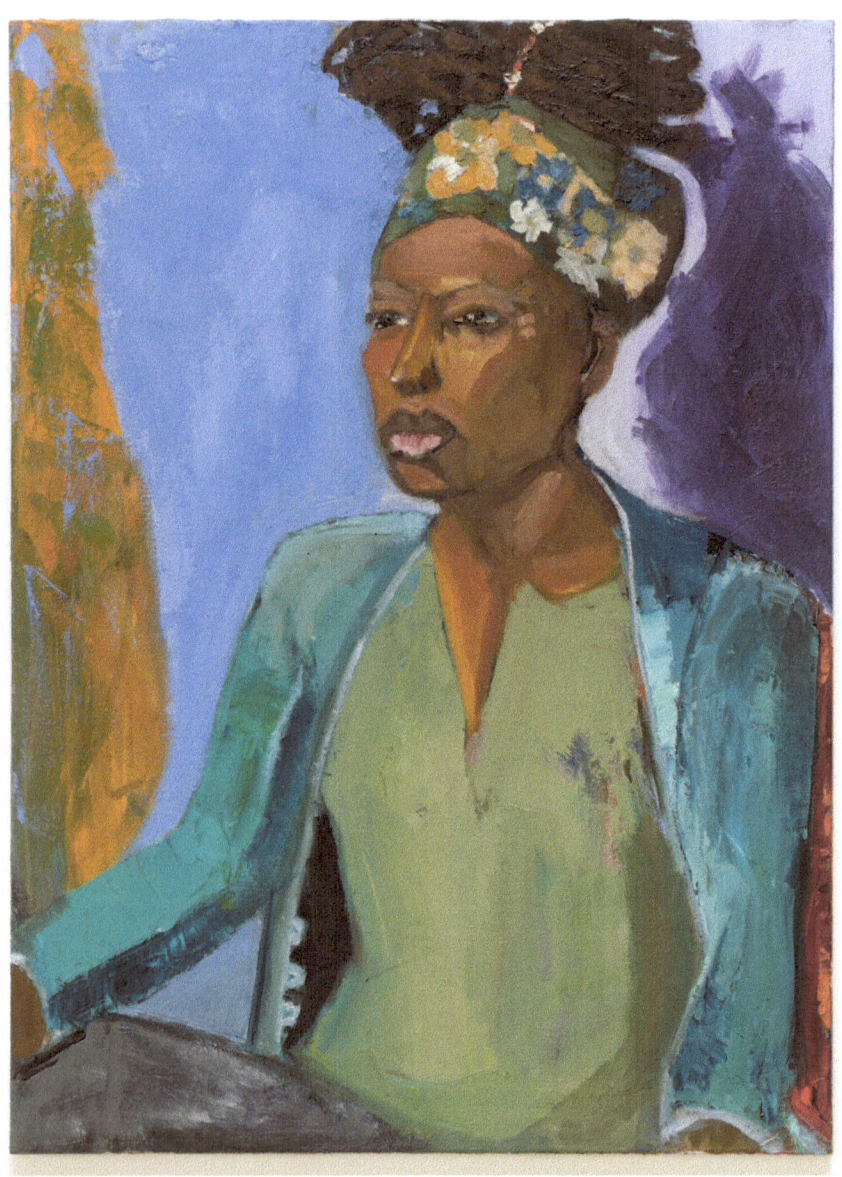

Figure 5.2 Blue Room. Oil on canvas. 20x24. McGleughlin

Part 2

The breach

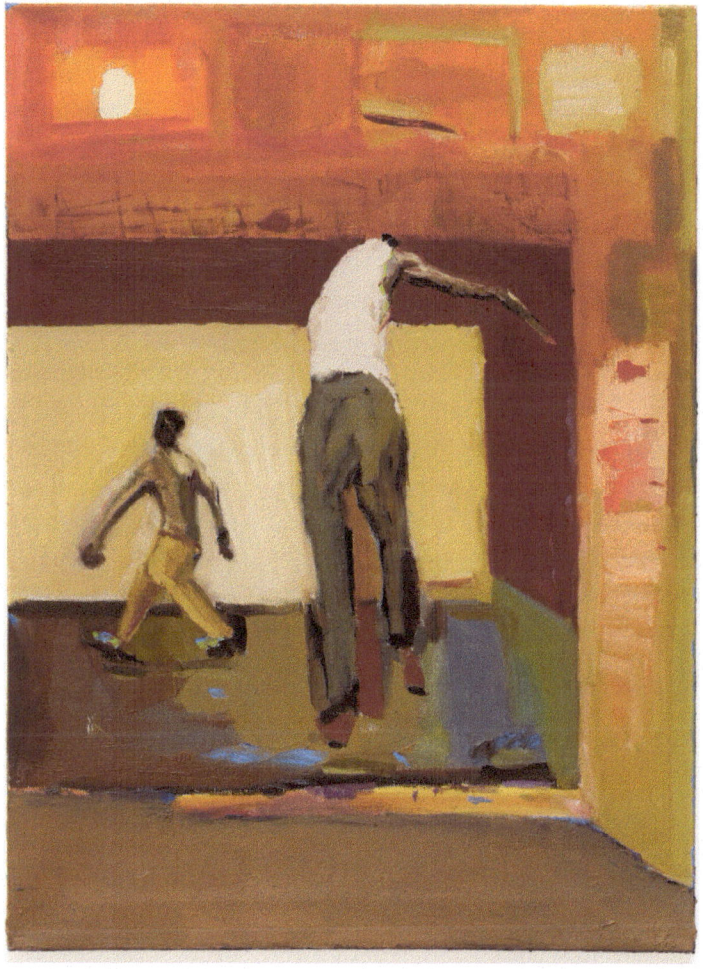

Figure PII.1 After Lichtenstein. Oil on canvas. 28x22. McGleughlin

DOI: 10.4324/9781032670348-8

Introduction

As analysts, our medium is language, yet so often it fails us—sometimes profoundly so, particularly when we are working with deeply traumatized patients. And how could it be otherwise, when the experience of these patients is rarely amenable to representation? Language also may buckle when we are grappling with the complexities of race and racism both within the treatment and in our attempts to understand and give form to the experiences of another while ensuring that we don't usurp their personhood and authority. How to work within and write about these spaces?

Part 2 continues an exploration of how what we rely on, speech and language, routinely can't hold all that is intended and experienced. This is true in analysis as well as the writing of analytic theory and practice, where the gap between experience and representation remains a struggle. In this part, I lean further into that previously mentioned disparaging remark by the British analyst, who, upon hearing a presentation of "The Raw Story," called it "performance art." My work as a form of performance art is intentional in the enactive writing I employ in the essay that constitutes the centerpiece of this part, "Do We Lose or Find Ourselves in the Negative?" But also, I intentionally appeal to the resources that art offers in our treatments themselves, in the ways we think about them, in our depictions of them, and sometimes simply as a resource with the person in the room. As analysts, we are cocreating new realities, new ways of seeing and being with our patients; how is this not a kind of art? Thus, in the essays here, I reflect upon what art like the portraits of Richard Avedon, for example, might teach us about how we practice our own work outside the bounds of language. In a similar vein, I draw upon the filmmaking of Alain Resnais to explore how a moment of punctum might offer a way of generatively entering the breach that trauma creates. And with regard to the dilemmas that cross-racial therapeutic work presents, I turn to insights and wisdom expressed in the art of Black writers.

In Chapter 6, "Do We Lose or Find Ourselves in the Negative?" (2015a), I revisit a treatment with a patient who taught me that my desire to say her name did violence to her experience of nonbeing. Where language fails, I turn to art, in this case to the photographs of Francesca Woodman. My patient and I immerse ourselves in a group of haunting images that Woodman created before she suicided at age 22. In looking together at these photos, we find ourselves able, for the first time, to perceive a kind of liminality that defines my patient's existence. These images, visually representing states of nonbeing, become a metaphor for my patient and me to create a new medium to communicate about the sequalae of her traumatic past without the reductive stamp of language.

Rather than create confusion around who is the analyst and who is the patient by offering my interior dialogue and sharing my vulnerabilities as I did in "the Raw Story," in this essay, I incorporate pieces of my own history into my patient's. I did this in part to protect confidentiality, but my more ambitious hope was that by presenting two minds as one, I might create a compelling case for taking seriously the claim that "minds are not located in our singular self" (McGleughlin 2015a). And I wanted to bring out the importance of listening from our own places of not knowing, or psychic breach.

The second paper in this section, "Answering Gestures" (Chapter 7), takes up the issues of psychoanalytic writing where the demand for clarity edits out chaos and, in exchange for giving the reader ballast, produces "the standard edition." In other words, by adding scaffolding, narrative storytelling, and chronology, the chaos of psychic trauma is replaced with a tidy story that can be the opposite of the traumatic experience described. I also respond to discussants who generously helped me clarify certain key concepts that appear and reappear throughout the book, like liminality, sovereignty, and the negative.

In the third paper, "When You Are in the Cellar, Am I Dead?" (Chapter 8), I engage Cathy Caruth's (1996) perceptive analysis of Resnais's (1959) film *Hiroshima mon amour* to illustrate my guiding belief that trauma can only be told dialogically: the patient needs an other to re-establish history and memory. Further, I suggest that the film makes the case that the patient can access the gap created by trauma with the other because the analyst undertakes a similar process herself within the treatment.

Hiroshima mon amour also allowed me to explore the limitations of a certain kind of empathy—a kind that calls for using one's own experience to enter into that of another, standard analytic attunement. I argue that traditional notions of empathy, where we step into the experience of another (putting oneself in their shoes) to understand their joy or pain often falls short of what is needed within a treatment. It relies on what we already know, not what exists within the breach, beyond our knowing. In the film, we see an empathy that challenges, even disrupts, another's story rather than joining it. So, too, in treatment we may need an interruption that surprises—invites some element of distinction, separateness, and bodily awareness to reintroduce time and the living body into an absent, or liminal state. This perspective highlights a critical shift away from the analyst as "healer," or even "witness," to a more *phenomenological experiencing together*.

At the end of that chapter, in a section titled "Interlude with Life and Death," I include a eulogy to my stepfather, who embodied the importance of having a real other in order to mourn what had been for me a kind of liminal grief about the death of my own father.

In Chapter 10, "white empathy," I ask whether the answers to the questions of empathy that were suggested by *Hiroshima mon amour* apply to our work in cross-racial dyads. I interrogate the idea that, simply as human beings, we can use and count on our own feelings to share another's feelings across the radical social divide of race, and I argue that in doing so we may inadvertently traumatize the patient. Drawing on Saidiya Hartman's (1997) work, I explore how the expression of a particular form of feeling, "empathy" can endow the recognizer as the arbiter of the other's experience and may actually disappear Black people when white people seek to understand them.

In response to this conundrum and my own desire to learn how it might be possible to tell the story of another without usurping that person's voice, erasing difference, or presuming to know what cannot be known, I turn again to the art world, more specifically to Black writers who address some of these issues. I extend my examination of the potential limits of an identificatory empathy and attend to how issues of power and vulnerability shape what is and is not possible within psychoanalytic writing and clinical practice. I close this chapter with the story of a clinical treatment with a boy called Fred, in which I think through possibilities and impossibilities and reflect upon the pitfalls of white empathy.

Through exploring the limits of both empathy and of language, and through engaging art's transformative power to shift our ways of seeing and being within our clinical practice, Part 2 seeks to extend the work begun in Part 1. That is to say, the chapters that follow aim to offer a more distinct shape and form to what an ontological psychoanalysis might look like in everyday practice.

Chapter 6

Do we find or lose ourselves in the negative?[1] (2015)

What is coming

When Walter Benjamin (1999) wrote,

> Language has unmistakably signified that memory is not an instrument of the exploration of the past, but rather its scene . . . memory must not proceed by way of narrative, much less by way of reports, but must rather assay its spade, epically and rhapsodically in the most rigorous sense, in ever new places and, in the old ones, to delve into ever deeper layers,

it is a guide post to psychoanalysts.

Trauma speaks in unknown languages, a confusion of tongues, enigmatic behaviors. What is unsymbolized hides, erupts, displaces, and confuses, creating interruptions, leaving gaps. The recognition of certain trauma is marked less by the trauma and its symbolic representation than by a gap trauma creates—what Cathy Caruth (1996) calls "a breach in the mind's experience of time, self, and the world" (p. 4). This breach, often experienced as a state of nonbeing, may be central to certain kinds of early trauma, because "the space of unconsciousness is what paradoxically, preserves the trauma" (p. 62). Unconsciousness or the breach itself, the breach in the mind comes to characterize our subjective experience.

How do we know or register a patient's states of nonbeing, or what I call present absence, and how do we clinically engage the phenomena? Our most familiar impulse is to understand, name, and represent trauma in language, but such an effort to close the gap of traumatic experience may be violating, a terrible erasure and misrecognition of patients who live the breach, whose present absence is a testimony to the gaps in their subjectivity. How do we

DOI: 10.4324/9781032670348-9

engage a self-state with little experience of body, time, or history? Is there a linguistic requiem for a psychic gap?

I had to unlearn my ability to see and name trauma as "something." Instead I entered what I call a negative enactment, which brought the experience of felt absence into reflective consciousness. In the language of Pontalis, I had to "permit the horizon of the object to appear in its immediacy, to allow the invisible to make its appearance through that which is visible" (Pontalis, in Abelin 1993, 898). Using the powerful imagery of Francesca Woodman, an artist who committed suicide at 22, leaving a body of ghostly photographs, my patient and I found a vehicle to recognize and represent the present absence that haunted her and her treatment and symbolized her suspension between life and death. Seeing Woodman's photographs in the context of our work together, my patient was able to register and later reflect with me on previously invisible aspects of her experience. I have included several of Woodman's photographs in an effort to participate with Woodman in "inventing an iconography of the invisible/unknowable" (Keller 2013, 177). This paper is also about a certain kind of listening this patient required, not listening *for* the breach but listening *from* the breach in my mind's experience.

To bring you into these experiences of a present absence and negative enactment, I have written about our clinical work partially in the "enactive mode" (Naiburg 2015), in which the text "performs or enacts its meaning" (p. xiii). For instance, I shift my patient's name (you will see naming is a crucial representation of coming into being) in order to evoke her shifting sense of selfhood. I imagined I'd use one name to denote what she had historically named herself and another for her emerging self-representation. But the convention did not capture her flux and multiplicity, so I interchanged them. I write this way, and with minimal narrative structure and scaffolding, not to frustrate you but in the hope that you might experience the mix-up between what is unsymbolized and what is beginning to be represented. I also use a collage of atmospheres, registers, and voices to convey my process of psychoanalytic witness to trauma, and I depart from familiar relational language and theorists to try to metaphorically (not necessarily theoretically) implant the idea of something that felt foreign.[2] Implicitly, this paper challenges, with Bromberg (1998), whether closing the gaps should be the therapeutic ambition. Instead, I gravitate toward a kind of *being with* that might require the summoning and bearing of one's own gaps and ghosts, as it did mine.

The case: what is represented

My patient comes to me about ten years ago. She does well in the world but feels little agency or subjectivity. I am her second important analyst in 25 years. She tells the story like this. When she is small, her father disappears, and a frantic search takes place. While they waited, time stood still, and she spun wildly around with her back pressed against a tilt of a world. She says she was sick with vertigo, alone. When he is tracked down months later, he is dead: he has blown his brains out. She is told he died of a heart attack, and he is rarely spoken of again. She doesn't remember him and doesn't care. Her mother is all that matters, her only horizon. She's a ship's cook and is gone at sea for long periods of time. When she comes back, she pronounces the world safe and leaves again. My patient cannot catch a breath with her mother's comings-and-goings. Her mother is a sailor who sailed the Seven Seas. She is no Helen. And the mud-filled flat she left her to is no Troy. Her mother is a cursing sailor but also the sirens' call. My patient knows that call, lies on that island in that sea, not tied to the mast, not tethered at all. She has no coordinates. She tells me, "I have only empty sacks." She has no home inside. No compass. No guide. The dead are not allowed to speak. They do not anchor an end. They cannot be located (Winterson 2011).[3] She tells me this history because she knows it matters; she's a shrink, but she's not much interested in dredging up the past.

The problem of naming/the first sign of the breach

I am disoriented from the beginning. My patient doesn't want me to say her name. If we name her, we will crush her. I learn over time that naming demarcates a presence that implies she's been here. If she signs something, like consent, it means she won't be here in the future (Derrida 1988). It's a dilemma. She's slightly out of all names, slightly out of the frame, like the lipstick of my favorite schizophrenic. I think it's not quite on her lips. Too bright, just slightly fuzzy. An old woman smoking from two mouths at once. But the pink colored outside the lines is on right. Tight. That's the funny thing, the rub. Or the stick. That's there too. The fag, the smoke. The pathos, doubled. The doublings of loss. Then and now? The doubleness of death—first her father, then, practically, her mother. It's worse than being cross-eyed. It's the face that smears, and smudges. The double.

She's ephemeral, ethereal. Just past my grasp. Every time I think I see her, she's gone. She is, there is, something always moving, sliding away. Now she tells me, ten years later, "Write the paper. Let's see what you can see."

"How do I call you?"

Unexpectedly, she says, "Call me Martin." Martin asks for this name for her disguise.

"Martin? It will be distracting. Gender is not at the center. They will think you are a boy or that the paper is somehow about—"

"About trans?"

I say, "Why confuse things?"

She says, "Don't be so literal. Aren't you the analyst? The paper *is* about trans. About crossings, crossings from the dead. Call me Martin with an (a)."

"Martan? Martina?"

She groans. Martin with an (a). Write it. But I write Marin. "What about that?"

"You wish," she says. "Marin. Like marine. Like the ocean, like blue, like water. Flow. It's Martin. With an (a). Make no mistake." She wants the (a) outside the name.

Now I write Matin without fail. It takes me a while to see it's French for morning. Matin. Our perpetual nonmourning. Later still, I realize in wanting to call her Matin, I have left out the "r." Without the capability to be. I am. You R. But she's not. That's the point. Or one of them. In the treatment, Martin with an (a) was never really there to be named. It's not just about this paper. As a child, she was called "Nay-Nay." As a noun, a denial or refusal. As a declarative, an emphatic form of NO. Nay-Nay. And in that singsong, childlike first rename, made by a sibling on a subway train (she insists she was named on the subway when her sister turned to see her carriage stuck in the door of the car and began shouting her unpronounceable name, "Nay-Nay"), the beloved nickname and what it signifies sit side by side.

She doesn't ever tell me the name before that name. Naming and constituting *are* the problem. It is taming, pinning down. It locates her as a thing, in the third person, out there in the grid of language. Without a name, Matin conveys her sense of not being. "To be without a name is to be without form or qualities, without shadows, without dreams, without imagination, without a soul" (Himes 2012, 16).

Now, all these years later, there is a firmness with which she wants Martin with an (a).

What's in clear (sight)

In my speech on graduating from psychoanalytic training in 2002, I write about Richard Avedon's exhibit at the Metropolitan Museum in New York, and the way he captures, in each photograph, something surprising, unfamiliar, not yet seen or known by either the subjects of his pictures or by us, the viewers, even as we contemplate familiar cultural icons (Hambourg and Fineman 2002). Each portrait is a transformation of someone we thought we knew redescribed and reconfigured. How did he invent, create, some might say find, these extraordinary vital parts we know without knowing?

We are told Avedon attends to his sitter with his whole being, watching and sensing viscerally, mirroring and responding to the slightest shifts in his body positioning, facial expression, and gesture. I thought then that portrait-making seemed like good relational psychoanalysis. "The portrait is always a solution of the objective and the subjective, the prepared and the improvised, the self and the other" (Hambourg and Fineman 2002, 16). Like the psychoanalyst, the portrait maker sees something, catches the element of surprise with his sitter, and then, with his vivid picture, shows what has been seen. Avedon's portraits seem to do this.

Something can be seen, new, within a single frame.

I am thinking with no shortage of my own omnipotence; I, too, will reach into the deepest parts of myself, like Avedon, and I will be fully alive and present to the meeting of Matin. I will, like a keen photographer, adjust the aperture, capture something surprising, unfamiliar, not yet seen or known. My picture-taking will show her *her* mind with my binocular bi-ocular

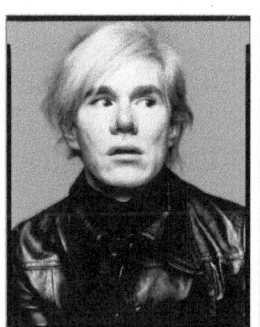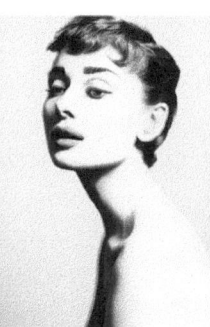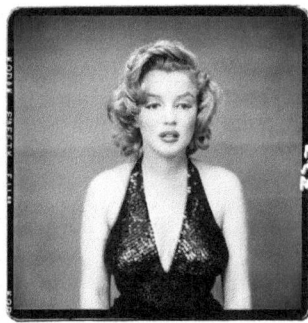

Figure 6.1 Screenshot collage of three Richard Avedon photographs, (left to right) Andy Warhol, artist, New York, August 14, 1969; Audrey Hepburn, actress, New York, December 18, 1953; Marilyn Monroe, actress, New York, May 6, 1957.

Photographs by Richard Avedon © The Richard Avedon Foundation vision such that we will transform, redescribe, and reconfigure her. We will hold the tension between what is seen and the potential life held by the unconscious. Avedon, with his sure frames and points of departure, with time and space neatly fixed and aligned, with a me and a you, a now and a then, can be bold in Black and white. Something else entirely between two people can take shape. But Martin with an (a) does not take shape. Nothing coheres. A certain indeterminacy of being—a liminality—something hard to see, to symbolize, exists between us. Something that cannot be seen returns to us again and again, a Möbius strip. A no scene. There is no portrait of Matin or Martin or Martin with an (a). Certainly no frame. I can't describe her, fix her, know her. And certainly I cannot show her.

Martin with an (a) is quite sped up really—more like a flip-book. Some images exist, haunt, but it's the pages moving quickly that give you the feel, the story line, the hurrying. A sense of her aura. Her orange aura.

Here is a condensed example from the very beginning of treatment. I cringe to read it. You will note how structured the dialogue is. Open-ended inquiries like "Tell me more" are not useful to Martin. Still, you can see the problem of my trying to "mirror" or "understand." Martin feels pinned like a bug.

In speaking about her mother, Martin with an (a) says, "I wanted to make her life better."

Me: "To be able to make her life better."
Martin: "No. Not able."
           I destabilize her when I extend her statements by even a word or two, and she bristles.
Martin: "No . . . not able to make it better. I didn't want to be able. It was too much. I felt relief when she remarried. I wasn't totally responsible for her. But then she was gone again with him."
Me: "Relief but gone again and lost to you."
Martin: "No. She was around. She was very involved with me. She was at the center of my life."
Me: "She was at the center. (Long pause.) She meant the world to you."
Martin: "No, not really. Well, we were very close. Her husband was angry I was so much like her."
Me: "Being close meant being like her?"
Martin: (*Glares*). "No. Jesus. (*Long pause. Martin goes blank.*) "It was about going to her. Being with her."

Me: "Being with her."
Martin: "No, not really. He was there." *(Dissociation.)*

Her negation does not feel like resistance, though it reads like it. She does not recognize a truth she opposes; she recognizes no truth in what I offer. She does not, indeed cannot, allow herself to see herself in a state of "alien action" (Green 1998, 651). The image would be too terrifying. She's not fighting me. She feels internally persecuted, pinned down and desperate. Each reflection terrifies her—is wrong, partial, enraging, can't be thought about. The effort to know or name through words is not yet possible. I wonder: has the breach caused a "radical denial of the primordial mind" (p. 652)? My reflection threatens her, as if I had erased something in my seeing and in establishing a thing to be seen. To "see" something definable, or any reflection that attempts to understand her experience, is to *not* understand the nothing within her. Before Martin with an (a) had a name, she cannot bear my "naming" her or her experience. Martin with an (a) wants an analyst who knows how to unname—to be with her both in and outside her experience of a present absence (Morris 2012, personal communication, drawn from Harold Bloom). She will teach me that naming trauma as a "what," as something that can be represented, is a betrayal. Trauma does not reside in events, but in "the breach in the mind's experience" (Caruth 1996, 4). And, it is also true that attunement betrays the profound singularity built into the experience of trauma (Stolorow 2007).

In a more everyday register, we never quite see ourselves (or each other). The seeing of one's self as a "what" is the problem. I am reminded of those disturbing double takes when I catch a glimpse of the reflection of my face in a store window, and the woman I see isn't me. This kind of double take occurs interpersonally when I dare to bring my solitary experience to another, and what I see reflected back surprises me, or is not the me I recognize. Martin with an (a) felt the same disconnect when the self I mirrored back to her was not the self she knew. When trauma's breach is suffered alone, when the wounding of catastrophe is constituted in isolation, any attempt to move it into intersubjective space betrays the experience of having been isolated. Intersubjectivity, then, was not only initially difficult but also, paradoxically, another betrayal (Nguyen 2012).

We are in a dilemma. Witnessing someone's story or no story can betray the profound singularity built into the experience of trauma. Yet, without an other to reconstitute an experience of selfhood, the rupture in human connection that is often at the core of profound trauma cannot be repaired. The dilemma is captured in our naming quandary. Being constituted in the mind of the other is a tyranny for Martin, yet naming holds the potential for her to constitute herself with me. We live in this paradox.

Martin longs to be constituted as Martin with an (a), but the name remains not quite complete, the (a) hanging off. She has no fixed identity or sense of subjectivity a name would imply. For now, she resists the power of the gaze to implicate a "her" that is not yet subjectively there. She wants to keep her aura. What then is the aura? "A strange tissue of space and time: the unique apparition of a distance, however near it may be" (Benjamin 1935/2008, 23). This aura suggests liminality of time and space that can't be reduced. She would think, like Barthes tells us in *Camera Lucida* (1980), in the very representation of the image itself, when the picture is taken, there is a death, including that of the aura. If I see her, it will feel like a kind of murder— "the stripping of a veil from the object, the destruction of the aura" (Benjamin 1935/2008, 23). Representing feels like robbing or, worse, death.

Treatment history

The treatment is rocky. First there is curiosity, then devaluing, contempt, scorn. A few years later a love develops, a hunger, but the longing is terrifying, and Matin slips away into deep retreat. The tumults of those years focus on her mother, on the emergence of that chaotic relationship into ours. Connecting moments are followed by her contempt, fear. My words often fail to reach her. The transference is positive, disrupted, negative. The treatment is rich, sometimes disastrous. But we survive, and in doing so, something else comes into being, delicate and ordinary. It's hard to recognize it as psychoanalysis, but I think we are laying down track, rigging the boat. Some might call this transitional space or a facilitating environment. The capacity for relating as two subjects is rare. Matin is not separate. There are few interpretations, not much reflective analytic process but a slow kind of simple daily life lived in the analytic frame. There is acknowledgment, witness, and shared rhythm. If we lived it in the world, we would be slowly walking side by side or cooking or maybe looking out together from a bench towards a sea. (For the missing mother?)

Perhaps we each know "the subtleness of the sea; how its most dreaded creatures glide under water, unapparent for the most part, and treacherously hidden beneath the loveliest tints of azure" (Melville 1851/1992, 301), but we talk of "where to store fur and how to treat hair" (St. Vincent Millay 1917, 41). I am containing, holding inside those monsters under the sea. I am thinking of Milner's concept, extended from Winnicott's ideas of unintegration, in which an environment must be reliably safe to allow the subject to flounder in "absence-mindedness" (Farhi 2010, 488). I am holding inside of me the image of Martin with an (a) beginning to *be*.

The image: what we do see

How do we represent what cannot be represented? As Proust writes, "A person, scattered in space and time, is no longer a woman but a series of events in which we can throw no light, a series of insoluble problems" (seen in Townsend 2006).

In the seventh year of the treatment, I go to the Guggenheim Museum to see Francesca Woodman's solo show. Woodman (1958–1981) has become a highly studied and influential photographer from the late twentieth century. She began photographing at 13 and committed suicide by jumping from a building when she was 22. In many of her photographs, Woodman is

> haunting the boundaries, edging out of or coming into the frame, almost slipping through the surface of representation, away from us, toward us, coming out of the back of the picture, blending into the walls like a maladroit tyro ghost.
>
> (Townsend 2006, 7)

Despite her perpetual presence in her photographs as model, Corey Keller writes: "Woodman is always on the verge of disappearance. Her face is most often obscured from the camera: on the rare occasion when she fixes us squarely in her gaze, the effect is riveting but disquietly unrevealing (Keller 2013, 178).

> Not only is she both subject and author in her works (as both the analyst and patient are), but also she intentionally alludes to the representation of self within pictures . . . while simultaneously suggesting a disjunction between the self and its identity, and between the body and the self.
>
> (p. 178)

I sense Martin with an (a), like Woodman's tyro ghosts, is also gliding, slipping into things, other self-states, other graves.

To see the Francesca woodman images that accompanied the original published version of the chapter please go to "Do We Find or Lose Ourselves in the Negative?" (2015) *Psychoanalytic Dialogues* 25 (2) 214–236.

Critics write that Woodman's work challenges the certainties of photography, "the fixing of time and space that might otherwise be understood as its most fundamental characteristic" (Townsend 2006, 7). She does this ironically, using a medium that is meant to represent what is most indisputably there. Yet Woodman's art is

> preoccupied with showing us that what is most indisputably there is uncertain, not fixed in time, filled with hesitation and the displacement of forms. . . .
> She is evading the fixity that technical limits of photography would impose.
> (Townsend 2006, 7)

In challenging the permeability of boundaries in actual space and time in visual representation, Woodman draws our attention to the liminality of personhood (Keller 2013, 177).

It is what Martin does, too.

Matin, like Woodman, seems to exude "a profound ambivalence—a simultaneous refusal and yearning to be constituted in the field of vision as an object of desire" (Sundell 2003, 53). For Martin with an (a) and for Woodman, being looked at and being seen emerge as boundary disturbances (Raymond 2010). Woodman conveys this through her manipulation of physical space. She is always moving our gaze, tilting the frame, obscuring, blurring the image, slowing the negative. Martin does it by shapeshifting, moving away. Each time I think we have come to shared meaning, I am wrong. If Woodman uses a medium that is meant to represent what is most indisputably there to show what is not there, Martin too creates this disjuncture in our experience of her by shifting self-states, disappearing from where she was just minutes earlier, erasing her mind, thinking of nothing, becoming blank.

One critic suggests Woodman's images are her own fort/da game[4]—an attempt to master her own state of nonbeing (my word): the casting out and reeling in of images that both grasp self-image and offer access to her own imagelessness (Phelan 2002).

Martin with an (a) plays fort/da, too. For both Woodman and Martin, psychoanalysis and photographic self-portraiture respectively could "promise *knowledge* of the self, [but] there is a resistant enigma of vision, a non-entity describing itself as an entity" (Phelan 2002, 987). Woodman's critics note, "In their paradoxical blurring and emphasizing of the body, Woodman's pictures pose questions about the limits of subjectivity in materiality" (Raymond 2010, 2). The aura of Martin with an (a) and the images in Woodman's self-portraits "obliterate our capacities as viewers to identify with them as subject(s)" (p. 987).

Like Freud's grandson, who is attempting to master his mother's departures and returns and hold a presymbolic image of presence in her absence, Woodman's and Martin's appearing/disappearing may be an attempt to represent and hold something that is just beginning to be developed and known: a sense of internal absence in presence. I am taken with the way both women seem to be drawing our attention to a kind of liminal presence that can look like fragmentation but might be pointing towards something else. Martin, for one, seems to be creating a way to represent an emergent sense of what's alien within her.

Woodman herself called some of her blurred motion figures "ghost pictures," and Raymond (2010) notes that one of her early curators, Alison Ferris, chose to exhibit her photos alongside the spirit photographs made in the nineteenth and early twentieth centuries. In these, glass plates were altered, and double exposures were used to trick mourners into believing that an image of the departing soul had been captured as proof of life after death. If Woodman is trying to photograph something that doesn't exist, as Kraus (1986) suggests, is Martin trying to signal the ways in which she doesn't exist and/or allude to how she is filled up, forced to live out the "devastating half life" of her dead (Abraham and Torok 1994, 167)? I had been thinking about Martin with an (a)'s shifting self-states or states of non-being in terms of her difficulty inhabiting herself. Now I begin to wonder if a second phenomenon is with us, that the ghosts of her father inhabit her. Does the (a) that hangs off Martin's name just represent her missing self-states, or could it also be Martin's ghost or phantom father? All this plays in my mind.

Certainly, Woodman's photographs seem to counter the idea of "photographs as documents of the past that bear witness . . . and substantiate the existence of experiences" (Blessing, Phelan, and Trotman 2010, 11). Instead they are spectral images that might, as Barthes (1980) suggests, be a rehearsal for death, allowing the viewer access to the ongoing psychic work of mourning. For me they also evoke the loss of never having come fully into being—of being neither dead nor alive.

It might be that ultimately Woodman is commanding the photograph not to destabilize identity, but rather to reveal identity's fractionary quality, as critic Keller (2013) notes. But I think there is more. Woodman inhabits another space. She herself writes that the task of her photographs was to allow her to locate "where I fit in this odd geometry of time" (Townsend 2006).[5] Hmmm.

The showing

Perhaps in unconscious association to the work that is between us (in the field), I mention to Martin that I have been to the Woodman show in New York. She decides to go see the show herself and has a powerful experience. She begins to photograph Woodman's photographs. In the following weeks, Martin and I look at those photographs and some books of Woodman's work. She brings me other images from the web. In session, we speak about what we see separately and together in the photographs. We wonder why Woodman's pictures are so liminal. Why is she ethereal, floating, ungrounded? What was Woodman trying to see; what space was she trying to inhabit?

Was Woodman haunted by ghosts? What happened before she jumped from the building? What is the meaning of how she plays with the boundaries between life and death?

We don't know if Woodman imagined her death, staged it, or if, in Barthes (1980) words, she wanted us to see a rehearsal for it. We don't know if her photographs speak to us from the grave, as he implies is possible. But I do believe Woodman has planted what Laplanche (1987) calls an enigmatic message (unconsciously, as is the case with all enigmatic messages) for those of us who wear her closely to decipher with our own afterwardness and, now that we know of her death,[6] our own understanding of what was happening before she suicided. Something stirs in our unconscious. Martin says she likes the indeterminacy of the photos, the way Woodman is never static and also always somewhere else. She tells me she objects to the world of reproductions, where the ephemeral is lost. It's why she doesn't like interpretations. She doesn't want to be anybody's picture, anybody's copy. In these photos, she sees something that interests her. Woodman's aura and her own. Martin's camera trained on Woodman's camera allows another vision.

Clearly, it is another nature, which speaks to the camera as compared to the eye. 'Other' above all in the sense that a space informed by

human consciousness gives way to a space informed by the unconscious . . . . It is through the camera that we first discover the optical
unconscious, just as we discover the instinctual unconscious through
psychoanalysis.

(Benjamin 1935/2008, 37)

What Woodman creates and Martin (a) and I see through the optical unconscious is a kind of ghost-like figure who cannot be stabilized or rooted. Is
Woodman a phantom? Is Martin? Am I? We don't know yet who we see,
who we feel, what we know. We feel how haunted Woodman was, and we
feel her haunting us.

Benjamin (1935/2008) notes:

Photography can bring out aspects of the original that are accessible
only to the lens (which is adjustable and can easily change viewpoint)
but not to the human eye. . . . With the close-up, space expands. With
slow motion, movement is extended and just as enlargement not merely
clarifies what we see . . . but brings to light entirely new structures of
matter, slow motion not only reveals familiar aspects of movements but
discloses quite unknown aspects within them—aspects which do not
appear as the retarding of natural movements, but has a curious gliding,
floating character of their own.

(p. 37)

Woodman has captured unknown aspects of Martin, what lies outside the
normal spectrum of sense impressions. Like a gift from a psychotic, ghost,
or angel, Woodman offers us another kind of real: the space between presence and absence. She has made the invisible visible and the shapeless a
form. When Martin sees Woodman's gliding, disappearing, fragmenting,
negative self, we come to know she sees something new.

The enactment

The more I read about Woodman, the more surprised I become. The body of
criticism on Woodman's work is curiously antipsychoanalytic. Biographi-
cal details are concrete, insubstantial, and provided as though without psychic relevance. Even the more psychoanalytic critics seem to disavow the
meaning of her death. In fact, in almost everything I've read, no reference
to her suicide is made, or else it is significantly underplayed. The focus is

on her genius, her aesthetics, "the question of whether aesthetic effects are tricks, illusions, or eruptive markers of the real" (Raymond 2010, 2).

Indeed, in the first catalogues and critical reviews of her work, a conscious decision was made not to mention her death (Phelan 2002, 984). Almost all of the critics plead for us not to interpret her art through her suicide or reduce art to autobiography or symptom. I understand. Still. It's as if repetitive, insistent images and themes of liminality have little meaning, and the psyche has no place. The various commentaries even refuse the idea that people who kill themselves are necessarily in some anguish. In the only piece about the meaning of death in Woodman's art, Phelan, a critic I greatly admire and who is critical of the denial of the meaning of Woodman's death for her art, indicates that her suicide did not necessarily signal a tragedy but a kind of tentative achievement, even her gift to us by helping us imagine a future in which she is no longer there (Phelan 2002, 984). With this exception, the more I read about Woodman, the more it seemed as if the critics seem to be trying to erase the difference between life and death.

When I tell this story to a colleague, he notes my big affect, my distress. He pushes me to think about why I am so disturbed. I cannot join the critics in this apparent disavowal of death.

If we think of these contrasting views, mine and the critics', as a visual scene, it is what Barthes (1980) calls the punctum,[7] the thing that sparks internal agitation, the detail that stands out, that punctures and pierces, that helps us see (Morris 2012, personal communication). Suddenly, the meaning of erasing the boundary between life and death registers inside of me like a shock that disturbs my dissociation of my own ghosts, of my liminality. While the disavowal, denial, or repression that Martin and I shared about the death of our fathers was relevant, it was not what was calling to us most. Metaphorically, it was her own difficulty inhabiting life, and maybe mine too. This punctum stunned me into seeing what had not been in my sight. Disturbed and awakened, I could begin to formulate from the site of my traumatic history my own liminality and Martin's. I had not been able to see how Martin hovered between life and death. The enactment with Woodman's critics catapulted me into reflection about my own grip of a sensory experience of present absence.

Knowing the difference between life and death

This moment in the treatment marks a turning point in the work. My moving away from known losses, Martin's and my own, into my own liminal state that changed what each of us could know. We leave the realm of "understanding," and enter the site of our unknown individual traumas, learning to forgo identification with the other to be with ourselves *and* each other in our "emphatic unsettlement" (LaCapra 2001). We are in a mode of "suggesting one might not know that one is dreaming, or that one might see only without knowing it" (Caruth 1996, 39).

What does this actually look like in the lived experience of the treatment?

It is very hard to say. I am not trying to place the experience beyond phenomenological description, but this kind of other-worldly transmission does not happen in language or event but punctum. The presence of Woodman's work hangs in the consulting room like ether. It permeates our space in waves, not quite mirage or image but atmosphere. Our much earlier version of "absence-mindedness" (Farhi 2010, 488), in which Martin and I were looking together from a bench towards the sea, has given way to something more gripping: we are now in that sea. Whatever was underwater, out of sight, is with us now as a palpable presence of absence, heavy and disruptive. The sessions are languid, drifty—hard to bear. Sometimes it means both of us, me behind the couch, her on the couch, are joined in a state of floating, somnolent, amorphous experience. I think of somatic reverie and drowning. I don't want to call it unconscious communication exactly, because I think we are creating something new that could not come into being until there was an intersubjective system to house the experience (Stolorow, Brandchaft, and Atwood 1987). We are embodying or enacting the absent past that couldn't be remembered or represented, because it was in excess of our frames of reference (Felman and Laub 1992). This is what I am calling a negative enactment: that which brings forward an invisible state of unformulated trauma like the negative of the photograph. When "we lose ourselves in the negative" (Pontalis, in Abelin 1993), something opens. As Caruth (1996) notes, the transmission of the unrepresentable happens when the listener is brought into the trauma, making us, in Dori Laub's language, "participants and co-owners of the traumatic event" (Leys 2000, 269).

Martin and I begin to know that wherever else she lives, she also lives in the shimmer, in the in-between, in the gap. This is as close to home as any state she knows. And I am a knowing guest.

If there is any concrete change, it's this: Over the next months as Martin and I hold Woodman's images between us, reveries about my dead father surfaces, and I think of my own failure to mark his death and the way that keeps me from fully inhabiting my subjectivity. Simultaneously, references to Martin's father emerge here and there in a dream or association. She might talk of missing, and I might say something like, "Your father went missing and has always been missing," and Martin acknowledges the psychic relevance. Or she dreams of herself lying on parchment paper, and if she shifts her weight, the paper will give way to a moving grave, carried on a conveyor belt below her suspended body. What had previously been invisible, unimaginable, increasingly emerges into images, feelings, and words. In the consulting room, time reasserts itself. There becomes a before and an after, a now and a then.

Soon her body, always foreign to her, will also emerge.

We talk. We come to live together the way her trauma was experienced too early to be fully known. We "feel" into what was cliché; that for my patient to lay claim to her own survival, she would have to lay her father to rest (Caruth 1996). She knows an unbridgeable gap where the missing father went missing and then was missing forever. In this story, missing the moment of his death, she is also unable to recognize the continuation of her life.[8] There was no body, no funeral, no grave, and no acknowledgment that her father was dead. There was no "then" or "after" that marked his death. If her father is not really dead, he cannot be mourned. But to claim life by grasping his death would be to remember him as a living being and lose him again (Caruth 1996). We wonder: has my patient made her father the part of her that escaped her (Pontalis)? The small (a)? Rather than experience identification with the dead father, in this frame my patient is possessed by this foreign body that "acquires from within a relentless power, the power of a drive. Words would break the continuity of that line—a total and final separation" (Pontalis, in Abelin 1993, 899). Representing the death in words kills the ghost and loses the object. Here is another dilemma.

My patient's act of survival is "the repeated confrontation with the necessity and impossibility of grasping the threat to her life" (Caruth 1996, 8), the threat that she has not known or has been rigidly disavowed. "Survival becomes, paradoxically, an endless testimony to the impossibility of living" (Caruth 1996, 8). Where memory might be, breach is.

The body brings terror

These shared understandings give way to terror. Now Martin with an (a) begins to feel how her disavowal of her father's suicide has impeded her ability to inhabit herself and how he has simultaneously possessed her.

Martin has existed in a kind of melancholic wandering in which no one cried out (Caruth 1996); no body was felt. Disembodied, there was no pain or pleasure. Now her body and the excruciating pain of the previously unconscious trauma return together. It starts with her breasts. Martin with an (a) tells me she feels her breasts for the first time. She can feel them as erotic objects. As soft shapes beneath her fingers. She never was a breast man. Now with the existence of a body, so do I become alive. She moves towards me.

She writes,
I wake up in the winter
I am wearing you tight
Across my chest where I have felt
Strange tingling for days and weeks now
And I mind just a little these pricks of soma rubbing
Into mind breasts chapped and almost straining across the room to you

The psychic cache of having breasts is unimaginable. With the breasts, the huge hole of their absence asserts itself. Now anxiety, symptoms, desire, longing. No one said breasts were just for fun. A direct relational element emerges. Can she use me? Am I real? Can she feel me? Will I stay? She thinks not. The return to bodily memory awakens relationality—and trauma.

At the site of Woodman's work, in our eighth year of treatment, Martin's drift gives way to terror. Suddenly Martin is shouting, trembling, sobbing. Martin with an (a)'s father's suicide begins to register through a terrible fear of the future. She begins to feel the terror she must have felt as a small girl as her world collapsed—feelings she could not know then. Each morning she awakens to the certain feeling that everyone she loves will disappear. Psychic reality trumps husband, children, me. We truly are abandoning her. She tells me I won't show up, won't come back, will evaporate. It's painful to separate, to know I will die. She wants promises. Assurances. To be part of my funeral or illness or any other departure she can imagine. She will not be on the outside of death again. She does not know if she can survive the future. The fear of it undoes her. It's not a loss she fears. It's a disaster. A whole world shattering. The catastrophe is back as if for the first time and only now in this strange place and time does it constitute itself. Martin with an (a) had not known the violence of her losses, and their return makes her sweat and shake. It is the traumatic awakening from death into life that is now upon her. My body/mind too feels dread. I hope it is the dread preceding surrender (Ghent 1990).

Discussion

What really allowed change? Working in the visual register allowed us to know about a state of nonbeing that did not exist in language and originally could not be represented in words. Without being fully conscious of what I was doing, I offered Martin a visual interpretation of her own (metaphoric) liminality. I see now this was an act of figurability in which the analyst "initiates and catalyzes processes that strengthen and/or integrate [the patient's] ability to think by strengthening and integrating weakly inscribed psychic elements or giving form to something that was previously unrepresented" (Levine 2012, 612). When I bring Woodman's images into the field, I am offering an unthought interpretation in the visual form, and new meaning is generated. I say an unthought interpretation, because I was not fully conscious of what I was introducing. Perhaps the images, ideas, and affects existed in a form that was pre-representable. When she and I see them together, something inchoate begins to form and be represented.

I want to notice at least two registers in which change happened. When Martin sees that I have seen a version of her experience of present-absence in Woodman's images, this allows her to accept outside sight, and see her reflection through my seeing her. My reflection is uncertain, partial, and tentative, and the images themselves suggest something inchoate, blurred, and lurking that feels reflective. These reflections give rise to Martin's unarticulated feelings about her own sense of nonbeing and makes mental space, emotional states, and their symbolization more possible. Martin then uses Woodman as a mirror to constitute an image of herself paradoxically as both a being and a nonbeing, so her "I" can see a version of her "me" (Seligman 2007, 336–37). We have created a space between Martin as subject and her experience of herself as someone who can be represented. And when we do, Martin is able to register her body, and the terror that accompanies the experience of being alive.

But what allows this use of me? Martin can do this, because she thinks that for me to see her as ghost or liminal being, I must have my own ghost(s).

This moves us into shared experience, which is necessary for witnessing trauma but not enough in itself. We have moved from object relating to transitional relating (Winnicott 1969). Martin has, without impingement, discovered her own motility. She reaches, creates, finds a "me" and a "you." Now something more like object use develops. Our relationship is real, vitalized, filled with love and hate.

If we believe trauma was experienced too early in Martin's life and too shockingly to be fully known by her, Martan needs an other with whom to constitute her traumatic history. I am interested anew in Freud's early trauma theory, as reviewed in Caruth (1996), not as theory but as metaphor. He tells us that what is truly striking about the train accident or trauma victim's experience of the event is not so much the forgetting that occurs afterward but that the person is never fully conscious during the event. Caruth emphasizes the temporal aspect of trauma, noting that the fright is not known because it registers a moment too late, when a breach has already occurred. Said another way, traumatic experience is not mediated through a mind and what it represses, because the mind has missed the event. This theory has holes (so to speak). In my view of trauma, moments of disavowal and acknowledgment oscillate; everything is registered, return is never literal, just (Morris 2012, personal communication[9]). Afterwardness confers meaning. Trauma lands and surfaces from the complexity of all we are and are becoming. Yet as metaphor, something calls in this outdated theory. The metaphor of nonbeing may be central to certain kinds of early trauma because the trauma is experienced only belatedly and indirectly. Because the patient does not own or possess the knowledge of the trauma, and our own truths continually escape us (Felman and Laub 1992), it is only in the engagement with an other that trauma becomes constituted. As Caruth (1996) notes, it is the fundamental incomprehensibility at the heart of trauma that necessitates that entanglement. Without fully grasping the other's or even our own trauma, Martin and I needed each other for each of us to create an opening to establish history and memory. "This speaking and listening, from the site of trauma does not rely . . . on what [we] simply know of each other, but on what [we] don't know of our own traumatic pasts" (1996, 56). I believe that it is our being in our *own* liminality rather than identifying liminality as a phenomenon we share that allows the intersubjective entanglement to give rise to the creation of memory and representation.

Being together, not coming together[10]

I want to emphasize this last point. When I am listening to Martin from my own corresponding history of loss, I potentially appropriate her story. I have been alive to the familiar issues of loss and disavowal regarding the death of my own father, but not alive to the way that disavowal left me, metaphorically in my own liminality. I colluded with Martin in not seeing how she has not been alive, because I was blind to an aspect of my own corresponding liminality.

By using our own known experience as a way to know the other, we may fail to create the necessary interruption in our patient's and our own looping self-narratives. We may need an interruption that surprises—something that is almost like a slap or shock that invites some element of distinction, separateness, and bodily awareness where absence and dissociation have been (Caruth 1996). The Woodman critics created this dissonance or shock for me and for Martin (a) by their negating the significance of her suicide, denying the difference between life and death.

As I wrote earlier (McGleughlin 2011), I continue to believe in accord with Slavin (2011) and Lombardi (2005) that when we are willing to travel back to the place of corresponding deficit within ourselves, to struggle with our own internal splits in our effort to reach the other, a channel toward change and transformation may open. I still believe alongside Harris (2009) and others that impasse may loosen when the analyst has access to unbearable affects and can metabolize, shift, grieve, change, and speak from this slightly altered state. Still, something more was highlighted in this work with Martin with an (a) that I have grasped in a new way. Then I wrote that we had to help our patients in those places we can't yet help ourselves, which I now understand to be our own places of potential. But perhaps it is equally true that our own absences need to be recognized and somehow represented. Martin with an (a) made a demand: to listen not from what I know about my own losses but from the place they have infected me and made me blank. There, where the "referential function of words begins to break down . . . what is transmitted is 'not the normalizing knowledge of the horror but the horror itself'" (Michaels 1996, 8).

Summary

Avedon showed us what we did not know in someone familiar. Woodman helped us recognize our need to see what is not yet there. Morris notes that acknowledging death depends on a willingness to be disturbed. Ultimately, it means being able to distinguish between life and death. Caruth (1996) emphasized the way in which one's own trauma is tied up with the trauma of another and that in the "very possibility and surprise of listening to another's wound," one is able to "bear witness" (p. 3) by creating a platform from which to enter the incomprehensible.

Martin with an (a) and I are still in process. Movement is not linear, more in and out. But we are in the grit of human relating. Yesterday she asks, in the language of Leanh Nguyen (2012), if I know real intimate contact with another mind/body who I have allowed to see me, smell me, know me in my abject fear and pathetic bodily functions. I nod. When I can feel your breath on my face, my terror smells ripe.

Notes

1 Derived from Pontalis 1999.
2 There is an extensive dialogue about unformulated experience most prominently explored by Stolorow, Brandchaft, and Atwood's (1987) who name the "prereflective unconscious," Bollas's (1987) as the "unthought known," and Stern's (1997) as "unformulated experience."
3 Winterson cites Romanian scholar Mircea Eliade's ontological as well as geographical notion of home. "Home," he tells us, "is the intersection of two lines—the vertical and the horizontal. The vertical plane has heaven, or the upper world, at one end, and the world of the dead at the other end. The horizontal plane is the traffic of this world, moving to and fro—our own traffic and that of teeming others." Winterson tells us, "Home was a place of order, a place where the order of things comes together—the living and the dead—the spirits of the ancestors and the present inhabitants, and the gathering up and stilling of all the to and fro. . . . At worst, a displaced person literally does not know which way is up, because there is no true north. No compass point. . . . For the refugee, for the homeless, this lack of crucial coordinate in the placing of the self has severe consequences" (p. 58).
4 Freud's writes about his grandson, who in an effort to master his mother's disappearance and return, creates a game where he casts a spool out and reels it backs in, a process critical to the development of continuity in absence. Freud calls this the fort/da game, and it was first discussed in *Beyond the Pleasure Principle* (1920).
5 The phrase appears in Woodman's text written below two photographs in *Some Disordered Interior Geometries*, reproduced in Chris Townsend, Francesca Woodman. Oxford: Phaidon Press, 2006 (p. 238).
6 Unlike Barthes (1980), who finds relief in his dead mother's photograph because it signals that she existed in a time before he was alive, and hence creates the

possibility that he can go on after her death, I find no mourning possibilities in these images. Woodman's indeterminacy, her refusal/inability/disinterest in capturing her own still life, her own portrait, a firmly rooted image of herself as alive or dead suggests something must precede our mourning.

7 Elsewhere I have described Barthes' concepts (1980) of studium and punctum in discussing a certain group of well-composed photographs (Chapter 2). Perhaps the critics view Woodman's work through the lens of what he calls studium. I want Woodman's critics to exist, not as spectators on the outside but as participants.

8 These are ideas formulated from Caruth's reading of the film *Hiroshima mon amour* (1961) in *Unclaimed Experience* (2006).

9 See Leys' (2000) critique of Caruth's reconceptualization of Freud.

10 Caruth 1996.

Chapter 7

Answering gestures

Further thoughts on "Do we find or lose ourselves in the negative?" (2015)

Ways of seeing, ways of being seen

Psychoanalytic writers have often erred on the side of studium (Barthes 1980), a way of seeing an image that bespeaks commitment or interest without true acuity, on the order of liking, not loving, an interest reflecting one's training or culture. I want to tell the story of my work with Martin with an (a), in "Do We Find or Lose Ourselves in the Negative?", with punctum: with the visual detail that stands out, disturbs, and creates "the pressure of the unspeakable that wants to be spoken" (Barthes 1980, 19). But how to do it?

My discussant Stephen Hartman helps frame my dilemma: "This is the double paradox of psychoanalytic reading: the anticipatory demand for clarification reproduces the standard edition" (2015). My paper is already more standard than I want. The editor suggested "a more usual format," with names, narratives, legends "that declare or thematize your intentions." I had to chuckle. He wants to steady readers, but such preemptive framing feels controlling and contradicts my invitation to the audience "to call up and bear your own gaps and ghosts." As Spivak tells us, the writer is always read, assigned, becomes a sign, and is not under the control of the person who speaks/writes (as cited in Johnson 2000, 79).

> By the time a description of a case is deemed fit to print, it is no longer the sole province of either the patient or analyst. The narrative has been subject to a rigorous round of edits and revisions. It makes an argument in a history of arguments and so it becomes a case about trauma with a kind of clarity that is precisely the opposite of trauma.
>
> (Hartman 2015)

DOI: 10.4324/9781032670348-10

I compromised what I thought was the enacted nature of the telling, but Hartman reminds us there can be no reading and writing without enactment. Writing/reading are fields and invite us to reflect more deeply on the kind of encounter we are always staging with an other. In Hartman's story of my story, we can parse more clearly the stakes of how a story is told and by whom as he separates all the Martins from Jade McGleughlin the writer, the psychoanalyst, and from the alluded-to missing patient. He notes not just the enigma of Woodman and Martin and McGleughlin's paper but also of Jade McGleughlin.

The personal part: I always want someone with me

Martin taught me the value in entropy, nonintegration, accumulating pieces, and as I did with Marie, stringing them together until a story emerges like a flip-book. As the writer, I want to bring you everywhere I've been, and if you live it with me, you can come to see it as I do. I am always in dialogue with you. I don't want to digest everything first and feed it to back to you. I am, of course, playing a little bit here—writing somewhat facetiously to prick the valorization of analytic containment. I don't solely believe in that style of politics or psychoanalysis. By reminding us that no language exists without a listener making it their own, the discussants revealed my unstated fantasy that you can be where I am. We can't live outside culture or language; there is no listening without our own ear. You have your own mind, internal objects, ways of anticipating, and this is necessarily so. Yet, like Martin, it's hard for me to accept your mirroring back, the difference of your mind. I want to give you the gift of implication (Smith 2013), to bring you to me.

   Zadie Smith (2013) introduces this concept in an art review about Signorelli's painting *Man with a Corpse*, pointing out the way in which sometimes we can fall prey to the fantasy that what we are viewing does not include *us*. Smith calls this nothing less than "a gorgeous illusion," an evocative description that belies the fact that there is something inherently problematic in the ways we fail to recognize ourselves in another's reality.

   [The painting] creates a triangular and unstable relationship—between you, the corpse, and the 'someone else.' Looking at it, I am not a woman looking at a man carrying a corpse. I am that corpse. . . . It's not me. But it will be me.

(Smith 2013)

By moving from represented to nonrepresented states, Martin forced us to surrender our illusion and encounter something hard to bear. Certain paintings and people do that by bringing us "to an intolerable, yet necessary place" (Smith 2013), the place to which Martin led us: our relationship to death.

And there are theoretical reasons.

Any representation always covers emptiness (Hartman 2015). It calls forward loss in whatever authorial direction one chooses. Focusing on the writing/reading enactments illuminates that the writer's decisions about how far to veer from the expected are theoretical *and* political. They involve hierarchies of power and inclusion: what kind of voice can and should be heard, whose name should be called? Strong prescriptive and regulatory forces exist in all healing practices and their tellings (Foucault 1980). Reading and writing enactments show we are being read.

The more readers praise my didactic writing, the less they cotton to being dragged along or, as Hartman nicely phrases it, my "curating" a more dialogic self. I understand. For the most part, we don't want to re-experience trauma; we want to be told its generative lessons. But I want a form of writing that reflects the mind prior to psychic organization: I don't want all depressive position, no punctum. Who else can afford to write in the voice of madness (Williams 1992)?

As Barbara Johnson (1998) wrote about the renegade Black feminist law professor Patricia Williams, her "writing possesses a logic that makes perceptible the realities of difference subordinated behind the rhetoric of neutrality . . . the style of her writing is not the sign of her identity but the enactment of her critique" (pp. 166–67). Williams exposes what Johnson calls the "network of constraints and censorship" (p. 168) that we employ when we edit out multiplicity, and then privilege, in the name of clarity, our objectivity, linearity, and one-person thinking—all of which I sought to disrupt. Our field lags behind others in challenging the way we force-feed scholarly writing as truth.

In earlier papers (2001, 2011), I consciously cultivated a mix-up between who is subject and who is object; who, patient and who, analyst. The necessity for this in clinical work is clear. But who is who? My discussant Melanie

Suchet (2015) takes this up when she asks if Martin gets to speak, and if I really listen to her. Am I helping to birth but also to negate something crucial about her self-representation, hence our name games? Is there genuine self-representation? As Suchet wisely asks, if I cannot ethically tell a story about Martin and this treatment without harming her but still have something important to convey, what is the right form? More radically, aside from the issue of confidentiality, if we took seriously that our minds are not located in our singular self, would we present two minds as one? When Suchet wonders about the impact of this writing on Martin, my first thought is "*I* gave consent." (Martin with an (a), did too!) It's more than a Freudian slip. It reveals my belief in the way analysts become engaged in the living of a case and, even more so, in its writing. Suchet (2015) observes,

> . . . is it the analyst herself that is represented in the adjoining piece? Is the 'a' a stand in for analyst, albeit a small one? If so, the analyst is co-joined, conjoined, she is the co-construction . . . adding a piece to the name is the recognition of the mutuality that the process of subjectivity entails.

Suchet intuits a deeper dynamic within my covering of my patient by incorporating pieces of my history in her case, blurring the frame. Who am I and who is Martin in this text? I am happy when Hartman (2015) notes that I want the blur, need the ambiguity to make the enigmatic legible, honoring the presence of the absent third.

It's no accident that the powerful body of Woodman's work that evoked/provoked the dream state my patient and I entered was about troubling "the conceptual and bodily threshold around the always elusive gesture of seeing" (Raymond 2010, 2). Could we cross boundaries of frame and personhood and still be operating with ethical responsibility as we conceptualize and communicate selected facts of a treatment? I have followed Gabbard's (1997) ethical principles: no details and no camouflaging that change the essential aspects of the treatment. Still, as Woodman showed us, photographs don't convey memory but *add* a new dimension. I write *not* to convey truth (Fuentes 2001) but to make a scene. I am with de Lauretis (1999) when she writes in reference to Freud:

> the case history belongs to its writer, not to its case: It is the history of a case, the reconstruction of a psychic trajectory, an interpretation, a

representation, a text of fiction, and not a 'true story'. . . . It is a text that bears the inscription of a subjectivity, a desire that is more its writer's . . . than its central characters.

(p. 38)

Would I be writing about the problem of being named if I had no trouble being seen?

Can patients stand to be expanded, multiplied in this way? Does the reader feel duped? If we are somewhere between believing the self exists only between people (and knowing it is an illusion) and that the self is housed in a mind or psyche, how do we show both in our writing? If, as Hartman (2015) says, I don't pretend that my investment in functioning in the abyss will aid a silent film star to mouth the script in a talkie film, what can I blur except "the lipstick that signifies the fallen diva's protest against talking?" Are these rhetorical choices, clinical decisions, hermeneutic reads, ethical principles?

Hartman (2015) joins me in the limits of field theory, writing that, as I learned from Avedon, "stations the analyst in the role of portrait maker and analysand in the role of model, roles that by definition reproduce exactly the images (photographer/model; container/contained) that their roles were functionally designed to produce" (p. 242). My earlier belief that I could be Avedon, the portrait maker, was more than just youthful naïveté. I followed a long line of thinkers, who, while doing something filled with creativity and brilliance, believed in finding something already there. (Think Caper 1999, who says our sole job is to show the other their mind.) When Hartman observes that, unlike field theorists, I allow entropy by taking up the analyst's not knowing, I am grateful. There is a *real* patient, also a missing patient, another patient, and the ghosts. This writing enactment asks something more than k-knots.

Jars, jugs, and pots

I can't resist this small quip. What is the deal with men and their containers? Johnson (1998) asks in "Muteness Envy":

Why does Keats write about his urn; Heidegger, a jug; Wallace Stevens, a jar; and Brooks, the well-wrought urn? Now Hartman writes of the pots of Bette Woodman! What is being symbolized? Johnson has lots of ideas about these containers. First and foremost, they are containers of ashes of the dead, becoming metaphors for the relation between form and content, body and soul, expression and intention. Like a human being, they have an inside and an outside.

(p. 142)

I haven't thought of myself as the container and Martin as the contained. I didn't think insides and outsides, more Möbius strip, orange aura. And I didn't read Martin as dead or empty, as interiorized femininity, void of presence. There's more on that, but there is this. Johnson (1998) writes that the speaker in Keats's poem "asks the urn for names, narratives, legends . . . the urn answers with chiasmus, tautology, abstraction. The speaker asks for history; the urn resists with theory" (p. 142). And we are back to the very writing dilemmas that plagued me at the onset.

What happens when we don't have enough words?

I want to take up Suchet's comments (2015) about the uses of dissociation (a customary way we think about trauma), from which I deliberately tried to steer away. Subtle conceptualizations can be hard to parse because of the paucity of language to describe states of present-absence, uncertainty about how the mind really works, and my "poetic" rather than precise metapsychological language. Yet Suchet's close tracking of my thoughts challenges me to be more nuanced in my thinking and phenomenological descriptions. I appreciated her understanding that entering into the state I call liminal, a present-absence, is part of the transformative arc of the case, and I feel her going there with me. When she is with me, I can think again. However, for me, the language of dissociation confuses rather than clarifies.

In using the term disavowal, not dissociation, I was noting a kind of refuting of the importance of something *towards or about one's objects*. Disavowal in this sense is a relational phenomenon (Morris, personal communication). I meant to capture something involving others/objects, but not a splitting of the self. I don't think a part of my self was bracketed. Suchet writes, "We witness McGleughlin discovering that she has *dissociated her own liminality*. She cannot come to know or accept M's liminality if she is disavowing her own." And later:

Another way to conceptualize this is that it is the breaking through of *dissociation as a defense* to enter into a type of *dissociated, deadened state*. And this deadened state is the medium from which the other can be known and reached.

Suchet suggests that I gain access to my own dissociated absent state, "the non-being that the analyst *knows from within,* which allows her a way to find the other through herself." She infers a kind of blind spot (Goldberger 1993) that did not allow me to conceptualize something potentially important in Martin's experience of herself—a now-familiar relational idea that potentially gives way to impasse (Harris 2009; Slavin 2011). I think I gave her that impression when I wrote I've been "alive to the familiar issues of loss and disavowal regarding the death of my own father, *but not alive* to the way that disavowal left me, metaphorically, in my own liminality." While we agree that an important state representing nonbeing was *with* us, I don't think it was the nonbeing *I knew*, or could come to know simply from my own experience. If we stay with the conception of trauma as beyond representation or borrow the Lacanian concept of the real, in which experiences occur but remain unrepresented except as aftereffects (as Suchet agrees), what do we have that would be split off? If in our state of present-absence we were evoking a primary terror, terror of loss of self and object, we were evoking a state in which our ability to use mind/body/affect (Smith 2013) as a processing instrument had broken down. If we approach the real and there is no self-representation, can a self dissociate?

I could not find M through the trauma *I knew* and was evoked by my dead father, her dead father; my missing mother, her missing mother; my liminality and hers. Instead, I am trying to talk about a presence of absence experienced as atmosphere that came to narrate something inchoate. I was suggesting that the feeling state of present-absence that we cocreated through long and complicated ways of being together, condensed and symbolized through the photographs of Woodman, gave rise to something that had not come into being and represented psychic rupture or an objectless state. Living in the emotional creation of what emerged between us generated the possibility for a kind of creative recognition, an act of figurability (Levine 2012). We made a narrative, a discursive way to organize, account for, and give meaning to an experience we cocreated. I would argue that I have not broken through my dissociation of my liminality as much as borrowed the concept of liminality to create an intersubjective scaffolding on which to build a psychic frame. I could not know liminality until we had created *the idea of liminality.*

I want to make sure you know Martin, the shrink, looks like us. She is a high-functioning person, although an aspect of her has not yet come into being. The language of not inhabiting oneself, or being caught between life and death, is an approximation, trying to steer us towards something about the difficulty of establishing history and memory. The liminality I speak of is both specific to Martin and me *and* a human phenomenon. Absence is what Ogden (2012) calls "the vital core of human experience" (p. 291) that is with us all. Trauma heightens our awareness by showing us what happens when there is no buffer, no disavowal of the presence of death. Humphrey Morris (personal communication) might say that disavowing/ acknowledging death is called living, and that oscillation is the condition of life's meaning.

Liminality is not deadness

I am afraid that in my efforts to describe liminality, sometimes calling it nonbeing or breach, I created confusion for my discussants. Hartman and Suchet heard emptiness and deadness, notions I did not intend. Liminality is a powerful affective experience, albeit on a border, neither here nor there, not a dissociated state. Suchet's casting what I am describing as a state of *deadened, dissociated* nonbeing captures the pull towards entropy but not the aliveness of the fight to survive. My closest association is to being kissed by the liminal beings called dementors in Harry Potter's world who suck the life force from you (Rowling 1997). This liminal state is omnipresent, disruptive, deadening, but *we were not deadened*. We are alive but *alone* in profound danger, because ultimately none of us can live in an objectless state. The state is urgent, gripping because we need to make contact with an other to survive. In the groping toward finding life and an other, the struggle to survive can give way to a certain framing, a scaffolding that holds. Two of us sharing aloneness allows for the recognition of an experiential gap. One might think of this state as the terrifying pull towards decathexis, the work of the negative (Green 1999) in which the only real thing becomes a "representation of the absence of representation" (Green 1999). Suchet's discussion helped me see the distinction I make from Green: I am not talking about dissociation, amnesia, repression, or, like Green, a pathological attachment to the negative. I am evoking liminality as a creative attempt to construct a sense of meaning out of meaninglessness, ultimately moving towards healing and growth (Slavin 2013).

In returning me to the Relational language of the intersubjective third, Suchet emphasized, as I did, that something new was cocreated, allowing meaning to develop. She notes that Martin's and my ability to do that is possible because we have established Gerson's (2009) intersubjective conditions for a "vital" or "live third." For the most part, I concur. However, I have one quibble. Intersubjectivity requires two subjects and the achievement of mutual *recognition* (Benjamin 1995). This concept of a third implies a level of development incongruent with the particular state I describe. "Vital," "live," and "mutual recognition" don't capture the entropy, the aloneness of that experience. Like Hartman's Scrabble, the letters are there but don't spell. A kind of catastrophic rupture in self-experience had happened but had yet to be experienced. And we went on being. I wrote, "We leave the realm of understanding, and each enter the site of our unknown individual trauma." That trauma has to be and always is, in some way, our encounter with death.

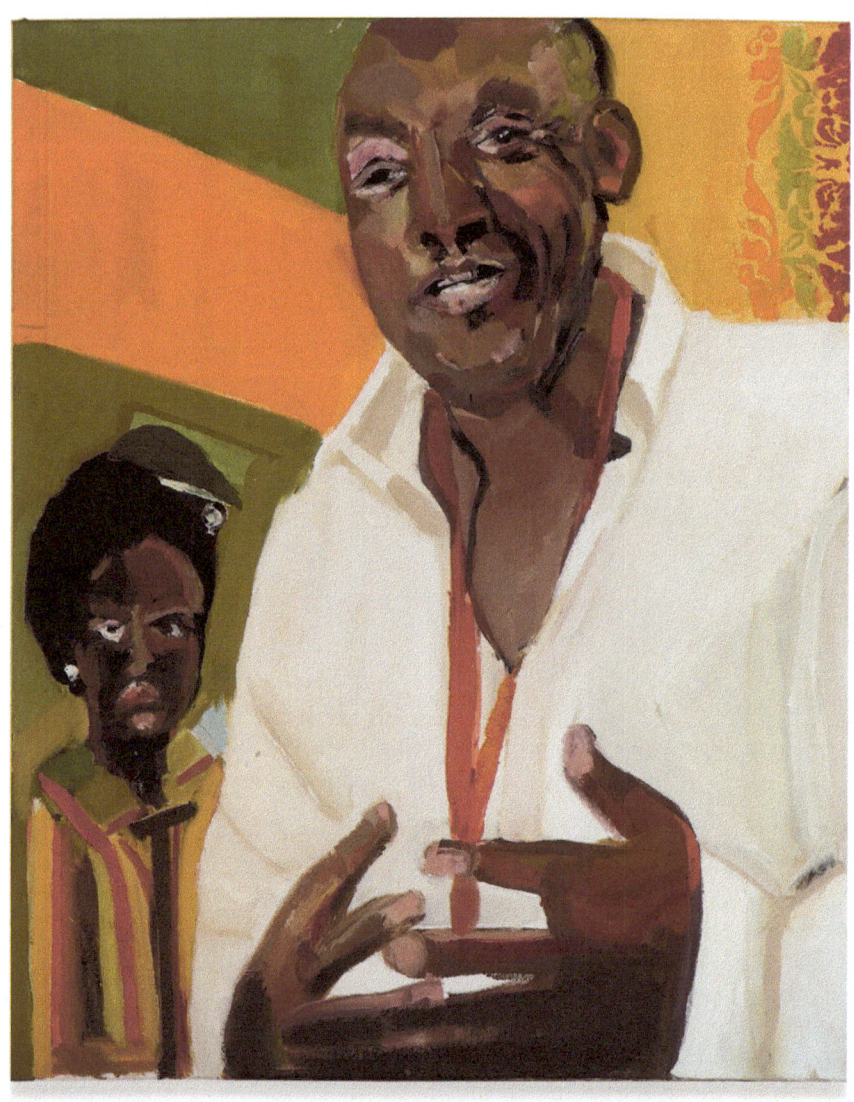

Figure 7.1 *Henry Taylor and his painting.* Oil on canvas 20x16. McGleughlin

Chapter 8

"When you are in the cellar, am I dead?"

Understanding the limits of empathy and the power of otherness through the film *Hiroshima mon amour* (2020)

It was not long after I wrote "Do We Find or Lose Ourselves in the Negative?" (2015a) when it happened: Watching Alain Resnais's and Marguerite Duras's film, *Hiroshima mon amour* (1959), I had another experience of punctum (Barthes 1980). As discussed in the introduction and Chapter 2, Barthes is writing about seeing and being seen prior to, or outside of language: studium and punctum are ways of looking and being looked at. They hold the tension between language and image. Suddenly, in one particularly visually arresting scene in the film, I felt something new about liminality. I found myself existing in a radical space of boundarylessness, where the lines between self and other, life and death, past and present were no longer so apparent. And in this liminal realm, something important emerged about the therapeutic action of my work with my patient Martin with an (a), something that had escaped my attempts to conceptualize the treatment through language. My mind existed outside my brain, in my body, and in the things and space around us.

Was it, as Walter Benjamin (1935/2008) writes, that "the camera not merely clarifies what we see . . . but brings to light entirely new structures of matter, . . . not only reveals familiar aspects of movements but discloses quite unknown aspects within them?" (p. 37). Benjamin calls this *the optical unconscious*, in contrast to *the psychoanalytic instinctual unconscious*, offering that it is clearly "another nature which speaks to the camera as compared to the eye" (p. 37). And, in fact, my body now "knew" in another way. Sense impressions flooded me—about memory, time, forgetting, none of which I can articulate. When punctum pierces, you see beyond what *is there* and feel something embodied that stands out, disturbs, provokes, or even shocks. So it was with Martin with an (a). I could see beyond what was there, affording new insights and understandings.[1]

DOI: 10.4324/9781032670348-11

The same experience of *nachträglichkeit* happened on another plane when I read Cathy Caruth's 1996 analysis of the film. Caruth examines it through the lens of studium; hers is a studied approach that helped me formulate what had remained inchoate in my own encounter with Martin. This led me to want to tell the story from one more angle, but not *just* to add to my understanding of this case. The film shows us a fresh way to encounter another, one beyond our usual way of seeing/feeling/being.

I want us to imagine its protagonists—the Japanese man, Lui, and the French woman, Elle—not as actors, but as analyst and patient, to further flesh out the ontological sensibility I outlined earlier in the book. Especially in cases of rupture and absence caused by trauma, transformation becomes possible not through accruing new knowledge but through an experience between two who "do not know" meeting in their blankness and liminality.

By analogy with the film, I suggest how we might rethink our therapeutic method in circumstances when conceptualizing trauma as a "what" can register as betrayal and when the patient's breach of mind alters time and hence the sense of having a coherent personal history. The film helps us see that when we use an empathy that draws on our own experience to enter into that of another, we may fail to perceive their otherness. And we may fail to create the necessary break in our patient's and our own looping self-narratives. By contrast, Lui, now conceived as the analyst, challenges rather than joins Elle's story; he speaks to her from his inner breach and "unsettled knowledge," and "live" from the sight of her frozen stalled trauma narrative. With Lui, we also witness an interruption that surprises—one that invites some element of separateness and bodily awareness where absence and dissociation have been.

While many of these ideas may by now be familiar, in choosing to use the film and its interpretation as ground, I hope to produce another layer of seeing/feeling/being as Anzaldúa does (1987) in her practices of border-crossing and metamorphosis. In particular, *Hiroshima mon amour* allows us to think about the ways we look and how this affects *what* we see. For, after all, seeing and being seen are central to the clinical problems with patients who suffer both developmental and catastrophic trauma.

The film plot

Hiroshima mon amour tells the story of a brief love affair between a French actress Elle ("She") and a Japanese architect Lui ("Him"). The two meet when Elle is in Japan to make a film about the World War II bombing of

Hiroshima, and for the first time she is able to tell her own traumatic war story. It goes like this: During the Nazi occupation of France, she fell in love with a young German soldier stationed in her hometown of Nevers. The two made plans to elope, only for the soldier to be shot and killed on the day they were to flee—which also happened to be the day the Allies liberated Nevers. Elle was publicly ostracized for the relationship and imprisoned in the cellar of her parents' home, where she went mad. As for Lui, we learn that he is a native of Hiroshima who'd been conscripted into the Imperial Japanese Army. When the bomb destroyed his family and his homes, he had been fighting elsewhere. In Elle's and Lui's telling of their respective stories of trauma, each comes to know something that they previously could not. How this occurs, and translates into change within the "therapeutic dyad," is what interests me. It is neither empathy nor understanding that prompts transformation, but rather disruption and a refusal to enter the other's story. Punctum. Rupture. A freighted collision between the protagonists.

Entering the film

Because so much of the theory of catastrophic trauma is formulated around the Holocaust and its aftermath (given the Eurocentric origins of psychoanalysis), it is easy to believe that trauma happens at a specific time and place, that it is indeed characterized by a "what" and a "when." Yet one of the gifts of *Hiroshima mon amour* is its cinematic unveiling of the limits of what we can see in ourselves, and what we can comprehend of another's trauma. The film opens with an extended prologue in which the man and the woman embrace each other amidst falling ash. Soon we learn that they have a major disagreement. The French woman has watched footage of the devastation caused by the atom bomb and asserts that she has seen and understood everything that happened there. This is resolutely and repeatedly denied by the Japanese man, no matter how explicit the evidence Elle offers, evidence that we viewers are shown on-screen. The couple's entwined bodies are intercut with news footage of the attack and archival footage of mutilated corpses, new war memorials, and the postwar urban landscape of Hiroshima.

Caruth suggests that the viewer might believe that Lui's denial of what the woman can see is, in fact, a powerful assertion of what *he* has seen—the pair are in Hiroshima, after all, his home. Yet this is not the case. Since he was not in the city when it was bombed, he has, in fact, "seen" nothing.

Lui's vehement reaction emerges from a more visceral place: The story told by images of the destruction cannot tell the story of *his* Hiroshima trauma, and what it will come to mean to him. His denial is not a matter of "empirical perception" (Caruth, p. 27) but a refusal of trauma as a "what": as something that *can* be seen. For the Japanese man, any attempt to understand Hiroshima as an event or series of events that are discrete or intelligible betrays the very nature of the trauma and its sequalae.

Moreover, Caruth proposes that Resnais's decision to use fiction to tell the story of Hiroshima, rather than the documentary he'd originally planned, accentuates the point that trauma can't be reduced to a "what." It does not reside in events, Caruth tells readers, following Freud, but in the "breach in the mind's experience of time, self, and the world" (p. 4),[2] something we as analysts now well know.

The aspect of the film that strikes Caruth as most important is how it dramatizes what happens when two absolutely alien experiences are brought together. The French woman insists that she is like the Japanese man: "Like you, I know what it is to forget. Like you, I have a memory"; he refutes this, over and over.

In these exchanges, Lui can be seen as *doing the absolute opposite* of what we as relational analysts are usually taught to do. That is to say, Lui utterly refuses to give Elle any sense that he grasps or empathizes with her traumatic experience. I am persuaded that Lui's refusal suggests his implicit (perhaps unconscious) recognition that *understanding through language is a misunderstanding, that it pins down the experience of the other, bypasses how trauma is frozen in time, and collapses meaning*, even when we are being invited to understand. To see, or even empathize with, something definable may erase trauma because the trauma actually is the mind's rupture.

I want to think about this moment of two alien experiences being brought together in a clinical setting. When the patient and analyst cannot find common ground, the result is often a crunch, (Russell 1983), or a relational knot (Pizer 2003). Words and meanings don't align, and each participant feels there is something enormous at stake that cannot be easily negotiated and leads to vertiginous confusion, not knowing who is doing what to whom. The difficulty of opening to the other's reality shows how we cleave to our own positions for psychic safety (Bromberg 1998), and it prompts a consideration of which alien self-states could be activated within us that would make it more or less dangerous to accept another's perceptions (Davies

2004). Such impasses are often highly affectively charged and conflictual before they may (or may not) yield something transformational.

Whether we think about crunches as destructive repetitions or generative enactments or both, we are taught as analysts that we have to be deeply psychically involved *and* reflect. It is often our job to locate a third position that gets the analytic couple out of a locked, antagonistic system. While actual resolution of impasse requires something less linear or unidirectional than I have space to describe, we are urged, at least at first, to set aside our own experience and enter more fully into our patients'. We work with ourselves to accept projections that feel intolerable, or to shift our own self states, or service the analytic field (Civitarese 2019)—to achieve a kind of empathic understanding where we figuratively try to slip into another's skin to see what they are seeing. If a patient is to feel seen, we learn that we must join with their point of view. However, not Lui. He eschews joining or identification or empathy as a means of working through an impasse caused by traumatic rupture. Instead, he beckons the French woman back to the point when she became frozen and lost time and memory. There, he joins her as a participant in her stalled narrative, a therapeutic possibility that I believe is worth our consideration.

A few words on empathy

Empathy invites a decentering from one's own experience, even when we recognize that the effort is inevitably filtered through the "sensibility and particularity of the therapist and a reality that is not simply 'internal' to the client but a function of the experience of therapist and client together as they interact" (Wachtel 2011, 4). Some consider the analyst's subjectivity merely unavoidable; others believe we must use ourselves in the treatment to achieve a deeper recognition. We are just beginning to write about how one's own psychic history affects the treatment (McGleughlin 2001, 2011, 2015a, 2020; Maroda 2022).

These evolving explorations of empathy highlight the importance of the analyst's unique subjectivity and otherness; they value not only points of conjunction but also points of collision. But in some instances, using standard analytic tools to negotiate experience between two separate subjectivities may be premature. For patients whose development have been thwarted, intersubjective relating may not a psychic possibility; instead, there may first be long periods in which experience is enacted, not reflected on. As discussed in Chapters 2 and 3, intersubjective relating is a developmental achievement, a hard-won capacity.

I've argued earlier that for patients with difficulty relating intersubjectively, empathic immersion in the other's point of view may be a necessary first step toward establishing a more separate, agentic self. Yet in this chapter, I'm exploring cases when *that* approach may fail, because it relies upon grasping what is in view—what we already know, not the breach that is beyond our knowing. Also, empathy can be predicated on the maintenance of the dualisms of self and other. It implies the confrontation of two separate and closed understandings.

Hiroshima mon amour gives us a way to imagine a clinical situation in which transformation becomes possible with neither empathic immersion, nor the negotiation of separate subjectivities. Ultimately, Elle has a transformational experience of being powerfully met through Lui's recognition *of the breach* and entry into it with her. His use of his otherness is crucial to her change.

By *otherness*, we usually mean our separate developed subjectivity, as discussed in both relational and self-psychological theories. Much clinical literature assumes or details the analyst's capacities as they negotiate therapeutic stalemates. What I'm talking about here is different: the place from which Lui reaches is a place inside himself that he had yet to experience, symbolize, and transform—implying by analogy the value in reaching from our own traumatic breach.

Caruth suggests that the Japanese man is denying not only what the woman has seen and remembered but, paradoxically, what she remembers *and* forgets. Recall that she is insistent that she knows her trauma—"Like you, I know what it is to forget. Like you, I have a memory." Lui's stance is a denial that Elle *can* know or even tell the difference between remembering and forgetting. The opposition of the man's "nothing" and woman's "everything" is not, then, simply about what Elle does or doesn't see with regard to Hiroshima (Caruth 1996), but rather about how trauma is conceptualized.

Traditionally, trauma has been thought of as either dissociated (in line with Janet) or repressed (in line with Freud), and therapy has been about achieving its conscious representation through a process of inference and interpretation. Elle thinks of her trauma as an event (remembered or forgotten), rather than the rupture of her sense of being, even her sense of being alive. When trauma's breach dominates, the trauma must be understood *dialogically*: it requires *an other* with whom the trauma can be reopened and reexperienced it in a new context. The French woman needs another person to re-constitute body, self, and time.

Originally conceptualized in Freud's sequence of repeating, remembering, and working through (Freud 1914), this formative psychoanalytic idea has been developed extensively through our elaboration of the concept of the repetition (Russell 1983). Historically, we have thought about transference and countertransference as opportunities for the repetition and subsequent representation of traumatic experience. In contemporary work, we might also talk about enactments—ongoing, bidirectional, affectively alive exchanges that allow what the patient has never experienced to come into being. Again, I am attending to a different aspect of what needs to be reopened when trauma makes itself known through breach. This requires conceptualizing both the patient and the analyst's places of opacity.

As clinicians, we are reminded that we, too, might not know when we're dreaming, or when we might see without our knowing it, or that what we see may itself constitute a form of not knowing (Caruth 1996). I am most familiar with such a muddying of sight when there is an amorphousness in the treatment's atmosphere, which I have come to think about as liminality. Something evokes/provokes a dream state that troubles "the conceptual and bodily threshold around the always elusive gesture of seeing" (Raymond 2010, 2). Liminality is a powerful *affective* experience, albeit on a border, neither here nor there, that confuses seeing.

But this troubled sight may be a very good thing indeed. As was true for the French woman, thinking we *know* the trauma may blind us to our own not seeing. My *knowing* through my identification with Martin with an (a) (Chapter 5) covered over the trauma that we each could not discern, something about our own liminality. In listening with the familiar language of trauma, I failed to recognize its strangeness and substituted my "knowledge" for what was beyond my understanding. Instead, I needed to be listening through what LaCapra calls unsettled knowledge (LaCapra 2001). Trauma is alive, shifting and circulating.

Liminality

One of the genius aspects of the film is that while we see in flashback the moment when the French woman's trauma occurred, what we come to feel most strongly is *the break in her going on being, not the event that induced the rupture.* When the woman finds her German lover during the war, she tells us he is wounded but not dead, and she covers his body with her own: She does not know the moment when he dies and can't even tell the difference between his dead body and hers. Caruth analyzes:

> Between the when of seeing his dying and the when of his actual death, there is an unbridgeable abyss, an inherent gap of knowing, the moment of the other's death. This missing of the when . . . is also experienced as a confusion of the body. For in missing the moment of his death, the woman is also unable to recognize the continuation of her life. "I couldn't feel the slightest difference between this dead body and mine," she tells her Japanese lover. "All I could find between this body and mine were obvious similarities." Then she plaintively asks him, "Do you understand?"
>
> (Caruth 1996, 38)

On some level Elle still does not "know" whether she is dead or alive (Caruth 1996), even after being freed from the cellar where she went "mad." Elle's inability to take in her lover's death has created a disembodied sense of herself, which persists in her dislocation from her body's sensations. In remaining liminal, in refusing her living body, she remains faithful to her dead lover but suspended in the moment of his dying. Elle cannot know her lover's death without losing him again, but by not knowing his death, she also can't know that she is alive. André Green's description of the "dead mother syndrome" (Green 1972) also includes this element of liminality: the individual internally preserves the tie to the lost or absent object at the cost of fully living.

What the Japanese man can teach us

In describing cases where what is repeated *is the breach itself*, an unknown and unknowable absence, I find that some of the most evocative clinical work comes from analysts who, in their own theory's language, suggest the analyst must "fall ill" at the corresponding level of the patient. Only then can the analyst join the liminal world of the person they're treating, a place where words might have little meaning (see Bion 1962; Civitarese 2008; Ferro 2009; Lombardi 2005; McGleughlin 2011, 2015a, 2020; Slavin 2011). Therapeutic action might then be conceived of as entering and undergoing a situation with a patient. My own thinking about what "falling ill" might look like often includes the analyst's allowing something to break open in herself that is enigmatic and disquieting—a step into her own breach. This is what the Japanese man, absent at the moment of his own loss, enacts. On reading Caruth, I have identified three things Lui does that give the French woman the capacity to know the difference between life and death and to reclaim her life—acts that I believe are clinically instructive.

The first: what we listen for

The Japanese man's ability to apprehend a message beyond the French woman's words is transformative. This is more than listening and translating the unconscious. Lui can sense, and we can viscerally feel—through the film's visual representations, musical score, and pacing—that the French woman is stuck in time. Despite her passion for Lui, some part of her has gone missing. In our clinical work, we may become sensitive to moments when our patients depart from their narrative or fail to inhabit it from the start. These are what I call negative enactments, (McGleughlin 2015a), where departure and absence bring us into an unknown realm. Sometimes we are enacting a state of liminality that, paradoxically, one can only know by leaving it—one cannot actually "live" there because liminality/absence does not reference something that has existed. (See Chapter 6.) But liminality is an idea about dwelling in a space between life and death. In this way, Elle's insistent "I saw everything" is not a claim to know everything about Hiroshima but an unconscious assertion to have faithfully remembered Nevers, her own story of catastrophe (Caruth 1996). In the Japanese man's *reorienting* the French woman to what happened there, he invites her into the site of her catastrophe.

The second: Lui becomes the other him

Lui asks a strange and wonderful question. He doesn't inquire about the death of Elle's lover as a fact she *could know*. Nor does he identify with her based on the recognition that they've each experienced loss or trauma. Instead, he assumes the position of her German lover and speaks *for* him. Lui speaks from the site of Elle's traumatic confusion, and from the time when she cannot *know* if her lover is dead or alive. He asks, "When you are in the cellar, am I dead?"

The effect Lui's question has on Elle suggests that what she needs to tell her story is not what she already knows of her trauma. Rather, it implies that she has not been able to mourn her lover because of a confusion over their bodies and her inability to perceive or absorb his death. When Elle affectively reenters the experience of her lover's dying, during which she couldn't tell who was dead or who was alive, she becomes able to tell her story. To know her German lover is dead, Caruth argues that the woman must address this story to *him*—now in the person of Lui. Moreover, it is only from the perspective of this death, taken on by the man who listens, that her story can be heard (Caruth 1996).

One idea we might have as clinicians is that by directing the French woman to comment on the "who" she was when her lover died, the Japanese man invites her to place a frame around her representation of that self-experience (or unrepresented experience), to allow other parts of herself to recognize that self. The *self in Nevers* becomes an object of study like any work of art. As Ogden says, "The individual (as object) is invisible to the self (as subject) until metaphors for 'I' (or in this case not I!) are used to describe/create 'me' so that 'I' can see myself" (Ogden 1997, 726). This might also be what Bromberg (2002) calls a process that requires a view of another mind experiencing one's own mind experiencing *the other*.

But this intervention does even more. By *refusing to understand*, the Japanese man creates the possibility of their connection because it frees him to become a new other: her German lover. The Japanese man's incredible question breaks down the rigid barriers and distinctions between self/other and inside/outside. (This is something that Caruth does not explicitly take up, but that field theorists achieve in their play with characters in the field, and that I'll address further in Chapter 9.) In this sense, the film suggests that when the *fallacy* of "self" and "other" is exposed, when we see that these do not exist *as absolutes* in opposing tension, we may move towards transcending this illusory dualism—and expand the ways we think about empathy.

Finally, I want to emphasize that it is not only the Japanese man's entrance as a real other that allows the French woman to establish her history and resume her life, but also as a real other *who genuinely does not know*. What is remarkable in the film, as Caruth observes, is that the Japanese man can join in the French woman's story *only because he can and perhaps, in some way, must* ask her the question of his *own* survival: "When you are in the cellar, am I dead?" Having fought on different soil, he too was absent; he doesn't know his history and questions his own continuing life.

This is not a technique. When, as described in Chapter 5, I enter from my own missing story (which, like the Japanese man, I never articulate), my patient and I can together enter a new one. The stance of the analyst might include permission to imagine that we, too, bring our own blank spots to work with patients, and that this bringing may be meaningful to them. As a field, we have not yet developed fully the need of the analyst to operate from this form of negative capacity.

The third: interrupting liminality

The third way the Japanese man helps to restore the woman's history and memory is to emphatically refuse her point of view. When Elle cries out for Lui to understand that she didn't know the difference between life and death, he slaps her.

The physicality and shock of the act seems to bring her back to her *living* body. The slap is experienced as violent but, simultaneously, an interruption of Elle's traumatized liminal state. Her not knowing the difference between life and death appeared to protect her from something even more horrible—losing her dead lover and the implicit betrayal of him. With the break in her closed self-referential narrative, Elle reenters life, and she and Lui come together within the breach that Caruth calls the very heart of their link to each other.

In borrowing the metaphor of the slap from the film, I am not suggesting that therapists engage in violence. Perhaps the word "slap" is its own shock to the analyst/reader, producing an interruption that we can equate with therapeutic action. Where empathy might aim to *understand or name* a patient's walled-off state, the slap transforms it by reintroducing the present moment and the physical body. It dramatically directs us away from individual insight toward acknowledging what cannot be understood in isolation. The slap is a vivid moment of punctum. Perhaps Bion's comment to his readers that he "died on the Amiens-Roye Road on August 8, 1918" is another example of a slap. The slap is necessarily provocative, interfering with the way we comprehend inside/outside and life and death.

Interventions that surprise

Certainly, an intervention that surprises is not new to psychoanalysis, but the film's slap gives us a visual way to understand this kind of therapeutic action. Some readers may put the slap in the same category as what Symington (1983) calls "the analyst's act of freedom," which he describes as something that allows him to shift his analytic stance and usher in his patient's transformations. However, in his 1996 paper "The Patient Makes the Analyst," he takes pains to note that he is not talking about an outward move on his part—an acting out of feeling or an enactment—but rather an *internal* shift. In effect, he slaps himself. While that may seem like Lui's move, it could as much be the opposite. When working in the breach, even deep creative processing that allows an internal shift can be a *misunderstanding* if it strengthens our internal *certainty*.

In their book *Dramatic Dialogues* (2018), Atlas and Aron discuss what might be interpreted as Mitchell's (1988) version of the slap: "clinical outbursts." These outbursts, even if unplanned, break through an impasse to arrest or change something where interpretation has fallen short. Interruptions of this kind are unique, highly context-dependent, and cannot be reproduced as technique. At the same time, they're not infrequent, and Mitchell claimed them as a meaningful form of therapeutic action. They have purpose, even though this may only be realized retrospectively.

Listening with Mitchell, we might theorize that in shattering a closed narrative or frozen state in this distinctive way (an act of freedom, a clinical outburst: that is, my translation of "slap") we confront the other with both their absorption in their own internal world and our otherness. But this formulation, which implies the analyst's capacity to know, ignores the analyst's *own opacity to himself.*

Since I originally published a very short version of this Hiroshima paper (McGleughlin 2015b), there has been new writing on the problem of the analyst's sovereignty. In their book, Atlas and Aron share my critique about the problem of the analyst's sovereignty (McGleughlin 2020), even in the groundbreaking theory of Mitchell.

Mitchell was a key shaper of relational therapists' belief in the importance of entering into an experience with a patient, or "the scene of catastrophe" in the language of this paper (Caruth 1996). In Mitchell's metaphor, we dance our patients' dance with them, but Atlas and Aron point out how analytic thinking at the time limited the use of this idea. The analyst wouldn't just join the dance; he would also act as the "teacher-observer who could determine what dance steps should be taught next, what steps were missing, and how next to elaborate the dance" (Atlas and Aron 2018, 70). Mitchell would later develop a theory of mutual unconscious participation of patient and therapist, but in 1988 he was not yet articulating a less consciously directed form of analytic joining.

While Atlas and Aaron's ideas are congruent with my critique of Mitchell's early work, they retain a sense of the importance of the analyst's intuitive knowing that I believe differs from my emphasis here on valuing a radical uncertainty. They tell us that Mitchell's outbursts were not tantrums or retaliations, that he "was simply adding new steps to the dance [by] his bursting out of himself" (Atlas and Aron 2018, 74–75). This casts the analyst's stance as thoughtful and intentional, not impulsive and sloppy, likely a preemptive response to the accusation that relational theory tends to idealize frame breaking (Greenberg 2001). But in doing so, the two authors underscore that Mitchell's "expertise as a therapist lay in his unconscious procedural knowledge of how to sense where a patient is going" (p. 75).[3] Atlas and Aaron write, "Good dancers are not consciously thinking about their steps but they are listening to the music and feeling, anticipating, and reacting to their partner's movements" (p. 75). Acting on implicit understanding is still a way of applying existing understanding. By positioning Mitchell's actions as knowledge-based and goal-oriented, even as they are intuitive and unthought, Atlas and Aaron differ from my argument: they reassert Mitchell's sovereignty and shy away from the implications of really not knowing.

I've tried to avoid likening the Japanese man to a receptive container, metabolizer, mirror, explorer, or interpreter of the patient's psychic content. Yet the slap, as I've depicted it, is like Mitchell's outburst. It *does* have a goal that is driven by conscious intention: to interrupt another's frozen narrative.

Still, the Japanese man does not meet the French woman's pain by hoping for something for her. He can only ask the question because, as already noted, it is a genuine one for him. He has allowed himself to call up his own gaps and ghosts, *not to identify with her, or distinguish himself, or to lead her somewhere but to join her*—each lost, alone, and liminal (not sovereign, or filled with capacity). What the film plays with, and what I believe is meaningful for clinical work, is *the analyst's* true opacity to himself. What the Japanese man cannot know, the way his own traumas have made him liminal, or blank, are at the core of his intervention. Clinically, one cannot intentionally create such a moment; one can only be open to its emergence. Similarly, for happenings that are as yet unthinkable, phenomenological experiencing together can allow *being* to coalesce, when knowing or narrating or grasping towards it prevents it.

It is now common to talk about undergoing a situation with our patients, as in living and working through intense enactments in which we are assigned a role via projective identification or becoming a character in the field (Ferro 2009). When we are invited to find a place of "hallucinosis" (Civitarese 2015) corresponding to our patients', or when we consider how the treatment might need "to infect us" to become useful, we are squarely in the realm of technique. In the vernacular of more classical analysis, we might imagine that the Japanese man/analyst is "working in the transference." Transference theory suggests that while we do not consciously invite our patients to cast us in a role, they inevitably will, and that when this occurs, we receive our patients' projections and then, ideally, metabolize them *with our higher-order functioning to interpret*. We might achieve a therapeutic shift by finding inside ourselves the truth of the patient's experience of us. Or we might enact new characters in the field (See Chapters 14, 15.) Or we might provide the recognition described in Winnicott and Benjamin's work, in which we use our separate subjectivity to offer a strong yet pliable other that permits the patient to experience her own self and reality. Even from those clinicians and theoreticians who most value the unconscious, interpenetrating mix-up of patient and analyst, the analyst is still the reader of the field.

But the kind of live participation in the film that was so moving and instructive to me was less these methods of addressing the other's experience, as if it was separate from us, than it was *a living through of the anguish of whatever liminal state or breach of subjectivity emerged in each participant within the interaction*. Our patients need our capacities, but most theories or methods neglect what can be fruitful in the places we are blank.

In the film and in Caruth's analysis of it, neither Elle nor Lui is fully developed, nor are their experiences understood through past determinants or transferences. Instead, the two characters come into being within a shared transformational field, in which they uniquely create *each other*. In this way of conceptualizing subjectivity, deep personal interdependence challenges individual selfhood, as well as analytic authority and asymmetry. Knowledge is not individual but springs from both separation and at-one-ment (Bion 1970).

Moving away from conceptions of therapeutic method as "understanding" is very much in keeping with a shift to a more ontological way of working. Here, perhaps, we interrogate our ability, or even need, to direct the "healing." This perspective might require loosening our idea of asymmetry, not in terms of responsibility to our patients but in terms of not holding on so hard to our separateness from them, or to our greater capacities. The breach of the patient and the breach of the analyst are places of symmetry. We might need to think more about the *missing* elements of our being/history, which may need to be constituted with the patient for something to transform. I am not talking here of a bright or blind spot (Goldberger 1993) but of the analyst's own place of implication.

Implication

In our viewing of *Hiroshima mon amour*, we are also invited to experience something of what Zadie Smith has called "the gift of implication" (2013) (Chapter 7). When art "works," or perhaps it is better to say, when art "works on us," there is a joining that takes place; we become implicated within the other's narrative. When the Japanese man sees the French woman, he is also her. When we see the film, we enter a version of what it means to live with (unseen) death. You may read at section's end, in an obituary I wrote for my stepfather, what it means for me to live with death that exists in liminal space, and how it centers my clinical experience.

The film does not have a happy end, if staying together would be that. As in analysis, there is no tying up of loose threads, no unambiguous change. Yet this does not discount the enormous movement in Lui and Elle, and the sense that something enigmatic and wonderful has transpired between the two. This ending gives us one possibility for what a more interconnected psychoanalysis might look like in terms of both frame and stance. The creation of an interpersonal context that challenges analytic authority suggests one more task for us: the willingness to live out loud with our blankness.

Cultural blindness and the limits of self-referential knowledge

We are inevitably limited in what we can see or know of another from our own experience. It is this facet of seeing that feels most important as I conclude this discussion of *Hiroshima* and anticipate exploring more of the complexities of race and racial trauma in the next essay. In closing, I want to draw attention to our failure to see, a failure in part emerging from our embeddedness in a psychosocial world replete with power imbalances and racism. In the film, as Caruth (1996) explains, the French woman believes Hiroshima marks the *end* of the war and the *beginning* of a new world peace, a view shaped by her own history and sociocultural location. Indeed, the bombing of Hiroshima can be understood as marking an end of World War II for the French, but the fact remains that it is only the *beginning* of ongoing suffering for the Japanese. Elle's perspective is founded in the erasure of continuing death, destruction, and trauma. Likewise, as Caruth notes, the international framing of this film as a story that becomes an *anonymous* narrative of *peace* registers in yet another key. It underlines the fact that it is possible to *not see* the actuality of catastrophe, seemingly in plain sight (Caruth 1996). These ideas become profoundly relevant for our understanding of an aspect of racial trauma in the United States in the following chapter.

Notes

1 This notion is well understood through the lens of *nachträglichkeit*, but what I'm seeking to highlight is the way it is brought about, that is, through a new way of seeing/sensing/experiencing the encounter that sets the process in motion.
2 Recall that Francesca Woodman's liminal photos do not record reality, and the story of my patient, Martin with an (a), cannot be told in facts (Chapter 5). In that treatment, feeling into the trauma required tolerating not knowing, non-integration, and, over time, accumulating pieces, and stringing them together until stories emerge like flip-books, creating pictures that we looked at and "saw" in new ways.
3 Procedural knowledge is a form of implicit knowledge and out-of-conscious awareness. Hence Mitchell would not have conscious intention, in this perspective. Nevertheless, this implies a form of automatic knowing, operating outside consciousness, but still a knowing based on personal experience.

Chapter 9

Interlude with life and death
Eulogy to my stepfather (2016)

My father was, in the beginning, the wicked stepfather. He wore a T-shirt, ghastly purple, lest anyone forget. It said, "Wicked Stepfather." He called me Chultz. I called him Spencer, a butler's name, shimmering right over the awkwardness of something formal or familiar. Besides, if he was going to take my mother from me, why shouldn't he serve me?

And he did. Three things stand out.

His most heartfelt gift to us, ever, were large print additions of *The New York Times* the day Nixon was impeached—laminated, well preserved, he wanted us to have them forever. The *Times*, his daily bible, had never used a bigger headline, and Lee had never felt such wicked pleasure. He relished politics. He hated crooks, bad guys, cheats, and stupid people, and he loved it when they got their comeuppance. He was high-minded in the best sense. Good. Humane. Decent. Brilliant. But didn't have to tell you. He had a moral compass. It guides me. We gave our son Max, Maxwell Lee, his name.

Then there's this.

He made my mother happy, not just, but very.

I was the youngest child, and I was home in the very beginning and home at the very end. I got to see real, ordinary, imperfect love.

We were not, any of the three of us, very graceful at the start. Everybody was jumpy, them with love, me with displacement.

But still the beginning was big, very big. Dee and Lee were giddy. Happy to have found this something comprised of words and food and body. And a deep daily rhythm. Dee settled, was pink-cheeked and mellow. Well, maybe mellow overstates. But she alighted. Was pleased. Very pleased.

Neither of them much liked to be told what to do or how to do it, but Lee bent Dee to the (very center) left, and Dee bent Lee to us, to family.

DOI: 10.4324/9781032670348-12

But first they were off. Big adventures, good life, beauty—and that was how they ended, too. To Pilar, Portugal, Paris, Provence and St Petersburg, Prague, Providence, Ptown, Paradise.

In truth, they didn't specialize in "P" places, but I feel Lee might like the alliteration. Or not. He used language artfully and inventively.

He was erudite. More than clever with words, he was precise, arch, mischievous, making words dance like he did the old ladies at the Alzheimer's day space where he would tap his cane and twinkle with newly remembered glee.

On his way downtown to said scene of regress (he was a snob, she married up, way up), Lee would translate the Latin on park benches and cruise his last flowers. His mother, Louise, had taught him the names. He loved lilacs. On our walks we wondered at the history each flower held. Water, weather, wind, breeding, good taste. He reveled in Central Park, next to school, next to home, the New York he liked best.

Louise also taught him Bridge. They were masters. "I'll listen," he would say echoing her own smarts. He kept his cards close to the chest and played them without hesitation, swiftly. There were no bad hands. He played what he had.

He knew where your cards were at all times, when to flush the queen, make good his four. I loved to play with him. A conversationalist, genuinely curious, he was generous to every learner I brought to the table. Sue said when she had had his trump when she was his partner, he made her feel like she had done something important rather than having been the beneficiary of the deal. Magnanimous, without quarrel or boast. A card shark without the shark. Vodka martini tinkling, later just wine. Pleasure.

Beyond Bridge, our go-to activities were the beach, Le Bernardin (I might be overstating our connection) and two laps of the reservoir, then later, one and last, just a trip to 92nd and Fifth.

Starting at about 50 (he died at 84) on every walk, and I mean every, he liked to complain about Dee's failure to get long-term health insurance. Long before he was sick, he was cursing my mother's stubborn refusal to believe in mortality. She held out till the end. Unwilling, she wrote. Unwilling.

And how could it be otherwise? It is very, very hard to watch someone whose world was mind, lose his. To have had something so vibrant with someone and be forced to live out your loss every day is a kind of shattering.

But Lee was right, she had a kind of refusal. The best kind. She believed in good living. He was her center, and she was very good to him, exasperated but tender, like we had never seen. He was happy at home with her; her cooking, watching, clearing paths, providing pussy cats. Not so very different for him except there were Peter and Norbi, beloved keepers as Dee liked to call them, but really magicians of gentle coaxing and firm command. He was still attending symphony rehearsals.

Actually, maybe the difference was when he was young and quite well, he didn't need the real symphony. You might find him still sitting in the car long after its arrival home, windows rolled up, absentmindedly conducting music in the air.

He was eating pâte caviar and chocolate ice cream right up until he couldn't swallow.

If you have to go, he did it in style. Well dressed (let's not talk about how long that might take) and twinkly until quiet stole him to her lair.

My brother said he had had his best Christmas in years watching us all. I showed him a painting I made for him, and in the first connected words he'd said in months, he looked up wondrously. "Is that me?"

Anne Michaels writes,

> The spirit in the body is like wine in a glass; when it spills, it seeps into air and earth and light. . . . It's a mistake to think it's the small things we control and not the large, it's the other way around! We can't stop the small accident, the tiny detail that conspires into fate: the extra moment you run back for something forgotten, a moment that saves you from an accident—or causes one. But we can assert the largest order, the large human values daily, (and Lee did that), the only order large enough to see.
>
> (Michaels 1997, Fugitive Pieces, p. 22)

Daily, yes. The everyday quotidian "roll up your sleeves and play your hand." Without diffidence or hesitation.

Dee taught and Lee benefited from our household mantra; living well is the best revenge. It is a kind of world order, never mind that life was lived on borrowed credit and the gigs long up.

Lee studied world orders. Especially fascism. He knew better than anyone that we are shaped as much by what doesn't happen as what does.

He had limits in what he could say—simple affection, words of love or apology; how much he loved his grandchildren Jesse, Max, Nicky, Octavia, Christian. He was a translator; Latin, Greek—of course. But also he moved from language to life. From books to love. Outside in. Private self, to reach.

And so here is the third thing—what in his own enigmatic way he translated for me.

Not the normal fatherly interest, or flattery, or paternal law (who could allow that?) but something else, a bit ephemeral.

My first father died when I was too young to know this death. The trauma was marked not by event but by breach—in my mind's experience of time self and the world. When you don't know the "when" of a death, or have a body to grieve, a certain liminality can crowd out life.

When you live with an absence, its presence is unseen and unmournable. It requires another to know its form, to come into being. It was because of Lee's solid presence in life that death could take shape, and what it means to have a father, and lose one, and find a father becomes meaningful, transformative.

It is silly to say, then, that Lee's death provided a body to mourn, a moment that death occurred. But indeed it did. There he was, his ox of a self, making mockery of those who hushed around a bed, would darken the room till at last he'd be dead. Dee wouldn't hear of that, and so she sat, we sat, she sat. More than one nurse mentioned Lee's good coloring—he looked better than anyone in the room—until he was ready and maybe we were ready too, free to mourn because here was a man, in life and death, that made that possible. That close-up, real-time end, that materiality, gives substance, shape to life, checks our omnipotence, establishes reality.

Like in life, here is Lee, this big beautiful man sure and steady—breathing, taking it as it came, on his timetable. No one could change or hurry Lee: not when we wanted but when he could. Like in life, here he was, providing this something none of us could quite name. Solid, stubborn, formidable background, charismatic, kind blurry foreground, in which we could come to know ourselves. Here he is. We will carry him forward.

Chapter 10

White empathy (2020)

In the previous chapter, "Psychoanalytic Technique as Understood through the Film *Hiroshima mon amour*," I began to think not just about empathy's potential for attunement but also how it may fail in a treatment, particularly in cases where extensive trauma impinges upon the formation of subjectivity. I offered that transformative work might happen when we *refuse* identification with the other's story and instead offer an interruption to the closed loop of self-narrative. In that case, the mark of attunement was the "analyst's" (the Japanese man's) negation of the other's understanding of a trauma that had become frozen in time. But what "worked" in the analytic pair in *Hiroshima mon amour* might not work in another. These are not techniques but ways we use ourselves, which we have often stumbled on unintentionally. Social context matters. And so does racism. Given the catastrophic trauma of racism in the United States and within psychoanalysis, a question arises: Can this reimagined therapeutic method hold up when white analysts treat patients of different races?

In the film, the Japanese man refuses identification with a French woman—but what if this were reversed? For a white Western analyst to *not* accept a story told by a person of color, much less *refuse identification*, may be mimetic of how white people have historically marginalized, shut out, and denied the experiences, voices, and humanity of people of other racial backgrounds.

This intervention could be redolent of the aggressive need of white people to disidentify with the Black other, something that Black psychoanalytic writers such as Michelle Stephens (2020) have traced using Frantz Fanon. Stephens (2020) quotes Fanon:

> One can have no further doubt that that the real Other for the white man is and will continue to be the Black man . . . the Other is perceived . . . absolutely as the not-self—that is, the unidentifiable, the unassimilable.
>
> (1986/1967, 161)

DOI: 10.4324/9781032670348-13

Given white people's need for people of color to hold shame, other-ness, and degradation, my clinical idea needs careful parsing. I want to make a clear distinction between a refusal to imagine a shared humanity across racial differences and a refusal to *use oneself* to identify with the other. The kind of disidentification I am suggesting is one in which white people identify not via their own referents, but rather by entering the story of a subject of another race as a participant—going into the person's experience, including their encounters with white people, potentially as oppressors.

In this chapter, I extend my examination of the limits of what I refer to as "identificatory empathy," but attend to how issues of power and vulnerabil-ity shape what is and is not possible in psychoanalytic writing and practice when working in white analyst/Black patient pairings.

Racism *is* specific, and it *is* structural. But a model that implies racism is only a trauma that can be seen, defined, named, and therefore eradicated (or compensated for)—what I call a "What-or-When" view of trauma—misses what is less symbolized. Racism is never *just* something definable. The his-torical and contemporary forces of negation that have shaped the lives of Black people in the US are also amorphous: determinant but sometimes residing in the absences and gaps, in the atmosphere, like the air we breathe (or can't breathe). In other words, racism, like other traumas, can also be a source of psychic breach—breach in time, linearity, memory, family story, archives—that creates states of absence and liminality. Here, too, empathy may prove futile because it relies upon grasping what is in view—*not* what is in the breach left by trauma, beyond our knowing. This is true for white peo-ple as well as Black, in different but crucial ways, where meanings of white-ness are dissociated or disavowed and can leave us in psychic breach. Work in the negative, where trauma can be known through the rupture in subjectiv-ity rather than events, requires something other than identificatory empathy.

I want to imagine modes of nonsovereign attunement that incorporate understandings I attributed to the Japanese protagonist in *Hiroshima* but that do not rely on the disruption of the patient's narrative. I explore a kind of live participation in which we phenomenologically live through some-thing together but which may be useful in the complex work across racially diverse dyads, with their inherent differences in power. The point is not nec-essarily to work through or understand better; it is to inhabit together but apart our different not knowing, grief, and blankness—the breach caused by trauma, including racism. It opens ourselves to the possibility of punctum, an experience of seeing and being seen prior to, or outside of language (Barthes 1980).

Caveat: Within psychoanalysis, we are finally recognizing what other disciplines have for decades: socially constructed racial categories are neither intrinsic nor immutable. Nor are they monolithic. Within racial categories, we each hold multiple shifting points of identification and difference that are fractal, often a mix-up of self and other configurations. So I approach identity groups as liminal constructs, a slide.

Even to talk about whiteness or Blackness without keeping the focus on how race is lived in different bodies, existing in different material realities and social locations, does not do justice to the concept of intersectionality, which I believe is an important theoretical lens for clinical work. How one comes to know and embody one's whiteness or Blackness is always already classed, gendered, and sexed. Each element of our intersectional identifications shapes the others. Approaching white and Black schematically (and as the only racial categories), as I do in this chapter, lacks nuance; but my interest here is in how anti-Black racism is a force in our psychoanalytic relationships.

I'm considering how particular ways of seeing and being for white clinicians may interfere with the establishment of empathy when working with Black patients; that is, if we understand *feeling with* as predicated on a kind of knowing by using oneself to understand the other. To better understand the sometimes-subtle perils of identificatory empathy—or what I call "white empathy"—I engage with the ideas of historian Saidiya Hartman and poet and playwright Claudia Rankine. I also consider examples from the art world about the danger of white representation of Black pain.

As far as clinical application, we need additional ways of knowing and perceiving than psychoanalytic theory routinely offers. Recognition theory, in contrast to empathy, holds out the potential for a two-way exchange, and thus could offer opportunities for a deeper sense of being with the other. Yet it may fall short if *only* the white analyst has the sanctioned authority to recognize the other and be recognized as someone who is more than her race. In appreciation of this risk, I offer additional frames to conceptualize connecting across difference, in part drawn from the work of feminist theorist of Black visual culture, Tina Campt, and in part from my own thinking on what I call the "generative force of the negative," (which I develop further in Chapter 15). These alternatives feel more hopeful than white empathy, and even its more complex cousin, recognition.

The paper closes with a discussion of a treatment I conducted in the 1980s with an 11-year-old Black boy I call Fred. There, I explore how I may have skirted some of the potential minefields created by my own white empathy, and possibly stumbled into a more transformational process.

Empathy's potentials and pitfalls

Empathy is, in many respects, essential to our work as clinicians. Fundamentally, it is a *joining with* in shared feeling. This idea—that we use ourselves to feel our way into something or someone unfamiliar—is ubiquitous. It might be the first way we learn to imagine the unknown. The realization that we're similar to another or share an identity or worldview can give way to intense feelings of connection. This, in turn, can circumvent notions of separate, enclosed selves, and the result can be generative and potentiating. At times, both inside and outside of the clinic, nothing is more powerful than someone entering our experience and seeing it as we do—a joyous "wow!" moment of feeling met. But building a bridge to another through our own experience may also usurp that of another.

Claudia Rankine (2015) writes compellingly about the impossibility of white people ever *really knowing* what it is to be Black in America, because of the gulf between white and Black experience:

> Though the white liberal imagination likes to feel temporarily bad about Black suffering, there really is no mode of empathy that can replicate the daily strain of knowing that as a Black person you can be killed for simply being Black: no hands in your pockets, no playing music, no sudden movements, no driving your car, no walking at night, no walking in the day, no turning onto this street, no entering this building, no standing your ground, no standing here, no standing there, no talking back, no playing with toy guns, no living while Black.

Rankine is questioning the possibility of white imagination, or of *feeling with* as a mode of understanding. In a similar vein, Saidiya Hartman, in her book *Scenes of Subjection (1997)*,

> points to how the experience of Black people may actually be disappeared when white people seek to understand them. White people cannot help but detail the African American experience of subjection through the telos of the white narrative that overwrites it. The result is that the

archive of Black subjection and suffering is fit to a white subjectivity and timeline. To wit, "we" (white America) have now come to a place in race relations where *we* have decided that *we* must reckon with *our* troubled racial history.

Hartman discusses letters that a white abolitionist wrote to his slave-holding brother urging him to free "his" slaves. To arouse his brother's empathy, the abolitionist recounts how he imagined himself and family in the place of the slave, narrating the humiliation, terror, and helplessness that he and his wife would feel in that circumstance. He then presses his brother to try the same thought experiment. While this must be an attempt to establish an ethical stance with regard to the other, Hartman (1997) wonders about "the repressive underside of an optics of morality that . . . must substitute the self for the other" (p. 20). How is it, Hartman asks, that the brother can't register the cruelty that befalls the enslaved person without using himself as the measure? Indeed, such is the insidious structural underpinning of white solipsism.

When I first read this, I was taken up short. In the therapeutic world, this intuitive move to use oneself to know the other is de rigueur. We feel our patient's pain through our own. How would an abolitionist possibly interest a slave holder—who, by definition, was unwilling to be affected by the experience of the slave—in any way *but* to call on him to put himself in the other's shoes?

But as Hartman describes, this form of empathy has a fundamental problem at its core: If the abolitionist brother must imagine himself in the condition of enslaved people, it reveals that he didn't believe they were human in the first place; he had to *elevate* them to that status (Hartman 1997). In fact, casting Black people as subhuman was a keyway that slavery was maintained; whites could believe that enslaved people did not feel the same pain or anguish that they did, never mind the same love or joy (Hartman 1997). As Du Bois (1935, 1968) wrote, Black people were not recognized *as citizens* under slavery except when they were punished according to white laws (1968). So while the abolitionist's empathy might be well-intentioned, it relies on substituting the white self, which Hartman argues annuls the experience of the enslaved person, whose body and voice are unseen, unheard, and displaced.[1]

Furthermore, white empathy is only given in recognition of Black pain, not to the whole Black person. That may extend humanity to Blacks,

Hartman writes, but paradoxically, it also effaces and restricts Black sentience *by making Black humanity contingent on that pain* (Hartman 1997):

> If the scene of beating readily lends itself to an identification with the enslaved, it does so at the risk of fixing and naturalizing this condition of pained embodiment and in defiance of [our] good intention, increases the difficulty of beholding Black suffering, since the endeavor to bring pain close exploits the spectacle of the body in pain and oddly confirms the spectral character of suffering and the inability to witness the captive's pain.
>
> (p. 20)

White focus on horrific acts of cruelty both obscures the constant quotidian insults to Black humanity and keeps Black resistance and joy unseen and uncelebrated (Hartman 1997). Hartman also unpacks white jouissance, the pleasure white witnesses are poised to take in the fetishization of Black pain. Is the "act of witnessing" always "entangled with the wielding of power?" she asks (p. 21). Can the "moral embrace of pain"—the kind the white abolitionist manifested—ever "extricate itself from pleasure born of subjection"? (p. 21)

Hartman's historical analysis isn't any less relevant today. As my colleague Eyal Rozmarin writes, "It took George Floyd's murder for his humanity to become legible to whites. But what is that legibility based on?" Black sentience becomes visible in death. Further, Rozmarin observes, "Floyd's death has endured the ritualistic performative aspect that unfolds with the full force of American show business media" (personal communication, 2020). But after that show has closed, how deep and sustained is our empathy?

White empathy in public view

Despite good intentions, recent attempts by white artists to step into the pain of Black people have been empathetic failures at best. Beyond the fact that, as Hartman would note, it is the rare white artist who creates public art about Black joy, the controversies I discuss below reflect an empathy that remains embedded in colonial relations. The recognition of the other relies on a white person projecting a white self into a Black body, *erasing* the experience of a real other and making the Black body fungible.

For example in March 2015, the white poet Kenneth Goldsmith delivered a conceptual piece about Michael Brown, the unarmed Black 18-year-old who'd been murdered seven months earlier by white police in Ferguson, Missouri. Brown's killing had sparked months of demonstrations during which police, often in full military gear, assaulted and arrested the protesters, further dehumanizing Black people. "Hands Up, Don't Shoot" became a rallying cry against police violence and helped galvanize the Black Lives Matter movement. Against this backdrop, Goldsmith presented "The Body of Michael Brown," reordering the teenager's autopsy report as a poem. Many considered Goldsmith's reading to be a spectacle in Hartman's sense, and they expressed their pain and anger on social media. Not only had Goldsmith exploited Black death for personal gain, critiques charged, but he has also failed to anticipate what it might mean to Black people to "have a thing" "made for a crowd" "out of a Black boy's dead body" (Kima Jones tweet)—to only see another white man holding the corpse of a Black child saying, "Look at what I made" (Flood 2015).

At the time, Claudia Rankine had not yet written her play *The white Card* (2019), but it offers an implicit commentary on what was pernicious in Goldsmith's work. Two of her characters are wealthy white art collectors, and their newest acquisition is a sculpture of the autopsy of Michael Brown. Turning the white gaze back on itself, the stage is configured so that the audience is forced to look not just at the performers but also at each other. Those of us who are white are thus made to see ourselves in the play's characters, to contemplate that *we are* the ones collecting Black pain for aesthetic enjoyment.

Shifting the usual power dynamics of who gets looked at and why, Rankine's work exemplifies what Tina Campt (2021) calls the "Black gaze": one that "refuses to reduce its subjects to objects or grant mastery or pleasure to a viewer at the expense of another" (pp. 38–39). Instead, Campt writes, a Black gaze "transforms viewers into witnesses and demands a confrontation" (p. 39). Discussing visual art in particular, she calls attention to images that "move us through our physical encounters with them and through our affective investments with which we imbue them," including the way they necessarily "implicate their viewers, their subjects and their makers" (p. 16). Among many meanings, I take Campt's words to be about work that requires our own vulnerability and accountability as makers and viewers.

The *way* we see and cannot see is enmeshed with both our subjectivity and history, something Goldsmith did not seem cognizant of. White people may be participating in a kind of erasure of the other's story when we stand outside it as observers and imagine we can tell it. From my perspective, the poet approached the murdered Michael Brown without his own vulnerability, or any obvious psychic investment that might have shifted the work.

Widespread objection also greeted the display of a painting called *Open Casket* by white artist Dana Schutz (2017). It portrayed Emmett Till, the Black 14-year-old from Chicago who was viciously brutalized and murdered in 1955 in Mississippi after a white woman falsely alleged that he had sexually assaulted her. (She recanted her accusation 62 years later.) Till's mother decided to have an open-casket funeral. She wanted all the world to see what racist murderers had done to her only son. Till's killing became a flash point for the Civil Rights Movement.

Schutz's painting of Till was hung in the Whitney Museum of American Art, a major institution where, historically, few Blacks have served as curators or even had their work shown. Her portrayal was experienced as making beautiful what was an abject horror—and set off large protests against the museum, which stood to profit from the spectacle of Black suffering (Artnet news, Muñoz-Alonso, March 21, 2017). Recalling Hartman's insights, when white people substitute ourselves as a means to understand those whose experience is vastly different from our own—whose brutal dehumanization is outside anything we've had to bear—we inevitably *mis*-understand. Using our subjectivity to inhabit (or project onto) the other turns what cannot be represented into a mimetic project: a production about who *we* are and what *we* know. If Schutz thought of herself as implicated (Campt 2021), the work might have been different.

Because both Brown and Till are sacred figures in the struggle for Black lives, the controversies over representation, appropriation, and cultural ownership set off by Schutz's and Goldsmith's pieces were particularly volatile. The two artists, based on their public explanations, thought they were exposing racism and honoring Black life. But not only did many Black people feel that their experience had been reduced or erased rather than revealed; once again, Black bodies were treated as *objects* to be consumed, named, owned, and profited from.

While the complications of a debate on "Who Owns Black Pain" (Smith 2017) are beyond the scope of this piece—these are not definitive thoughts on representation or cross-race storytelling—the reactions to the poem and painting underline my skepticism about telling clinical stories of our patients as if they are not really the stories of ourselves.

White people *cannot* imagine, as several authors have underscored. And yet as clinicians who may be working across the racial divide, we also must find our way to *being* with the other, raising fundamental questions about how we can use ourselves. Our stories and the clinical work we do require us to own both our vulnerability and implication.

Therapeutic work is different from historical analysis or cultural reproduction because we "live" with another person in an intimate relationship. Multiple interpsychic and intersubjective communications take place on conscious and unconscious planes, and we are positioned in a bidirectional field. In fact, a stronger empathy or recognition always relies on understandings achieved through a two-way exchange of affects, thoughts, and enactments, including transference/countertransference, that are shaped in relation. But how do empathy and recognition work if we rethink these theories through the lenses of power?

Empathy again

Freud understood that empathy is intricately involved with countertransference, as have most clinicians following him (Bolognini 2004). The analyst's affects provide access to empathy, but, as Bolognini notes, affects are highly complex and notoriously unpredictable. Whether negative or positive in valence, they may arouse identification in the analyst or, as easily, unconscious conflicts that undermine her ability to feel with the patient or to think about those feelings (2004). Dissociated whiteness might be one such conflict.

Layton (2020) suggests that empathy exists not just psychically inside a subject but entails a complex negotiation among subjects. However it is defined, empathy's shifting definitions are always an encounter with alterity. The extent of one's empathy, she writes, can be traced to "the adherent's level of comfort with the degree of fusion and/or separateness from the suffering other" (p. 178) and is thus social and political. In other words, Layton notes that empathy tends to be accorded to people who are most like us, meaning it is bracketed by "normative unconscious" demands for conformity (Layton 2020). We have been loath to acknowledge that empathy and relationality are influenced by our (often invisible) ideological commitments that shape our psychic lives—lessons we have learned looking at class, or sexuality and gender.

If we are white, as Sheehi (2020) points out, we are embedded within a system of whiteness—marked by language, rules, and behaviors—that may create an ideological orientation for colonizing relations, which manifests in what we see and feel. As a white person, I can and do operate within a discourse[2] but also from a "standpoint": "a concept intended to capture both *unanalyzed* structural advantage and social position in the material environment, as well as a conscious and critical apprehension of whiteness and its location in relation to the systems we inhabit" (Harstock, as seen in Frankenberg (1993), p 265). I am white (unconscious, unanalyzed), but also a white anti-racist person (conscious, intentional). Both positions are operative, which means I assume what I may, knowingly and unknowingly.

Recognition theory

Theories of empathy evolve. Psychoanalytical thinkers after Winnicott (1971a) have built on his idea that to be genuinely seen and known—and establish subjectivity—the infant needs space to feel her feelings and a separate other strong enough to recognize that experience as the child's own (Benjamin 2004). In therapy, these processes are thought to occur in the transitional space, where the analyst recognizes the desires the patient comes to feel. Recognition here remains unidirectional.

If we take recognition as potentiating but also think with Hartman (1997), white analysts are challenged to trouble a theory that relies on *our* recognition to make the experience of the Black patient knowable, understandable, or valid. The analyst's presumption of her own subjectivity and superior capacity to do the recognizing may be a kind of white ruse. If I, a white person in the dominant culture, have the license to define good and bad, right and wrong, even whether you are human, as Hartman helped us to see, my empathy for you may not encompass you, but more my imagination of you. This form of white empathy, imbued with the power of not only analytic authority but also what correct living means, consumes the very idea it proclaims. Instead, if we think of ourselves as "involved in another's harm by virtue of (our) participation in collective forms of agency that enable injury, exploitation, and domination but that frequently remain in the shadow" (Rothberg, McKay 2019,

1), we can appreciate the way race may warp an intersubjective process of recognition.

Building an argument that contrasts empathy and recognition, psycho-analyst Rachel McKay (2019) writes about the deeply intertwined nature of empathy necessary for psychic safety, as well as the process of a *two-way recognition*, which may capture the more intersubjective yearning to be known by a separate subject:

> We may have entered the interaction, or the therapeutic relationship, believing that what we needed was for the other person to understand our experience, but in the moment in which we suddenly are part of something more than we could have known to wish for, another person reaching from inside herself to grasp something of who we are, there is the potential for simultaneously knowing [ourself] and being known. . . . Each person feels both more oneself and no longer the same as we were.
>
> (p. 76)

Empathic recognition is worked toward *from a place of not knowing*. If white analysts were to speak from all we do not understand, including the dissociated and disavowed meanings of whiteness, and the places that racial trauma has left us in the breach,[3] our stance toward the other would have to change. Then we are not just containers or witnesses or interpreters or storytellers, but fellow sufferers undergoing an experience with another.[4] That way, we might participate in a genuine search with patients for our own missing histories and meanings, including the way we are involved in the oppression of the very patients we treat.[5] Within the system of white hegemony and in the analytic field and in ourselves, we are each psychi-cally vulnerable. But we are not equally vulnerable.

Campt offers a concept, which she names "hapticity," that strengthens my thinking about how to work across unequal playing fields. She defines "hapticity" as "an *effortful* practice of *exertion* and an *active* form of strug-gle . . . to remain in relation to, contact or connection with another" (italics added, p. 103). Where white empathy relies on identification with someone "less fortunate, less secure or utterly precarious," hapticity relies on *physi-cally* feeling and experiencing the discomfort across space and distance. Campt notes that hapticity is "not about sharing the pain or suffering of differently racialized subjects. It is recognizing the disparity between your position and theirs and *working* to address it."

To achieve this way of being with others, Campt leans upon our relationship to images and art, "requir(ing) we actively inhabit a [perceptual] state ranging from disorientation and unease to implication and vulnerability" (p. 18). This resonates with McKay's intersubjective empathy and with the clinical position I described in other essays, where I argue that the goal of therapeutic action is to build a connection through shared but separate (perceptual) experiences of "non-understanding," which require the analyst's vulnerability.

To adopt a position of "non-understanding" does not set us apart from our own racism, nor give us a pass. Our work is "the labor of feeling beyond the security of one's own situation" (p. 104) and continuing to go on. Rather than colonize, fetishize, or collapse the other's experience, when the analyst becomes a participant undergoing something with the patient, something new may happen.

Nevertheless, language like "feeling across difference" and "laboring" to arrive at meaning can suggest a relational negotiation or intersubjective exchange that bridges the self/other divide. As crucial as work on this level is, especially when we approach it with our nonsovereignty, I believe relationality and intersubjectivity incline toward maintaining separateness between patient and analyst.

A second challenge to a theory that relies on our agency to confer recognition proceeds from the premise that the self is not singular, not isolated from the psychic/social/relational world or intersubjective space. Then we can say that memory, meaning, and history exist *between* us. Knowledge is not held individually but is emergent within an intersubjective field inflected with social structure as well as psychic structure, and perhaps not lodged in language.

While recognition theory suggests "each person feels both *more* oneself and no longer the same as we were" (McKay p. 76), I think there are times, as you will see with my patient Fred, that together we become not more of ourselves but less; we are de-structured rather than pulled together. I am suggesting that this might be a good thing, and it is what I refer to as "the generative force of the negative." Here, transformation can occur through a deep interconnectedness that is best described not as the meeting of minds but more as something that arises in an embodied living through together.

Neither outside of power relations, nor occluded by an effort to understand the other, this potentially *transformational empathy* is a pocket between analyst and patient. Through the dissolution as opposed to bolstering of individual subjectivity, a *psychic* symmetry may emerge that yields another kind of "being with" or "feeling across." Such phenomenological experiencing, involving two people who each *do not know*, can allow *being* to constitute in a way that knowing, or narrating, tends to crush. This use of self may be particularly useful in cross-racial dyads where the catastrophe of slavery and its afterlife makes itself known. I am not sure, but that is my hope.

With Hartman's arguments about the *jouissance of the role of witness* and problems of white empathy in mind, I look back on clinical work I did in the 1980s with a Black 11-year-old patient I call Fred. At the time I was a newly minted 24-year-old social worker with little theoretical scaffolding to understand what I might be feeling in the swirl of the treatment. But in my backward glance, I see I might have happened upon a kind of work I can now both appreciate and imagine with real caution. My patient did not have words to negotiate his experience. Nor did I—my words now have the benefit of my acquired meanings and sensibilities (*nachträglichkeit*). Inadvertently, I learned without knowing it.

Fred

Fred, a Black 11-year-old boy, came to our busy city children's hospital clinic because his school had filed a series of reports with the state alleging that his grandmother's boyfriend might have sexually abused him. Someone had called the school anonymously and given a great deal of detail about the alleged abuse that they had reportedly witnessed. While most of the children in the outpatient psychiatry department where I worked were Black or brown, most of the referrals to our sexual abuse team were for white kids, an interesting phenomenon itself, as if children of color did not suffer sexual abuse. Or their maltreatment went unrecognized— a story white people didn't bother to see, or Black people refused to tell because they couldn't trust that it would be handled without racist presumptions.

Fred's evaluation yielded few answers. He was quiet. I imagined he was terrified. While our evaluation clinic was tasked with establishing a reasonable idea of whether a child had been abused or neglected, as clinicians we knew that the child's conscious story rarely reveals how they have been hurt. Instead we were trained to look at whether a child could play (Winnicott 1971b) and to distinguish spontaneous, flexible, and fun play from a rigid, repetitive, post-traumatic sort. Fred did not play at all during the assessment period. He had, after all, just been removed from his home. I never knew whether he felt any relief at being apart from his grandmother's boyfriend or just shock about what he'd lost, what was to come, and how he had no place to be. At home and away from home, he was (it seemed to me) in harm's way.

Fred's evaluation ended, but he surprisingly chose to stay on for therapy. While his social worker had brought him to the assessment sessions, he subsequently came alone. The clinic made some rudimentary attempts to pair kids of color with therapists of the same race, but there were only two Black clinicians, both without openings, so Fred stayed with me. Treatment meant that I could stop "looking in" on Fred in an effort to "know" what might have happened. Instead, I could simply learn to be with him.

My first psychoanalytic supervisor at the hospital taught me a lot. He told me that it didn't matter what I said, it mattered how I was—and how a child and I could be together. So that was on my mind, yet I couldn't tell exactly how Fred and I were together. Not knowing didn't mean we were nothing, though. We felt like something. Winnicott (1971b) suggests, "Psychotherapy takes place in the overlap of two areas of playing, the patient and the therapist" and "where playing is not possible, then the work done by the therapist is directed towards bringing the patient from a state of not being able to play into a state of being able to play" (p. 38). I wondered whether I'd ever manage to bring Fred to that state, but I kept hoping.

Over a period of some months, Fred agreed to play basketball with me. He would shoot. His movements were awkward, as if he were shooting in slow motion. It wasn't that he seemed too cool to try, but like there was no effort for him to make. He had no jump shot or proto-dunk, no fake or fast dribble, no speed. But, somehow, he almost always got the ball in. I was adequate neither as defender nor shooter. Fred would pass me the ball, and I would always miss. And he would pass it again. I was terrible, I mean really terrible. Fred didn't help me explicitly, but he watched closely. He wasn't playing against me or with me. Maybe it was akin to parallel play, but it seemed like more. We didn't take turns, but there was something about fairness in the air, almost like he could see I needed another chance, despite the fact that I would surely miss again. He might have picked up on my awkwardness or vulnerability or even felt sorry for me. This was a kind of reversal of usual play therapy, where the therapist might throw a game or give an extra turn but was in command. We hardly spoke, but in this way a certain uneven companionship developed, or so it felt to me. If I knew enough to raise something relevant about basketball players, he would make a spare comment or two. I tried to learn. I read the sports page so I could ask. We had some kind of rhythm going. And some kind of fun.

Soon, our building's configuration changed, and we couldn't play basketball anymore. Fred would sit across from me in my very small office with his hands on his knees, staring ahead. The play space was gone. He didn't want to do much after that but always wanted to come. Often Fred seemed to be listening to something in his head, maybe music, maybe voices, I didn't know, but most lines of inquiry went nowhere. Medicines were tried and discarded; meetings were had. I rolled up my sleeves with all the various teams and consultants, worked in all the ways I knew, but I felt an awful helplessness. The precarity of Fred's situation felt like a crime, and I feared I was part of it.

It seemed like Fred and I were enacting something (at least) about having had something and losing it, and the gaping void that follows. The quiet felt like our loss and all the others'. Sometimes Fred would offer something of his own, but more often he waited for me. Intuitively I knew to stop asking questions, though if I mused aloud, not expecting any reply, Fred would usually nod or smile in response to something I said. It might have been compliance, but it didn't feel like just that. Sometimes we laughed a lot. We might converse about a change in the office, the weather—hardly ever about school and never about home—but our action wasn't in words. The quiet felt connected, but I was also anxious that I wasn't "helping." I never felt Fred's silence as refusal, more as internal protection, like he was trying to survive inside his head. I did wonder, would he have wanted to say more if I were Black?

I was acutely affected by these hours with Fred. I cried from the beginning of every session until the end for the entire year. Whether playing basketball or sitting still or talking. Not sobbed or gulped, but tears continuously dripped from both eyes.

But that is not to say I was feeling *something*. I was awash *without* the feeling. The tears felt affectless, flat, unlinked, out of my control. There was something deeply unconscious or dissociated going on. Disavowed.

I couldn't make them stop. I was humiliated and worried about impinging.

Fred never commented on my crying. I wasn't sure he noticed. He hardly ever looked at my face, exactly. He was, I thought then, completely uninvolved with the spectacle of this almost-grown white lady's emoting. My tears might have paled in comparison to the kind of atrocities he'd known or endured from adults, but I feared what I was communicating to Fred and what he had to pretend not to see: that he made me too sad, that I was a lightweight in the face of suffering, that I couldn't bear the reality he had to bear.

A few times I tried to ask him if he could help me think about why I might be crying. It was a crazy question to ask him, I knew. I suggested a few ideas, but even I wasn't persuaded. In the years that followed, I kept trying to translate within myself the message of those enigmatic tears. It would have been easy to think my tears were the result of empathy: for the loss of his family; or the likely abuse or trauma he'd suffered; or his isolation and aloneness (which is always very painful for me)—all of which *did* disturb me, and make me very, very sad. But those explanations didn't fully explain my tears, given that I saw lots of gravely traumatized kids at the clinic. I didn't cry.

My own aunt had schizophrenia, and I wondered if what I imagined Fred heard made me feel especially close to his possible suffering. I thought that perhaps the stark sadness of my aunt's life, her loneliness, might explain the way Fred moved me, but this too was not wholly persuasive. I wasn't sure if Fred's being Black was involved. I saw mostly Black kids at the hospital, so why it would matter particularly here? But the mix-up of all that was Fred, and all that wasn't happening for him, stunned me.

The tears were on my mind as time passed because they were in some way the most access I had to Fred. I thought I might be unconsciously giving expression to Fred's experience, housing his sorrow, metabolizing something, but I didn't know what I could give back without knowing, naming, or pinning him down. Certainly, Fred's sadness was beaming into me and activating my own bottomless loss, absence, and terror—and the defenses against it. I didn't know what the interpenetrating mix-up was between us, or what kind of unconscious communication was ricocheting back and forth, but this is where we met.

The phrase that comes to me now is "crying machine," I was like a "crying machine." Or a whiteness machine. The almost mechanical falling of my tears might point to Fred's traumatic shock, or to my own mimetic defense against shock, or against my own horror and what that might mean for how I would fail Fred. I didn't know. I imagine that in that moment in his life, Fred felt like an object, moved along with almost no human involvement. It was as if he wasn't a person. He seemed to convey this understanding in his business-as-usual shrug whenever another insult or cruelty occurred. Fred might have felt his vast insignificance. I know I felt mine in my inability to help.

But back then, I didn't think about the tears quite as much as I am writing about them now. They were also strangely and achingly matter-of-fact, if you can imagine. Just like that, without explanation or meaning, there was Jade's crying. It was part of what was, like the big window in my office that couldn't be opened, or the huge, dirty stuffed bear where other kids sat but Fred didn't, or the untouched broken toy soldiers, or the way Fred was shuttled from foster home to foster home, usually without the Department of Social Services even having a conversation with him about why he was being moved, or where he was going. Or the tears were just mine, the pain of whiteness, not of a Black boy, or not reflecting his actual personal experiences at all.

One day Fred didn't show up, and I never saw him again. I thought he had been moved to another catchment area, but his grandmother might have taken him somewhere, out of his foster family, out of the reach of state power, maybe to protect him from that, or maybe not, maybe in search of something else. But he was gone. And nobody could find him, although all of us, including his school and the Department of Social Services, and probably the police, looked for him. I looked for a long time. I was crazy with worry and helplessness and fear, but that was it. I was at a dead end. I couldn't believe that he was gone.

Maybe 12 years after Fred had disappeared, about a week before I left the psychiatry department after 15 years, already nostalgic for what and who I would lose in leaving the hospital to become a psychoanalyst, the woman at the front desk called me. An adult was here to see me, but he didn't have an appointment, and he was nervous. Could I come? I came out just a few minutes later, but Fred was already gone. He left a crumpled paper on that front desk. It read,

"mrs. j. your crying was everything. Fred." And then on the next line, "me too."

Trying to make sense/abandoning sense

I have carried this story for 25 years. How can I give it to you without pathos, without aestheticizing it, without cheapening it to a story of the good white lady and the hard-to-reach Black boy? Without white savior complex when the actuality of Fred's life is completely unknown to me except in imagined worry? Who would even believe me? I hardly believe myself by now. But Fred had come back, briefly. I tried hard to find him again, but that was it, again.

Is there any way for me, as a white analyst, to present this work without potentially engaging in some form of racial voyeurism, of making Fred's pain spectacle? I am wondering now about how relieved and gratified I felt by the note. I was so happy. Happy he was alive and "better," and happy that the work we did made a difference. And that he could now cry, too. I couldn't believe it.

Embarrassed by my pain, and then my pleasure in Fred's note, I have never talked about Fred, except in a general way: to describe the systemic failure of Black children by what was then called the Department of Social Services, or how "helping" agencies have destroyed the integrity of the Black family over generations (Roberts 2022). As a mostly white hospital psychiatric department, we are implicated in this failure by our involvement with a (white) child welfare system that severed Fred from his Black communities—and then couldn't find him. What had I done to help across the long years that Fred had gone missing and was maybe in danger?

But now, my story of Fred and me seems appropriate as a means to engage the questions of this essay and book. We are always telling a story of ourselves when we tell a story of the other. When I tell this one, in the almost laconic rhythm of how we played basketball, I find myself immediately bound up with the problem of white empathy. While my tears remain enigmatic to me, I do know that my specific whiteness shapes what I feel and leads me to see and paint a particular portrait, to make the cut, consciously and unconsciously, in particular ways. And the work also had a kind of integrity that I can stand behind. Fred and I were deeply connected—and that mattered. Who was mrs. j?

If I consider that my own whiteness, pain, and absence shape my telling, I could be displacing some more Fred-oriented way to tell the story. I don't want to talk about Fred's internal world here or tell a story that would be diagnostic or mere conjecture, but I can say that his profound sorrow and the horrific nature and precarity of his situation—alone, moved around like a cog in a cruel machine, cut off from himself, family, and community—was beyond comprehension for each of us. I was living in bafflement, unlinked affects, somnolent states where language breaks down. I was, I imagine, living in some aspects of Fred's unlanguaged psychic state and, I'd later come to understand, my own.

Can I bring a Black gaze (Campt (2021) where I feel across difference from my vulnerability to see Fred as a subject "refusing to grant mastery or pleasure to a viewer at the expense of another" (pp. 38–39)? Can my writing about Fred "transform myself, much less viewers, into witnesses and demand a confrontation" (Campt, p. 39)? How to confront myself, make myself accountable, and also bring forth the very real intimacy Fred and I created?

While I do not think the form of aesthetics that Campt is advocating via the Black gaze is something only achievable by a Black artist, I nevertheless wonder how a Black clinician might tell the story of Fred. Not only might they tell a hundred other stories I might not even fathom, but they also would have had a whole other experience with Fred in treatment. He might have spoken more freely with someone whom he perceived as more like him, someone with whom he perhaps felt more readily at home. But I am not sure what home was for Fred.

An enormously brilliant novelist such as Toni Morrison would create for her reader an entirely different experience of Fred, not only because she is Black but also because of what she can do with language. Her searching, kaleidoscope approach takes us right up close to her characters' humanity without reduction or political correctness. Morrison never allows a single aesthetic or political value to define her characters.

Psychoanalytic writing has its own aesthetics, invisible but no less political for being so (Johnson 1998). The way we live and write our ideas can pin down subjects and keep us separate from them. For Morrison, humanity is cast not against external morality but unearthed as her characters' (and readers') experiences collide with multiple, shifting systems of psyche, knowledge, and power (Morris, personal communication). The reader grasps being human as something not easily synthesized, not any one thing or event, but as expressed through someone's mosaic of engagement with various worlds. This, in psychoanalyst Humphry Morris's words, is "acknowledgment that lies beyond empathy, what narrative complexity and fragmentation open up" (Morris, personal communication). There is something crucial about being able to think about, and express in writing, the complexity and fragmented experience that are the texture of our multiplicitous lives and treatments.

Given my other writings (2011, 2015a, 2020), I am of course wondering about the ways Fred and I were "separately together" during that long, hushed interlude. Perhaps what I sometimes refer to as a kind of "present absence"—how trauma's impact upon an individual hampers the formation of intersubjective relationality within the therapeutic dyad—was caused by Fred's specific experiences, and/or the trauma of racism. Or maybe my familiar frame of present-absence obscures that Fred's quiet was about his refusal to engage with another white person working in a system whose paternalism may have cost him his home. Or maybe he spoke sparingly because he felt "out of place," that he did "not have the right to a place?" (pp. 308–9), as white analyst Stephen Knoblauch (2020) observes in discussing his Black patient's experience. Or, drawing from Sheehi's (2020) commentary on Knoblauch's case, a Black patient's silence may be a refusal to submit to the invisibility of being seen through a white gaze. Citing Moten (2003), Sheehi underscores that the social construction of the "mark of invisibility" is a

> racial mark . . . a function of the ideological gaze, notably that practiced by Whiteness. To be invisible is to be seen, instantly and fascinatingly recognized as the unrecognizable, as the abject, as the absence of individual self-consciousness, as a transparent vessel of meanings.
>
> (p. 68)

We are missing Fred's voice.

I appreciate Sheehi's point. How can I not rethink the "present absence" construction I often write about when trauma has created breach, now through the lens of race? Race theory, and theory in general, function differently for subjects with and without firsthand experiential knowledge. When you have endured racism, theory may provide a way to narrate the raw experience of being rendered absent by a white gaze. But when experience of racial trauma is (consciously) absent or disavowed, theory can only operate as a structuring fantasy, with all the dangers of subsuming the *affective reality* this implies.

In talking about a "we" and what we experienced, I am inevitably fantasizing about Fred. But I am trying to express that being in my own present-absence with Fred, rather than identifying his, allowed me to reach to something unknown inside me and to be in that with Fred, perhaps a haptic notion? I like that possibility born of hindsight. I think we were in a region of interaffectivity, but I can't be sure. When Fred credited my crying as "everything," I felt hopeful we were. Exploring the tears—and more widely, our phenomenological *experiencing together*—might move us beyond the dichotomy I created earlier by pitting a more "Fred-oriented way of telling this story" against the way in which "my own pain and absence" informed my narration. It might challenge any easy read on self and other.

Making meaning, or failing to

Fred and I *did not make meaning* together at the time of treatment. We did not reach that singular space where emotion, imagination, and reflection combine to enable both patient and analyst to achieve a profound understanding of what is happening between them (Bolognini 2004). But something powerful occurred. My search to *know* (nominally about the abuse) and my failure to do so; our attempt at play and all that was between us then; the loss of that play and the long, still months that followed; and how we each held that space, separately, and together—all these beats had meaning. Fred and I *experienced something together*.

In play therapy, we take our lead from the child and play the roles they assign us. We may recognize something in the child or the play, mirror it, change a sequence, introduce another outcome, imagine something forward. These kinds of standard therapeutic methods suggest we are using ourselves, our emotions, imaginations, and minds to enter the scene of the play: to hold, contain, enact, and interpret the intersubjective field with the goal of metabolizing the other's trauma. As clinicians in this story, we have capacity. In fact with Fred, I did have some capacity. There is an argument to be made that I was simply employing the play therapy toolkit. But it was also my incapacity that allowed our intimate connection. Often the best child work is about experiencing/being together.

I don't mean just accompaniment, though I do believe that witnessing the story of another can lay the groundwork for affectively charged moments to become alive (Stern 2012). And increasingly psychoanalysts are theorizing the importance of witnessing, often when interpretation or mirroring fail in the face of catastrophic trauma.

But witness locates me as observer, charged with seeing what the patient can show. Even while witnessing can shift from looking *at* the other to looking *with*, *through*, and *alongside* (Campt 2021), it leaves us separate, as those who peer in. Yet I don't believe Fred or I thought of me as outside whatever the situation was, or as the only one able to see.

As much as witnessing, I was being witnessed in my helplessness: I too was under observation, with all the exposure of one who doesn't know. I think Fred felt this. My vulnerability, apparent from the first in my basketball playing, but certainly in my tears, was a kind of (unknowing) surrender to a shameful part of myself that arose in response to Fred's pain and my own. Being willing to be seen and impacted by Fred, and enduring our mutual helplessness, might have offered a different kind of recognition. We move toward one another in ways that matter but that we often can't see. I believe Fred and I shared experiences of unmetabolized traumas, never represented but experienced in real time.

Today I think the flatness of my tears were their own kind of shape. Fred, like Martin with an (a) in "Do We Lose or Find Ourselves in the Negative?" required me to listen not from what I knew about my own losses but from the place they have infected me and made me blank (McGleughlin 2015a). The tears were, and are, a kind of enigmatic message that I am translating and retranslating. We can't and don't make sense to ourselves, yet the message inside of us is a force that sustains our momentum.

Working in the breach

Like the Japanese analyst and the French women in *Hiroshima*, Fred and I were engaging from the site of the trauma, from some incomprehensible liminal place. Those were not constructs that I knew or felt at the time, but now I might say that our mutual blankness gave way to states that were marked less by images or pictures or thoughts and more by lived sensation and rhythm: unlinked states. Void. We were each in the breach; we were in the breach together. But how can I be sure there is a "we"? Ever?

So I am tempted by the idea that we shared a state of nonbeing (a necessary oxymoron)—its own kind of intersubjective entanglement that later gave rise to the creation of memory, meaning, and representation, in Fred. I think his note meant that.

One thing seems true: If there was mirroring, symmetry, it was to something nonrepresentational, not identifiable. It was not that we shared trauma that connected us, though Fred and I both had experienced catastrophic parental loss in childhood. Those losses are specific to each of us across distinct and vastly unequal lives, and maybe, too, psychic circumstances—on some level, we were unimaginable to the other. What might have been more symmetrical was how our respective traumas registered, not just as events but as ruptures in our psyches.

Something of the real might have been signaled by the constant outbreak of my tears that could not be narrated but was simply endured by us both. Or maybe my tears functioned like the slap in *Hiroshima*, interrupting our experience and commanding attention. They surprised over and over again, conjuring something startling that could not be described or understood. As I have tried to show elsewhere, there was something in my incapacity, my *unknowing* and not translating, that seemed to matter most.

It's hard to know how race figured exactly, but to come to another with our *vulnerability and our not knowing* is a form of empathy, respect, and connection. Analyst and patient being together, rather than in more asymmetrical positions, may open space shut down by racism's constraints, including binary frames: inside/outside, represented/unrepresented, self/other, or analyst/patient. The likelihood of usurping the other's voice or shaping their experience through our own could substantially diminish. And other possibilities may emerge, including our seeing how we are seen.

Still, whatever my ideas, beyond what one can learn in the liminal space of the negative, there is Fred's vivid trauma, the horrific state of affairs for him. I was not able to intervene in the material reality of his life. And I know whatever difference I might have made was one piece in a life filled with unimaginable obstacles and suffering—and, I hope, pleasures and joys.

And there is also something so extraordinary in Fred, that in the 12 years before he made his way back to my office, he was able to use me and our time together—the potential space we held—to make his way in the world. His decision to let me know that our work had an impact suggests gratitude but also a desire for a certain kind of pleasurable mutuality, signaling relational growth (McKay 2019). I have rarely been so moved by "me too."

I do notice how often I narrate cases in which a patient comes back, and I've had quite a few: other kids I treated who return to me as adults, Fred who brings the note, my patient whose treatment ends but still I "know" when her mother dies and I find her. I want to tell you about all the things that happen after the end, as if no one and nothing really dies. I am always waiting, willing the resurrection, the moving of the stone.

I dream about Fred sometimes—that he is the avant-garde musician Benjamin Clementine riffing, and so I paint Clementine and think of Fred. He shows up in other portraits too. Maybe it is the gift he gave me of that crumpled up note that keeps me so involved. Maybe my psychic involvement was a gift to him. Maybe it is the pull of impossible returns that become possible.

I think I'll "know" Fred again, somehow. I feel toward him now, whatever that is worth.

There is something about the way the world must end and come again (Du Bois 1920/2001).

Notes

1 Paul Gilroy's work, in *The Black Atlantic* (1993), notes the transformative role in upending the white story of the abolitionist movement when slaves communicate their own story through song and music. Music played a crucial role for slaves in surviving the conditions of slavery through "simultaneous self-creation and self-emancipation" (p. 69).

2 A discourse is "a historically constituted body of ideas providing conceptual frameworks for individuals, made material in the design and creation of institutions and shaping daily practices, interpersonal interactions, and social relations" (Frankenberg 1993, 265).

3 Here I distinguish dissociation as a process of separating off experience in another self-state outside current awareness, whereas breach interrupts the continuity of self-experience, personal history and time.

4 In aesthetic theory from which the concept of *Einfühlung* (Lanzoni 2018) hints at two-way process: The viewer alters the art and the art alters the viewer (I am altered by the art; the altered "me" alters the art I perceive, changing it as well).

5 I think here of Lauren Levine's (2022) careful work (in press) where she becomes emboldened to carefully track the meaning of her whiteness on her patients of color.

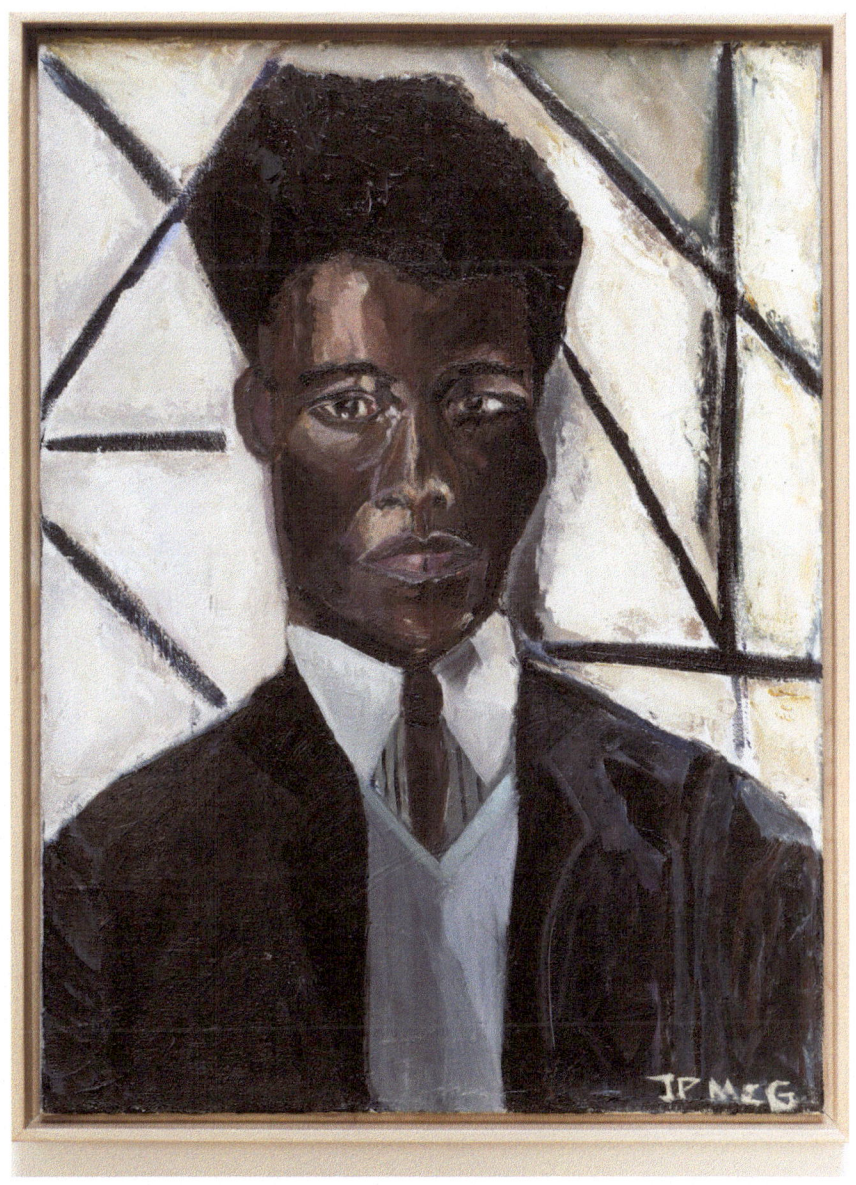

Figure 10.1 Benjamin Clementine. Oil on canvas. 24x18. McGleughlin

Part 3

The problem of telling the story of another

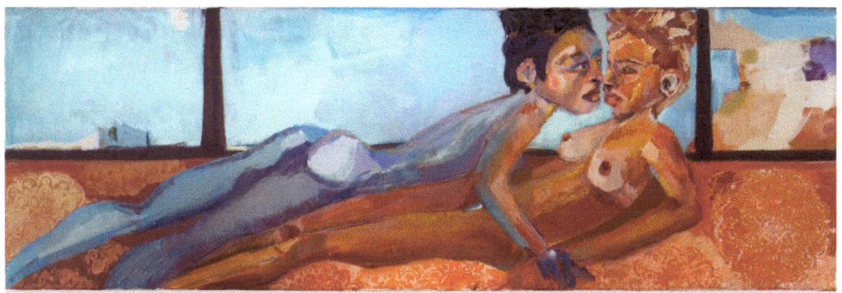

Figure PIII.1 Vital. Oil on canvas. 36x 12. McGleughlin

Introduction to part 3

The question of belief always enters clinical writing and perhaps never more urgently than when one's subject resists vision and may not be "really there" at all. Like . . . the distortions of forgetting which infect memories, and the blind spots laced through the visual field, a believable image is the product of a negotiation with the unverifiable real. As a representation of the real, the image is always partial, phantasmatic. In doubting the authenticity of the image, one questions as well the veracity of she who makes and describes it. To doubt the subject seized by the eye is to doubt the subjectivity of the seeing "I" (P. 1).

Clinician as (reliable/unreliable?) narrator

Rather than use my own cases as I did in Parts 1 and 2, here I examine the work of several authors to look at forms of storytelling that might usurp the other: when one narrator speaks for two; when old psychoanalytic

DOI: 10.4324/9781032670348-14

stories shape what we can see; and when normative psychoanalytic theory is imposed on subjects who live outside its bounds. I pay attention to which narrators appear credible and whether they actually are, and I include a story of my mother, where I try to upend psychoanalytic ways of looking.

As analysts and analytic writers, we always want to speak a truth about a patient's experience, but we necessarily fail. There are issues of consent, authorship, confidentiality, but there is more to it than that. No matter how closely we attempt to represent a patient's story, it bears an inscription of our own subjectivity and desire as a writer (de Lauretis 1999). It remains *our* story. To convey clinical material is to distort it. And yet can it be otherwise? Storytelling is our bread and butter, our way of thinking, containing, communicating, teaching, surviving. But we deal in narrative, not historical truth. We write and listen from our commitments and, in so doing, may go so far as to erase the other. For some patients, being represented in words flies in the face of inexpressible aspects of their subjectivity, and is even experienced as annihilation, as we will see in Elena Ferrante's Neapolitan Novels.

In less stark circumstances, these risks remain. Sometimes erasure occurs subtly, enactments at the sentence level. An example: a colleague uses diminutive adjectives to describe quite dramatic moments in a treatment. She is "a bit" concerned by the patient's writhing on the couch; the patient had "brief" convulsive episodes, which lasted up to 15 minutes. With these minimizations, I think my colleague was speaking out of her need to present quotidian work; she didn't want to tell the all-too-familiar, capital-E Enactment story. She was working her own discursive paradigm and performing her own theoretical commitments, enacting her own rejection of the drama that occurred. This is what I call a "refusal of story," one that will "always enact the story of its refusal" (Berlant and Edelman 2014, 3). Yet, paradoxically, downplaying the behavior of her patient actually *amplified* it. In each paper, we will look at whose story might be refused.

Because we tell clinical stories in language, we privilege aspects of subjectivity that can be captured in words often neglecting what we don't know and what is enigmatic, as when something unsymbolized emerges between patient and analyst in the gaps of representation. For me, the real import of my colleague's case was transmitted unconsciously in what was not on the page. While I suggested this to her, my comments could never capture the complexity of what *actually* occurred within the analytic couple. What I offered was refracted through my theories, ways of listening, and attachments. And our listening enacts its *own* performance. We hear what we know already, what we have ears to hear.

As clinicians, we wield language such that we legitimize some ways of being and unknowingly constrict, collapse, and even disappear others. How we narrate—how a story is told, who tells it, the language used, who is made visible and invisible—involves implicit theoretical and political decisions about what exists within or outside of a world, a world whose stories normalize some behaviors at the expense of others (Bruhm and Hurley 2004).

As example, we write old developmental theory as if there were not new or alternative narratives that could enrich it, or we insist on normative ways of viewing another, despite their own experience. This can make our stories inured to time, as static and unchanging as the ideas we draw on. We want to make our points, and we unfold narratives that confirm those points and promise progress toward meaning.

To illustrate these dangers in clinical storytelling, and the harm it can do to the subjects we write about, I take up three texts and explore the potential commitments of the authors, and what, if we are close readers, we can see emerging in the gaps in narration. I want us to doubt the one who creates the image, who is nothing more than the artist at hand, who tells a tale unchecked by the other's story as *they* might tell it. As Phelan writes, when "exposing the blind spot within the theoretical frame itself (the singular narration of how we tell a clinical story for two), it may be possible to construct a way of knowing which does not take surveillance of the object, visible or otherwise, as its chief aim" (1994, 2). By refraining from telling a story about another as if they are separate from us, we can interrogate our own (possibly distorting) investments and perhaps discover new insights. In this section, following Phelan (1994), I try to expose the ways that in each text a "visible real is employed as a truth effect," and to ask what unarticulated discursive truth remains unquestioned.

Our first text (Chapter 11) is Elena Ferrante's Neapolitan Quartet, whose narrator, Lenù, tells the extraordinary epic tale of her "terrible and dazzling" friend Lila. While Ferrante's chronicling (through Lenù) of the women's experiences is riveting, the author also demonstrates how telling the story of another can inadvertently erase the other. In the "The Promise of Radical Relationality in Elena Ferrante's Novels" I ask what is told, who tells it, and from what place of truth? How can we psychoanalysts depict, as Ferrante does, the power of the unconscious force of the enigmatic message? If ruptures and gaps surface the unsymbolized, how might we intentionally create an experience of tears in the fabric of being, of the breach through which trauma is registered? One answer is suggested by the paintings of Marlene Dumas, a white South African artist whose work is centrally involved with issues of representation. Through her work, we see that it is you, the viewer, who is being surveyed and viewed. This turning of the tables is something we might apply in our clinical writing. Viewing art forces me to face myself.

In the Ferrante paper, I also look to fiction to move beyond traditional psychoanalytic models, namely Oedipal theory, and offer a glimpse of another kind of imaginary. In the books, the two girls'/women's relationship—primary, primal, erotically charged, and enigmatic—is the fulcrum for their development; it creates a kind of transitional space that holds the potential for growth and transformation. Rather than restrict subject formation to the family, or even a unitary mind, Ferrante stages a relational subject—no "I" without a "you." Subjectivity develops in and through relationality between the girls and in the break from stultifying family forms. We see desire and identity installed as we experience the way sexuality and mind are inextricably bound. New kinds of kinship networks engender other modes of being, feeling, and knowing—creating internal constructions that can also constitute "health."

The use of authentic and self-revealing voices to establish reliability can be misleading, as I highlight in discussing the Neapolitan novels and, in a subsequent essay, a paper by Alessandra Lemma titled "Trans-itory Identities: Some Psychoanalytic Reflections on Transgender Identities (2018)" (Lemma 2018). Writing about a patient called "Jane," Lemma does what we ask a narrator to do: she anchors her theory, locates her own social and identity position, and is transparent about her point of view. I argue, however, that she does these things not so much to reveal the limits of her own understanding but to assert her objectivity and credibility as a narrator. Like all of our psychoanalytic stories, Lemma's is imbued with her perspective, which, given her stature in the field, carries great sway. But for this reader, a gap emerged in the persistent disparity between the rhetoric of transgender acceptance and *the application of an unquestioned normative theory* that undermines transgender life.

In fact, the risks of storytelling for another is nowhere more apparent than when we measure our patients' experiences against regulatory norms superimposed on those who live outside of them. How we think about gender and sexuality and what we write about it can masquerade as truth, obscuring the ideology in any of our work. Here, too, if we think about the blind spot within the theoretical frame (Phelan 1994), disavowed allegiances to normativity suggest the unreliability of the tale we are being told. And if we ask, with Edelman, about what stories we are being led towards and from, I suggest that we are being led from queerness to the hope of heteronormativity. We may need to listen, not just to the words we are offered but to an untold story that exists in the absences, gaps, and ellipses of the story: I am alerted to the potential disappearance of Jane/Jake as subject illuminating the deeper scars of the traumatic failure to be seen and loved by the other.

When, as analysts, we repeatedly doubt that which doesn't fit with our own point of view, we impose a way of seeing the other that contradicts their own sense of self. For some patients, like Jane/Jake in Lemma's case, the act of representing oneself in words involves a struggle to be seen, even to prove the reality of one's experience. Lemma's persistent disbelief in Jane's experience is presented as if it were just "good old psychoanalytic thought."

The third paper, Chapter 13, "Thinking outside the Oedipus box," challenges our wish to hold on to concepts like the Oedipal even as we recognize that normative developmental theory of sex and gender fails us when it comes to producing a new imaginary. I critique psychoanalytic models of developmental for their insistence upon viewing subject formation and queer life through "stabilizing frameworks of coherence imposed on thought and lived experience" (Berlant and Edelman 2014, xxii). Instead, I posit that the kinds of special intimacies, loyalties, and capacities some narrate as possible only through the successful-enough navigation of Oedipal issues may happen in multiple ways.

But we need new metaphors and new conceptualizations to imagine them. Ferrante's novels offered one possibility, through the girls' relationship. In this paper I look at the sexual agency (some women) women were able to develop as part of the second-wave Women's Liberation Movement. I suggest that sexuality is not just a private phenomenon shaped exclusively within the family but also a social phenomenon developed in and through our engagement in community and within the public sphere. I argue that a collective movement could and should be considered an intersubjective space as powerful as the triadic space of Oedipal models.

Absent new developmental stories to draw from, and with clinicians regularly looking to traditional psychoanalytic theory to understand subject formation, I argue that we will continue to produce mimetic narratives that substitute ideology and/or metatheory for close observation of our patients, ourselves, and our realities.

In the last paper, "Translation: A Mother Story," I explore the possibility of breaking certain norms as they "exercise the power to craft us" (Butler 2015), through the intervention of countervailing ways of seeing and being. I use Halberstam's *Queer Art of Failure* (2011) as a way to play with a version of my mother's life that took her "failures" and reimagined them outside of a normative developmental story. In psychoanalytic terms, my mother was not Winnicott's "good enough mother," but, I argued, her failures in right living, her refusals and disruptions, created a wedge in which new forms of kinship could develop. This opened space for my queerness to grow. By "delinking the supposedly organic and *immutable forms* of family and inheritance" from the force of historical progress (Halberstam, p. 70), my mother escaped from "the reproduction of mothering" (Chodorow 1978), from the generational transmission of who she or I could be.

Halberstam's "urging [us] to think in terms of the negation of the subject rather than formation," "the disruption of lineage rather than its continuation," and "the undoing of self rather than its consolidation" (Halberstam, p. 126) liberates us from fixed ideas about generational inheritances. It also unsettles what otherwise become mimetic understandings of health in the name of universals. Thinking with Laplanche and Queer theory, I try to refigure our discussions of desire and health outside of a frame of identifications/failed identifications and Oedipal family drama, in order to imagine new ways to live and love.

Storytelling again

In my Ferrante and Lemma essays, I focus on the hazards of storytelling and the way it may impinge or erase the other. If my mother were to read my reimagining of her "failures" as the route to expanded possibilities for me, she might feel similarly ill-used. I intend to offer her tribute, love, even reparation, but my story (unchecked by the reality of her voice) will necessarily rankle, may even be felt as erasure. It's my portrait, my cut. Like our patients who are the primary "objects" of our gaze, my actual mother is both a vivid presence and haunting absence. When I write my mother as separate from me, as if *my gaze* does not make her an *object* for you to see, as if she is apart from the me who makes her, I do disservice. I think of the story as one of as much fiction as it is fact.

What would it mean to think and write without naming, pinning down? Without assuming our stories are "true?" Without relying on temporality to make meaning, without looking to the future to give value to the present? Without making a point? A self-conscious acknowledgment of performance upends our telling of the other's story as if it were theirs. By thinking of writing as something we are staging, rather than about a person we are surveying (often ourselves in disguised forms), we allow a different kind of play, a play of discontinuities, blank spots, and instability.

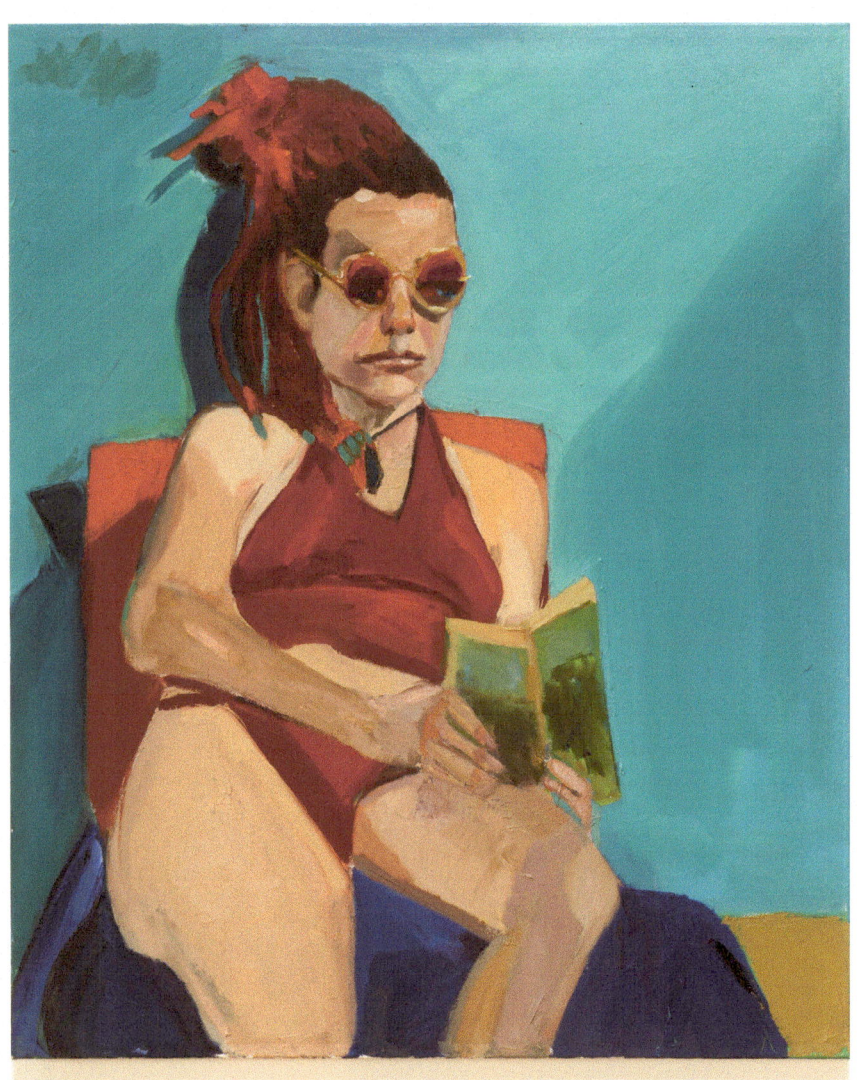

Figure PIII.2 The swimmer. Oil on canvas. 24x 20. McGleughlin

Chapter 11

The promise of radical relationality in Elena Ferrante's novels (2015)

Obsession is the sacrifice of light
to the richness of submergence.
But love is separation,
the membrane of the orange dividing itself,
the surface of silver
that turns glass into a mirror.

—Anne Michaels,
Modersohn-Becker 2001

One day in college, a keenly smart professor said, "If anybody wants to see an example of a perfect essay, see Ann's." Instantly I felt as if were the main character in John Sayles's movie *Lianna*, when suddenly all women light up as erotic possibilities. At the market, on the playground; old women, young women—each instantly becomes alive, libidinized in a way the character had never imagined. POW! at the old woman at the store! POP! at the girl on the swing. POW! POW! when my teacher recognized the mind of a quiet, awkward woman, who came alive for me, cathected, eroticized, given the mark of what it meant to be smart.

The power of this moment starts with my mother and the shame I carried about my mind—a shame she never knew she had about hers. This shame was intertwined with others we couldn't speak of in order to survive. I wanted to be the mind my mother wanted, which had everything to do with the phallus she didn't have. And I wanted a powerful other, who would be eroticized, to recognize it. Fundamentally, I could not find a home in my mother's mind. Like an irritant she tried to work out, sometimes explosively, my mother spit out my attempts to cozy up to her. This kind of hostility and homelessness sent me searching for protection in a containing

DOI: 10.4324/9781032670348-15

relationship. "To have a place within another's mind," Spezzano (2007) writes, "is to be protected from the threat of chaos" (p. 1566).

Ann saw me, she met my hunger to be seen and recognized by a powerful mind. It wasn't just that her big mind recognized mine, but that in allowing me to think with her, to use her mind to find my own, we became not life partners but lifelong collaborators in thought. Mind becomes accessible for me in dialogue whether internal or actual. Thinking and making meaning reflectively together are crucial to feeling secure in the world (Seligman 2007). So imagine my delight, kinship even, in discovering Ferrante's incisive description of one girl's embodied and fierce use of another to build a mind of her own.

This engagement between girls, where sexuality and mind are inextricably bound, offers psychoanalysts a rare chance to see a site of subject formation beyond the family. Lenù and Lila's relationship is a kind of transitional space that holds the potential for growth, transformation, and the development of subjectivity. It also interrupts our sense of a unitary self. If we are somewhere between believing that the self exists only between people (and knowing it is an illusion) and that it's housed in an individual psyche, here is vivid portrait of the way body and mind need two bodies, two minds, to be.

Sadly, however, this collaborative vision is undermined. Suspicion, envy, and alienation crowd out desire, connection, and expansiveness. While critics often cite the intense competition between the girls as central to their friendship, I believe a formative love story comes first. I want to show how the promise of radical relationality gets rerouted, dooming subjectivity and intersubjectivity, ultimately disappearing Lila. I suggest that because desire has no place, it becomes alienated, turning into envy.

First, let me comment on how Ferrante tells her story. The four Neapolitan novels rush breathlessly through five decades of Italian political and social transformation, from post-World War II to the late 1980s. The story of modernization is instantiated in the entwined lives of two characters. Lenù, the narrator, struggles against tradition and male authority to leave the old neighborhood, change social classes, and become a person with her own mind. Meanwhile, the ferociously creative Lila, Lenù's "terrible and dazzling" (p. 47) friend, is denied education and remains rooted in the neighborhood, where she is entrapped but still resists the weight of old-world traditional Italian culture.

The specificity and epic sweep of history grounds us in the real world. But Ferrante's rhythmic storytelling moves us into another time register—characteristic of clinical process—in which past, present, and future are collapsed, and we enter ever-deeper layers of memory and trauma. This kind of narration lends itself to identifications and fantasy. We experience Lenù's mind and inner life as if our patient's, or our own, and with the hyperfocus and actual pace people process emotional experience. Temporality is not forward-moving, or not only that. As with music, there are repetitions, elaborations, and even reversals.

Movement into psychic time carries its own enigmatic message. Lulled, even seduced, we believe Lenù's narration as historical truth because she is comprehensive, brutally self-revealing, and self-effacing as she traces the microscopic effects of her love, envy, and rage. Yet as Lenù's storytelling unfolds, we realize we have become accomplices in an act of erasure. We have listened to the story like an analytic hour and been taken in by the way Ferrante has kept us close to the sensorial with the force of her language, blinding us to Lila's disappearance as real subject.

"Vibrant and lethal like a dart," Lila emerges and fades like an image or apparition, not because we don't hear about her but because she exists in the gaps. What is unknowable and unrepresented is evoked in us rather than told. And she is "at once an externalized version of [Lenù's] 'I' and an ambiguous part of the 'I'" (Johnson 2014, xxii), a vivid presence and haunting absence.

At quartet's end, Ferrante claims resolution, peace, and subjectivity for Lenù, but I think the author unconsciously transmits a different truth: when the cost of having a self is the destruction of the other, only a defensive autonomy is achieved. With Lenù our only narrator, the refusal of Lila's story will always enact "the story of its refusal" (Berlant and Edelman 2014, 3). But I am getting ahead of myself.

To trace how the relationality that holds such potential ultimately falters, I look at Lila through three lenses: as signifier of an enigmatic message, as transitional object, and as love object denied. And I think about the problem of one narrator speaking for two.

The enigmatic message

I want to start with Lenù's relationship with her mother to put the girl's development in the context of her deprivations, as well as to illustrate how her longing for Lila is set in motion by what Laplanche (1987) calls the enigmatic message. The enigmatic message, which leaks from the care-taker's unconscious, is necessarily sexualized and installed in our bodies, felt but unknowable. As is the nature of enigmatic messages, we cannot recognize a "what" so much as a "where." Lenù's quest to bind herself to Lila—like mine toward Ann—has the power and punch of striving toward that message, which, because we cannot process it, becomes repressed and remains as the unconscious core of our subjectivity, disrupting psychological life, signifying something important but elusive and eroticized. This is one version of how subjectivity evolves from sexuality. Lenù is dogged by her need to translate the enigmatic message passed by her mother and signified in the enigma that is Lila. This drives the story. And it reorients us as psychoanalysts away from the oedipal as central to identity formation, and toward something else where sexuality is at the fore.

Early in the first book, we learn that Lenù cannot find home in her mother's body/mind, which is repulsive to her. Her mother, in turn, finds Lenù meaningless in her life. Neither was agreeable to the other. Instead, Lenù finds solace in school. Lenù relies on her teacher's recognition until she learns that Lila is actually the one most capable of pleasing her. Lenù's first-grader's pride in knowing her alphabet and reciting her letters is only ordinary striving or overachieving. In contrast, the skinny girl—who, "like a salted anchovy" (2012, p. 52), gives off an odor of wildness—is effortlessly brilliant. Lenù realizes she will never eclipse Lila, who becomes for her a force of nature: "Her quickness of mind was like a hiss, a dart, a lethal bite" (p. 48). To manage her envy, Lenù tells us, she makes peace with being second.

As my professor's recognition of Ann ignited a fierce erotic desire, so, too, with Lila and Lenù. As Lila becomes the mind that Lenù needs, Lenù devotes herself to studying so she is able to keep up with her. If she could stay with Lila, Lenù felt "my mother's limp, which had entered into my brain . . ., would stop threatening me" (p. 46). She decided to model herself on Lila and never let her out of her sight. To leave Lila, Lenù says, would be for Lila to have something of hers that she would never give back. Boundaries blur. Lenù's pleasure in Lila and need for her are inextricable.

In Lacanian terms, we might say Lenù's desire is for recognition. But it is also the desire for what we believe the other desires; it is the desire of the one from whom we want recognition—first the mother, then the teacher, then Lila. If desire is another word for lack, Lenù's hunger pivots on this lack, which cannot be satisfied (Lacan online). In this read, what Lenù is missing fuels fantasy and the effort to be the mind her mother doesn't have, and have it recognized by its signifier, Lila. Lila holds the promise of a better life. This, in Berlant's (2011) terms, is optimism.

Transitional object

There is a powerful iconic story that frames the beginning of the first volume. The girls are 6, in the midst of parallel play, when Lenù offers to let Lila hold her precious doll, Tina. It is her first gesture of friendship. Lila cruelly and unhesitatingly pushes Tina down a grate, essentially throwing her away. Lila's murderous impulse leaves Lenù powerless to assert her omnipotence over the capriciousness of parental care. The loss of Tina, who was "alive" for Lenù (2012, p. 57), feels like "an unbearable sorrow," "collapsing space" and causing "a malaise" that would last for years (p. 57).

Tina is what Winnicott (1969) calls a subjective object. The infant takes what she has found outside of herself and transforms it into a carrier of personal meaning, taking the first steps in demarcating a transitional space between herself and her mother (Modell 1970). As Barbara Johnson says, "No human can be formed, can become individuated, without establishing a space that is neither inside nor outside" (Johnson 2014, xix).

Lenù learns to hold back her despair, a skill, she says, that she sharpens over time. Eventually she would come to feel violent pain, but she senses that the pain of quarrelling would be even harder to bear. "I was as if strangled by two agonies, one already happening, the loss of my doll, and one possible, the loss of Lila" (p. 54). Later, when she is separated from Lila, Lenù will suffer a similar bodily sensation, a feeling of deflation and emptiness in the space between skin and bone. Our empathy for Lenù builds. And we are alerted to the powerful effect of the two girls as one.

First use of the other

Thinking with Winnicott (1969), when Lila tosses Lenù's transitional object away, she establishes herself in the doll's place. Lila becomes for her the transitional object, neither wholly inside or outside of her. This further sets the stage for the girls' deep, embodied, fated entwinement. From that moment, Lenù feels the magnetic draw and abandonment to the pleasure that is Lila, now both the carrier of the enigmatic message and transitional object for Lenù. She sees Lila as superior, extraordinary, transformative.

> I felt as if she had everything in her head ordered in such a way that the world around us would never be able to create disorder. . . . I remember a soft light that seemed to come not from the sky, but from the depths of the earth, even though on the surface, it was poor and ugly.
>
> (p. 76)

Walking hand and hand with her, Lenù feels "the pleasure of being free" (p. 76).

Love is an elixir. Reflected in the gleam of our lover's eyes, we see our most desired and desirable self. We and the world become more radiant. Love transforms both lovers; its magic soothes old wounds and produces new growth. But its loss threatens the core of the self. Lenù pursues Lila for all the healing bounty love brings—and to avert dangers its loss entails.

Loss comes when Lila, unable to pay for middle school, must drop out. Infuriated at the waste of Lila's mind, the teacher vents her anger at Lila, withdrawing her recognition. Lila's trauma is sealed when her father, enraged at his daughter's efforts to stay in school, throws Lila out a window, echoing the tossing of the doll. Lila denies the impact of this trauma until 22 years later, when she tells Lenù that it precipitated her first episode of "dissolving margins."

Without diluting the specific horror of the violence Lila endures, Ferrante brilliantly makes another point: one about the fate of girls for whom these are *ordinary* traumas, or what Berlant and Edelman (2014) calls "crises of accommodation" to the cultural and historical circumstances girls find themselves in. Routinely beaten by her brother and father, Lila must accommodate to her family. She gets sick, is sent to a stenography program, flunks out, and looks like a child who "had eaten poisonous berries" (p. 91). Lila looks vulnerable for the first time.

Blinded by her own loss of Lila, Lenù disavows Lila's. Her vision of seizing the world with Lila is diverted into a destructive route, jouissance: "The uneasiness of discovering Lila's vulnerability was transformed by secret pathways into a need of my own to be superior" (p. 92).

Lenù looks forward, not only to being at school without Lila where she might finally become the best student but to telling her as well. Yet, she is transfixed. Without the other girl beside her, Lenù's interests and ambitions flag. Things she did by herself failed to excite her. "[I]f her voice withdrew from things, the things got dirty, dusty" (p. 100). Although she excels academically, Lenù knows she is not really first. The girls are separated by "time-honored ways that barriers to desire, sanctions on women's aggression, and the structure of differential mobility and access to power under patriarchy play out in conscious and unconscious life" (Harris 1997, 213). Educational and class divides create a kind of "intimate estrangement" (Berlant and Edelman 2014) that haunts the girls, ultimately pushing them apart.

The books trace the rhythm of rupture and repair. When the girls fight, Lenù is bereft. When, after their first estrangement, they reconcile, Lenù begins to be able to think again. Even in Book Four, despite decades of searing rifts, when the two connect, Lenù still feels a charge, as something from Lila "that enthralled me, stimulating my brain as it always had, helping me reflect" (Ferrante 2015, 269).

After her ouster from school, Lila remains resourceful but withdraws to the neighborhood, where she marries and continues to assert a wild brilliance and influence. Unable to bear being separate from Lila, and her friend's flourishing without her, Lenù denigrates Lila. In one of the subtle erasures of Lila that continue through the books, Lenù ignores the psychological and material conditions of Lila's life and turns to the Lila of her fantasy: she persists in imagining their jointly writing novels, becoming rich and escaping the neighborhood together. Lenù still hopes for the transformation that Lila symbolizes, but she is insensible to her pain.

The same thing happens in an exceptional moment in which Lila has her own voice and reveals vulnerability. She tells Lenù, whose article she has edited and made a success, that she never again wants to read anything she has written. When Lenù hears this, she is consumed by fear that without Lila she'll lose access to her own mind. She does not notice the suffering implicit in her friend's words: Lila is no longer a part of what was once a shared world.

At another point, Lila writes Lenù a letter describing a terrifying incident in which she exploded a copper pot with her mind, suggesting a psychotic break. Instead of registering Lila's perilous psychological state, Lenù focuses on the magnificence of her prose and ability to give life to objects by depositing a sensation of threat in them.

> I thought again of that wonderful passage of the letter, of the cracked and crumbled copper . . . was an image that I used all the time, whenever I noticed a fracture in her or in me. I knew—perhaps I had hoped—that no form could ever contain Lila and that sooner or later, she would break everything again.
>
> (2012, p. 266)

Foreshadowed in Book One, Lenù's blindness to Lila's plight is driven home in Book Four. There, guided by shame and feelings of diminishment, Lenù continues to nurse her own fantasies at the expense of seeing that

Lila is in mortal danger. Lenù's inability to respond to Lila's suffering is heartbreaking.

A word on love

Some read the friendship between Lenù and Lila "not as boring lesbian plot" but as one of "entrustment"—an Italian concept "in which one woman . . . entrusts herself symbolically to another woman, who . . . becomes her guide, mentor, or point of reference" (Tortorici 2015). But I find this description devoid of jouissance. Lenù's attachment to Lila is too powerful, contested, and shot through with destructive and libidinous pleasures to fit this frame. I prefer to read as Johnson (1998) does in "Lesbian Spectacles: Reading Sula, Passing, Thelma and Louise and The Accused." She finds evidence of crypto-lesbian plots in relationships between women that are overvalued and underexplained—fascinating, ambivalent, and irresistible. I suggest that Lila's power over Lenù comes in part from the other girl's status as unruly signifier of the enigmatic message, imbuing their encounters with a frank eroticism. Listen.

The erotic gaze

From childhood, Lenù recounts, Lila "lighted up like a holy warrior. Her cheeks flushed, the sign of a flame released by every corner of her" (2012, p. 52). Lenù's sexuality revs up before Lila's, but Lenù still answers to her friend. Even when she feels "the magnetic force that my body exercised over men," she realizes the force of how Lila acts on her, "like a demanding ghost" (p. 96). Later, seeing Lila naked for the first time, Lenù is on fire. The particular pleasure of gazing on the 16-year-old's beauty led to a state of not being able to avert the gaze or remove the hand without turmoil,

> without expressing by that rejection the violent emotion that overwhelms you, so that it forces you to stay, to rest your gaze on the childish shoulders, on the breasts and stiffly cold nipples, on the narrow hips and the tense buttocks, on the Black sex, on the long legs, on the tender knees, on the curved ankles, on the elegant feet; and to act as if it's nothing, when instead everything is here . . . and your heart is agitated, your veins inflamed.
>
> (pp. 312–13)

What Johnson might consider clues for a (non-reductive) lesbian read are everywhere. Mind and body merge, and Lenù feels enhanced by Lila's recognition. Dancing together, with Lila in the man's place, is pure exuberance. She describes her desire through the neighborhood boys' eyes as "an energy that dazed them, like the swelling sound of beauty arriving" (p. 143). Lenù revels in Lila's body. Her fantasy of future togetherness is equally charged: "I pretended . . . I, I and Lila, we two with that capacity that together—only together—had to seize the mass of colors, sounds, things, and people, and express it and give it power" (p. 138).

The first time Lenù goes out of town, she fears losing the meaning in her own life if she cannot keep track of Lila. Their reunion after a summer apart is particularly sweet; Lenù is overwhelmed by Lila's affection, how close they now were, and the force of Lila's delicate beauty, comparing this to "the tremor of an earthquake" (p 133).

Lenù's attraction has no place to go as the inevitability of heterosexuality asserts itself. She is experiencing something in the realm of the libidinal that "involves the shock of discontinuity and the encounter with non-knowledge" (Berlant and Edelman 2014, 4). While the trauma of class is pivotal in alienating the girls from each other, the "repression of desire as a consequence of gender arrangements" (Harris 2000, 156) exacts a toll, too. Compulsory heterosexuality continues the intimate estrangement that class divides began (Berlant and Edelman, 2014).

Love turns

Lenù's childhood fear that losing Lila will alienate her from her own mind finds a new expression when Lila begins to bow to the conventions of family, class, and heterosexuality: Lenù decides to shed Lila as collaborator and coconspirator. "As if to chase away the feeling of revulsion" (2012, p. 132) that she would lose Lila to a man, she tells Lila that she is going to high school in order to make her jealous. "I wanted her to realize I was special . . . to feel she was losing something of me . . . I exaggerated" (p. 133).

Lenù's conflict about loving Lila is what in Berlant's terms (2014) we might call an encounter with "negativity," where "unbearable, often unknowable, psychic conflicts constitute the subject to the social forms of negation that also, but differently, produce subjectivity" (p. xxii). Lenù ends up becoming the subject she fears: jealous, petty, solipsistic. Where solidarity was, fear of loss produces aggression. What looks like boasting to stir envy also contains Lenù's wish to remain close and loved. As Lenù bests Lila to shield herself, she imagines Lila is trying to outdo her, yet Ferrante takes pains to show that Lenù misinterprets what are actually Lila's efforts to protect her. Harris (2000) warns, "Love forbidden and erased can still boil into its potent opposites" (p. 156).

Desire becomes murky, tainted, threaded with rivalry and projection, because all routes to erotic love are foreclosed. Envy is the unconscious solution to a longing for surrender (Ghent, as seen in Harris 1997). The unconscious trauma of repressing desire in deference to cultural expectations (Harris 2000) does damage.

What might have happened if Lenù and Lila could have loved each other freely? Following Harris' (2000) lead, I "inquire after the loves and longings spoiled but not given up" (p. 156). What is the fate of female homosexuality for women who identify as heterosexual? Harris asks. Where, she wonders, drawing on Butler (1990), do heterosexual women mourn same-sex desires? How, besides being thwarted, is a woman's homosexual desire sealed or organized (p. 156)? I do not suggest that Lenù and Lila were lesbians in some essentialist sense, but that prohibition can foreclose possibility, not just of sexual love but of reciprocity, collaboration, and intersubjective engagement.

Displaced heterosexuality

Ferrante's story does not offer a model of fulfilled female heterosexuality. Lila's sexuality is almost impossible to know. She is wholly independent, almost devoid of needing the other, springing from nowhere with a preternatural sense of people and their foibles. Her relationships with men appear to be instrumental, the next man solving the problem of the one before. Beautiful and charismatic, she takes no pleasure in her own sexual power. She is almost portrayed as asexual. While she shows an unusual agency and will, a strong inner conviction, she challenges any easy gender identity. She is set up as so much of a woman as to be not quite one. In another time, we might call her queer in the sense of someone who "resists political and social order and indulgently refuses all systemic complicity" (Bianco, online). Lila is an outlier.

Lenù's heterosexuality is instrumental, too. When she thinks of getting involved with a boy, it's the prestige she would acquire in Lila's eyes that has meaning. She pines for Nino, but when Lila starts dating him, she grieves more for losing Lila than Nino. Later, in the face of being replaced by Lila's fiancé, Stephano, Lenù despairs and feels her body as ugly, shabby. Her relationship with her own boyfriend, Antonio, seems to be about keeping up with Lila. When she has sex with the boyfriend, Lenù's first thought is: Does Lila do these things with Stephano?

Before Lila's wedding, Lenù doesn't know if she should "embrace her, weep with her, kiss her, pull her hair, laugh, pretend to sexual experience and instruct her in a learned voice, distancing her with words just at the moment of greatest closeness" (p. 313). Lenù feels she is washing Lila only for Stephano to sully her, and she imagines her entwined with her husband, "his violent flesh entered her with a sharp blow like a cork pushed by the palm into the neck of a wine bottle" (p. 313). Her remedy is to imagine Antonio doing the same thing to her at the same time.

By the fourth book, Lenù tells us that Nino, who'd become her romantic obsession, had never been able to fulfill the expectations of desire set up by Antonio—which we know is about her desire for Lila—"because it was an expectation without a definite object, it was the hope of pleasure, the hardest to fulfill" (2015, 251).

Envy denies sight

Perhaps because Lenù's fantasy of Lila's wedding night is a premonition of her friend's rape by her husband (in Book Two), it is hard to square Lenù's envy with the reality of Lila's life. By Book Four, Lila has lost her child and become physically and psychologically debilitated. Yet Lenù reveals her outlandish belief that Lila is writing and secreting away a great book that will outshine Lenù's—in fact, annihilate her—reducing her success to simply an effort to escape her low-class origins. Worse, she fears that Lila's memory will endure after death, and she, Lenù, will be forgotten, all her achievements for nothing. While at moments she knows that this is a fantasy, she obsessively perseverates on this idea. She feels better only when she further demeans Lila, noting she couldn't really write a book because she does not love herself enough to sign her name to one. Lenù projects all the destruction she cannot own. Unmoved by the changing circumstances of her own power and of Lila's decline, Lenù's identity as narrator of Lila's story is fixed in a fantasy inured to time. The jouissance Lenù experiences is lethal. Here is schadenfreude.

What goes awry? So much indeed became possible for Lenù because she tied herself to Lila, harnessing her brilliance to form a mind of her own, that it is still possible to sense Ferrante's radical vision. Transitional relating is a vital lifelong project bridging fantasy and materiality, an arena of meaning composed of both creating the object and finding it. Yet as the story progresses, a needling suspicion enters the reader's mind. Idealized or devalued, Lila has little articulated subjectivity of her own. Lenù cannot recognize Lila as a separate person whose actual existence could check Lenù's omnipotence. Ultimately, Lenù is not able to make the transition from what Winnicott calls *object relating* to *object use* (1969).

Unlike Lacan, who believed lack propels subjectivity by forcing the child to assert his or her own need, Winnicott (1969) thought that the child needs a recognizing other to see and know herself as subject. For Lenù, this other could be Lila. But for an object to become useable in this way—that is, as a separate entity outside the child's omnipotent control—the object has first to establish that separateness. The recognizing other has to survive an attempt to be destroyed without retaliating or withdrawing. If able to do this, the object is established as a real (not projected) other whose subjectivity is acknowledged. But if the other does not survive, the child suffers from an endless sense of ruinous power, as Lenù does first with her mother and then Lila.

Lila resists being seen and is unable or unwilling to contain Lenù's projections. As the story is narrated by Lenù, Lila does not push back with her own reality, much as she doesn't outright resist her family's cruelty. She does remain involved—and so does not withdraw in that way—but in the face of Lenù's inability to tolerate her subjectivity, Lila cannot assert her own. Nor can Lila counter Lenù's murder of her in fantasy. When Lila's powerlessness breaks through—for instance, when she has a psychotic break following the earthquake—Lenù's paranoia about her friend's intentions lessen, and potential for growth reemerges. But it is not enough. Lila remains only a bundle of projections for Lenù—and the possibility of intersubjectivity is foreclosed.

Incapable of encountering the separateness of Lila, Lenù has no room to mourn her loss. Butler asks, "Is the life that is mourned, the 'you,' finally separable from the 'I' at all" (Johnson, p. xxii)? Lenù, our narrator, lives in a state of "suspended animation":

> If conventional forms of apostrophe assume the distinctness between the "I" who utters the address and the "you" to whom the address is uttered, that distinction breaks down when the "you" turns out to be of one's own flesh and blood. It is not that the two figures effectively merge, but that "the you" is at once an externalized version of the "I" and an ambiguous part of the "I"—more an object of projection than subject in her own right.
>
> (Johnson, p. xxii)

Without recognizing Lila as real, Lenù cannot use her for self-reflection; ultimately, without being able to see herself, she is frozen in time, her own image suspect.

What we learn from the way Lenù tells her story

Why am I surprised when I realize that there is so much projection in Lenù's telling of Lila's story? Surely, we are all guilty of this when we tell our clinical stories. Peggy Phelan (1994) offers us a cautionary note about our writing that applies here:

> The question of belief always enters clinical writing, never more urgently than when one subject resists vision and may not really be there at all. Like distortions of forgetting which infect memories and the blind spots laced through the visual field, a believable image is the product of a negotiation with the unverifiable real. As a representation of the real, the image is always partially phantasmatic. In doubting the authenticity of the image, one questions the veracity of she who makes and describes it. To doubt the subject seized by the eye is to doubt the subjectivity of the seeing I.
>
> (p. 1)

Is this portrait of Lila a reliable one? As Lenù's delusional fear and self-referential view are increasingly exposed, we are left with ruptures. Doubt about the seeing "I"/eye begins to infect this Ferrante reader; the gaps create an opening that surfaces an idea of Lila as Lenù's creation, more mythical then real. Ferrante retains her vision of one mind being inextricably bound to the other, but now the darker side of merger reveals itself.

Who then is Lenù, whose vulnerability we have entered, whose ambitions we have felt, whose sorrows have been ours; who is the Lenù who now feels that she is the creator? Who saves Lila by writing the story that disappears her? While we begin to question the story as "truth," nothing makes her more believable and complex then her own struggle with the unreliability of her narrative. "Lila is not in these words. There is only what I have been able to put down. Unless by imagining what she would write and how, . . . I am no longer able to distinguish what's mine and what's hers" (2015, 469). Ferrante's genius is to both draw our attention to the problem of Lenù as narrator and retain her as an honest storyteller who grasps the double edge of writing.

Lenù herself is aware of this paradox:

> So either I tend to pass over my own affairs to recapture Lila and all the complications she brings with her or worse I let myself be carried away by the events of my life, only because it's easier to write them but I have to avoid this choice. I mustn't take the first path on which, if I set myself aside, I would end up finding fewer traces of Lila since the very nature of our relationship dictates that I can meet her only by passing through myself. But I shouldn't take the second either. That in fact, I speak my experience in increasingly greater detail is just what she would favor . . . . I'm scribble on scribble, completely unsuitable for one of your books; forget it Lenù. One doesn't tell the story of an erasure.
>
> (2015, 25)

As reflective as Lenù's comments are, including her admission of her need to travel through Lila to find herself, which Lila is she referencing? Her words seem to contain a sharp disavowal. She simultaneously acknowledges her wish to be free of Lila and repudiates the consequences of that wish. She assigns to Lila the words that *one shouldn't tell the story of an erasure*, as if Lila's desire to be erased is the only determining reality. Her own contribution to blotting out Lila is articulated but not understood. "Of course, I knew I was violating an unwritten agreement. . . . I also knew she wouldn't tolerate it" (2015, 463). Lenù even acknowledges her wish for envious revenge: "everything that came from her . . . had seemed to me . . . more meaningful, more promising, than what came from me" (p. 463). But, ultimately, she denies her own aggression.

We are hopeful when Lenù writes, "Only she can say if in fact she has managed to insert herself into this extremely long chain of words to modify my text, to purposely supply the missing links, . . . to say of me more than I want, more than I'm able to say" (2015, 2). But that hope dissipates when she admits that she had hoped for this intrusion "ever since I began to write our story" (2015, 2). Yet Lenù has already let us know that she is affronted and diminished by Lila's reflections back to her. For instance, earlier in the quartet, when Lenù publishes a book exposing people in the neighborhood, Ferrante foreshadows the disaster of her writing *Friendship*. Lila, breaking with her usual detachment, is furious about the damage Lenù has done to them to advance her career. Lila is critical again when Lenù writes about Naples and fictionalizes the stories of actual events and people. Lenù does not heed these warnings, and when the book meets with academic success, she believes that she has won and Lila has lost: "From childhood I had given her too much importance and now I felt as if unburdened. Finally, it was clear that what I was wasn't her and vice versa" (2015, 260). With *Friendship*, she uses the same self-serving analysis, despite her promise to Lila, following the bleak life and death of a mutual friend, that she would never write about her.

Lenù is persecuted by the Lila of her imagination as the real Lila disintegrates. She imagines herself as a kind of savior of Lila, that in writing about her she preserved her for history. Lenù writes, "I could make space for her in me and give her an enduring form" (p. 371). There is no mention here that the "enduring form" of the book comes at great cost to Lila. When Lenù says "I loved Lila. I wanted her to last. But wanted it to be me that made her last" (2015, 463), her grandiosity is laid bare. The real Lila disappears against this fantasy of reparation, and we hear Frankenstein. Lenù's difficulty bearing Lila's fragility continues a kind of nonseeing of her that ends their friendship.

Ferrante, who is narrating Lenù's solipsism and omnipotence, is aware of their dangers. Yet at the end of Book Four, Ferrante's point of view is hard to decipher: Does she truly believe it is possible that Lenù has freed herself from Lila's power? As Lila vanishes, Lenù claims autonomy and subjectivity, but Lenù's story is not a story of one "I" confronting another "I," or of Lenù mourning Lila and establishing herself. Lenù remains an "I" unmoved by the changing circumstances of her own power and Lila's decline. In fact,

I want to contest Lenù's sense that she is finally an "I," because I believe there is no "I" without a "you."

Art critic Richard Shiff (2008) writes about painter Marlene Dumas's work:

> One associates subjectivity with the capacity to use the pronoun 'I.' When Dumas spoke of her interest in two subjects confronting each other, she and DeKooning, she and a lover, she and a line, she may have associated the status of "subject" with the capacity to use the pronoun "I." This would be natural; if you have a serious encounter with a line, you may feel that the line says, 'I am aware and conscious.' It is an I you are an I. Because the association of the I with subjectivity is so natural, it is also, as Dumas might say, 'suspect' because of its allegiance to and preservation of its own image. . . . In contrast, the pronoun "me" is less suspect, because it is more susceptible to change, more responsive to contingencies. . . . The I, isolated and untouchable, creates a fixed self-image, like a photographic pose. It repeats itself becoming unreceptive to changing conditions insisting on acting in character. The Me is less like an image (dead), more like a mark (less dead). It has its own character but is forever affected by the marks surrounding it.
>
> (p. 171)

Lenù is the isolated, untouchable "I," less affected by contingencies, not a "me" who is subject to change in a real relationship with an other. When Ferrante implies that Lenù has been released from Lila's power to influence her, it's as if Lenù has lost track of the mark of Lila and sees a dead image, a frozen "I" in the other. Lenù's own riveting fear of losing love keeps her insecure, alienated, without a sturdy "I" of her own. As we've seen, the promise that Lenù's and Lila's relationship held for both of them to thrive is never fulfilled. Optimism does not hold (Berlant 2011).

What, then, are the meanings of Ferrante's story? In the language of Berlant and Edelman (2014), we could say Ferrante expands "the field of affective potentialities, . . . and infrastructures for how to live beyond survival toward flourishing" (p. 5). Both Lenù and Lila defy conventions of motherhood, sexuality, and womanhood, "survive the dominations of power," and transform "the experience of de-legitimating being" (p. 7). Yet if the women are trying to "detach from lives that don't work" and "from worlds that negate the subjects that produce them" (Berlant and Edelman 2014,

5), neither succeeds, because the cost of their survival is each other. We might imagine a "different world-building potential" if these girls could have emerged into a future in which the ways they relied on each other, sometimes as necessary kin, also allowed for the real use of the other in Winnicott's sense (1969). Instead, Lenù's story leads from the possibility of radical relationality to defensive autonomy as self-proclaimed success.

Relentlessly hopeful, I longed for this story to include the imaginary where two women claimed a life of meaning with each other and flourished in the subversive power of their connection. But Lila is an enigma, losing time and boundaries, shattering, and finally disappearing, not a subject in her own right. In Lenù's failure to recognize her as such, a great tragedy unfolds.

Psychoanalytic storytelling/disrupting the law of the gaze

"A story implies a direction," Edelman (2014) writes. "It signals as story a movement that leads to some payoff or profit, some comprehension or closure, however open-ended." "This leading toward," he continues, "necessarily entails a correlated leading from" (p. 3) What then does Ferrante want us to make of the story of Lila's life? Lenù would have us believe hers is a life of achievement cast against the failed life of Lila. But what would Lila's own story of hope and disappointment, attachment and rupture, accommodation and liberation be? If we believe with Edelman that the story Lenù writes that leads from Lila's "refusal of story" will "always enact the story of its refusal" (p. 3), a very different tale than the one we are told potentially emerges. In Lenù's story of Lila's downfall, set against her own bourgeois, middle-class life, an unarticulated discursive truth remains unquestioned. Doesn't Lila's life offer a critique of the stultifying conventions she has been subject to? Lila's disappearance tells more than one story.

Ferrante offers us, then, a cautionary tale about the dangers of storytelling when one purports to tell the story of another unfettered by the reality of the other's different story. Given these dangers, Edelman asks, "What are alternatives to narrative knowledge and knowledge as narrative?" (2014, 3).

While Ferrante conveys an implicit understanding of the risks of narrativizing another's story, she also demonstrates what it means to tell a story in which an untold version exists in the absences, gaps, and ellipses. This emerges in the disquiet of the reader, provoking uncertainty and the chance of another vision. Ferrante has sent her readers an enigmatic message. By engaging us in the register of psychic time, she invites us to notice our own enigmatic messages. Her work, so ordinary in its dailiness and microstories, seeks our deeper translation.

For some patients, like Lila, the act of representing the self in words is a denial, even a violation, of inexpressible aspects of their subjectivity (McGleughlin 2015a). What if we intentionally rather than inadvertently create for our readers, as Ferrante does, an experience of tears in the fabric of being through which trauma is registered? As Lenù's tale becomes progressively more unreliable, as she herself understands, we are alerted to the disappearance of Lila as subject. In the negative space, Lenù's copious confessions obscure the deeper scars of trauma, the failure to see the other.

In telling our clinical stories, we could more self-consciously turn our gaze back on ourselves and allow what is unsymbolized to emerge in the listener's experience, like the pow of the enigmatic message and allure of the enigmatic signifier. Forms of art and artistic forms of writing can privilege what we don't know. They can allow for emergent possibility.

Chapter 12

Transgender imagining and the danger of normative theory (2019)

Black scholar Sylvia Wynter (1995) writes,

> human beings are magical. Bios and Logos. Words made flesh, muscle and bone animated by hope and desire, belief materialized in deeds, deeds which crystallize our actualities. . . . And the maps of spring always have to be redrawn again, in undared forms.

(p. 35)

I am especially interested in using her poetically imagined "maps of spring" to inspire change in psychoanalysts' habits of storytelling. When we in the psychoanalytic mainstream measure the lives of our flesh-and-blood patients against a set of regulatory norms that reinforce the idea that there are better and worse ways to live, we risk annulling the poignant human experience of the people who come to us for help. This danger looms especially large when we're presented with "undared forms" in gender and sexuality, because *how* we think and write, often presented as truth, can impose a way of being on our patients while obscuring the ideology implicit in any of our work. Specifically, I want to think about how our psychoanalytic communities narrativize about transgender people, as well as work with them—and to underscore that this conversation *requires a deeper challenge to psychoanalytic theorizing about gender and sexuality.*

The last two decades have brought an increasing focus on gender—in popular culture, academia, and, of course, in psychoanalysis. Entire categories of gender are being transformed by people whose gender assigned at birth does not conform with who they feel themselves to be. Though gender was certainly already "soft assembly" (Harris 2008), and gender queers were at the forefront of gay liberation struggles before and

DOI: 10.4324/9781032670348-16

after Stonewall, the male/female binary had yet to be exploded. This new movement, lively and vigorous, seeks to free people from the idea that biology is destiny. Many no longer assume that gender is constituted by "woman" and "man," or that it's a destination rather than a shifting configuration of desire and identity (Halberstam 2018), multiply determined, mobile and fractal.

This evolution has sparked fierce anxiety and backlash. In the U.S., hundreds of bills have been proposed—and many have been enacted—that limit transgender people's rights. This includes laws that prohibit medical professionals from providing transition care for adolescents, in contravention of every major medical organization in the country. In tandem with this legislative assault, data show that acts of anti-LGBTQ+ violence have risen sharply, more than tripling between 2021 and 2022. Transgender people's very humanity is on the line.

As I update this paper from its 2019 original talk, the backlash is growing in psychoanalysis (Saketopoulou 2022a). Deeply conservative texts have been published, often in the guise of empathy or even as efforts to protect transgender people replicating our field's errors in the treatment of homosexuality. This is happening despite decades of movement-building that swept away the justifications for pathologizing and excluding LGBTQ+ people from full participation in the field—we came into psychoanalysis and made it our own. But while psychoanalysis has granted a kind of legitimacy to some of us queer analysts, others are still being written out—namely, transgender subjects. We do not want to be the good gay "in-crowd," cast against ever more marginalized groups. Yet psychoanalysis aligns us with the social hierarchy against which we rebel. To be outside the proper story of psychoanalysis is to be a mistake, a deviation.

The longing to belong and the problem of tolerance

The wish to belong is powerful. On entering analytic training in 2000, I routinely turned down opportunities to teach and speak on gender and sexuality. I wanted to be free to think about other things having thought about sexuality in all my other work. It wasn't shame about being out—I have loved and lived with my partner of nearly 40 years, have birthed and raised two children with her, and became the first openly lesbian president of a psychoanalytic institute. And even though I believe, and celebrate, that abjection within the social order often leads to the most potent transformations of it, and even though I wanted my institute to change, I did my political work as a queer activist elsewhere. I didn't want to begin training in my usual outsider position. I wanted to be a credible analyst, not a credible *lesbian* analyst. I wanted you to find home in my mind (Spezzano 2007) and mine in yours. That can require that I look like you. While I formed a rich intellectual community, my queer self was subtly but culturally not quite right.

Even so, acceptance for LGBTQ+ people is only one step toward fundamental change. Despite game-changing theory by queer and feminist analysts and people of color, palpable exclusion persists because institutional psychoanalysis has failed to challenge its old normative theories. For instance, developmental stories that make sense of the diversity of Black lives have been left out, even as we move to models of "diversity and inclusion." And biases in favor of cis-gendered white heterosexuality remain deeply embedded, as evidenced by the profession's current surveillance and critique of transgender and nonbinary individuals. The intractability of racism, heteronormativity, and gender normativity in psychoanalysis is like plaque—you scrape at it, it thins, but ultimately it comes back, distorting your mind.

Attachment to normative theory can be especially destructive when it implies that those who are different aren't capable of defining their own subjectivity or creating the lives they want. Such judgments violate fundamental psychoanalytic principles and curtail an understanding of the many ways human beings live, create families, build community, and even imagine. Yet psychoanalysis lags behind other mental health professions in recognizing the right of transgender people to define their identities. The American Psychological Association's guidelines, for one, view conversion or reparative therapy as unethical and urge members to provide trans-affirmative care.

While struggles to articulate a queer life are as relevant to those who live within gender and sex norms as without, critiques of universalizing thought often come from people who have been denied personhood by the social and political order, whose agency is unrecognized, delegitimated, and suppressed. We form identity groups to resist dominant power. But we can find ourselves in a double bind. When "feminist" or "queer" or "BIPOC" psychoanalysts organize to challenge a universal notion of what it means to be human, this very process can reify an old psychoanalytic narrative, because these categories are produced *in relation to* a perspective and history that still defines us as "other" (Wynter 2015).

Rather than seek inclusion in the psychoanalytic story (and the human story) as second-class citizens, we need to create new knowledge that unsettles and reimagines personhood (Wynter 2015). And transgender practitioners in the analytic world *are* writing their own stories (Hansbury 2017). They're making inroads by speaking and acting in opposition to the system of gender oppression. Theirs is not a teleological vision—moving from psychoanalytic origin story to emancipatory story (McKittrick 2015)—but rather the building of narratives that include those who've been excluded from the psychoanalytic norm. The imperative to tell new developmental stories, to lay those side by side with other stories, expands the notions of Bios and Logos (Wynter 2015).

Psychoanalysts need to understand people on their own terms, not as a lesser version of normative living. Otherwise, we usurp intrinsic freedom. It matters, now more than ever, that psychoanalysts not only accept transgender people as people like them, but also show that the field is willing to change, to draw on transgender experience to imagine new ways to live and love.

Lemma's paper

I will use Alessandra Lemma's paper "Trans-itory Identities: Some Psychoanalytic Reflections on Transgender Identities" (2018), published in the IJP, as an anchoring text to focus on the hazards of psychoanalytic storytelling about transgender subjects. I use it as a foil to ask questions of psychoanalysis about its theorizing about gender.

I choose Lemma's work specifically because she is reflective, nuanced, and open-minded. She has a well-deserved reputation internationally as a thinker, theoretician, and clinician, one who's treated transgender patients for many years. Her aim is to explore "premature embracement of the empowering potential of the transgendered identification for under 18-year-olds who are seeking medical intervention for gender dysphoria" (2018, 1092).

Importantly, Lemma is not discussing all transgender people. She carefully carves out a certain class of transgender person—ironically those most distrusted to speak for themselves—and assures us that she does not consider transgender life to be inherently pathological. She cautions her fellow therapists against entering treatment with a predetermined goal, or regarding the decision to have surgery as "an indicator of pathology" (p. 1101).

"Psychoanalysis should never be used as a tool of coercion or conversion—however subtle—when it comes to individual choices about how to live one's life," she states, referring to the profession's invidious history of prejudice against homosexuality (p. 1104). Finally, Lemma brings us right into the vexing issues of identity—she acknowledges that the position she writes from as a "cis-gendered" (matching her natal sex) woman has no more certainty than a transgendered person's.

This is all to say that Lemma does exactly what we ask a socially conscious person to do: she establishes her relation to a text, considers the context of her work, and makes her own investments known. So I was hopeful that we could meet the challenge that historian Ann Holder (2018) offers:

> Can scholars and intellectuals cease to be what Wynter calls the "grammarians" of the institutional order—even under the seductive guise of being its critics?. . . . Can we let go of the desire for mastery of the past and present, in order to participate in imagining a citizenship after or beyond domination?
>
> (Wynter 2015, 2)

However, the more I delved into Lemma's work, the more upset I became that the paper would not advance us in our psychoanalytic treatment of transgendered people. While Lemma's rhetoric was trans-friendly, her reliance on normative theory told another, more distressing story: one that undermined appreciation for transgender life. Further, when authors position themselves as discerning—as the opposite of homophobic or transphobic—it is easy for readers to accept their storytelling as thoughtful, even progressive.

As an example, Lemma invites us to trust her experience and to join in her belief that she, in particular, may be able to discern "good trans" (legitimate trans)—that is, to discern those who might genuinely need surgery or body modification (what she calls "the best compromise under the circumstances") and those who don't. Reading her paper underscores a need to challenge a psychoanalytic view that employs an approach that imagines a fixed and "authentic" gender identity as something that could ever or should be discerned by an outside other.

My goal, however, isn't to single out Lemma or any particular colleague. Rather, I want to use her work to raise questions about how we as psychoanalysts may harm people when we unquestioningly apply normative theory. When we tell a clinical story of another—never more so than when a patient's and analyst's understanding are at odds—we are not presenting the truth but an (ideological) version of it, one which, intentionally or not, demonstrates our own theories. Even with the good intentions of caring clinicians like Lemma, normative assumptions color what we see, hear, and think, to the detriment of too many patients. More broadly, when psychoanalysts adhere to standard developmental and gender theory as the undisputed model, we don't only risk hurting the people in front of us. Whether we mean to or not, we add one more link to the long chain reaffirming that there is one "right" way to live.

The case

Lemma tells the story of Jane, a 17-year-old whose parents send her to psychoanalysis after Jane has declared that she is a boy, with an attraction to girls. She is seeking to (partially) transition. Lemma uses Jane's case to illustrate her theory that a growing number of young people who identify as "trans" and who may not intend to "fully transition" (p. 1092), but are nevertheless keen to customize their body, are performing a "psychic surgery" (p. 1092) through enduring modifications of the body, or fantasies about its modification. Lemma believes that their issues are not primarily about gender at all.

In discussing her work with Jane, Lemma's bias is both disavowed and laid bare. She reports—"descriptively and not as an indicator of a successful outcome" (p. 1098)—that upon conclusion of their work, Jane, now 21, no longer needed to transition medically or otherwise. Lemma also informs us that Jane has a burgeoning interest in boys, although she began a sexual relationship with a girl during the treatment and is still in it when the case ends. "We do well to wonder what might have happened if Jane had just been validated by the transgender community," Lemma writes, "or been seen by a therapist who only mirrored *what* she felt without engaging her in making sense of *why* she felt this way" (p. 1098). The clear implication is that, had Jane been seen by a psychoanalyst in the queer or transgender community, she would have been in danger (Kelleher 2004): she might have changed her female body, transitioned, liked only girls. In this view, if you "fix" the gender, heterosexuality will follow (Langer 2019).

This story is reminiscent of "successful" analytic treatments in which the analyst is said to have helped the homosexual patient show sexual restraint.

We return to the familiar idea that heterosexuality is the natural order of things. Gender variation is not atypical yet healthy, but at best a symptom, at worst, pathology or not even "true." It is always less than, a second choice. Despite her assurances to the contrary, Lemma seems to believe a cis heterosexual life is a better life.

The analyst and identity

It's rare that we psychoanalysts talk about our own subject position or sexual identity, possibly because we've believed that people cannot use us as blank screens if we do. But, of course, we each have sexual identities. And, of course, we are presumed to be heterosexual and cis: coupled, monogamous, with children. This is how the idea of normal is promulgated. As healthy analysts, we are all alike. Lemma draws attention to her own identity ostensibly to take responsibility for how her status as a cis-gendered woman might limit her, but the revelation ends up being employed to bolster her credibility. For example, the corollary to her claim that Jane might have been harmed had she been seen by a member of the LGBTQ+ community is that therapists who *aren't* transgender, like her, are the only ones capable of providing clear-eyed care.

Lemma's framing suggests a neutrality that I don't think exists for any analyst. It also strikes at the integrity of LGBTQ+ psychoanalysts: They're somehow dubious, unable to thoughtfully detect what she can, which is, not incidentally, the route back to *normal*. Reading Lemma, I can't help feel confirmed in my belief that suspicion follows if "I don't look like you." If I tell you I am queer, are my 30 years of work with adolescents and transgender kids in private practice and in the psychiatric department of a children's hospital less valuable than those of a heterosexual colleague? But why does Lemma assume that queer psychoanalysts would *not* carefully reflect on what might help patients become more of who they want to be?

I agree with Lemma that analysis often involves slowing down with a patient, exploring the "subjective experience of embodiment" and or the "unconscious investments" of the body and psyche (2018, 1091), but wouldn't any good psychoanalyst do just that? To not refute a patient's stated identity is not to gloss over the painful psychic work required to establish what any identity means to a young person and work with that. In fact, an affirming stance may facilitate a deep dive into meaning making. Lemma's paper helps us think through what, if anything, about the analyst's identity is useful in our therapeutic stance. Does being outside an identity group guarantee neutrality, or does it merely align you with the dominant culture? Would we want to say that an African American analyst should not treat an African American patient because the therapist may be biased in their favor, colluding with their assumptions? Just as white psychoanalysts in the United States are eager for Black colleagues to help address the field's history of racism, so, too, LGBTQ+ clinicians might be embraced as resources for work within their communities.

Psychanalytic thinkers seeking to restrict gender transitioning suggest that those who protest the profession's normative assumptions are being unpsychoanalytic and politically correct. Adopting the language of the oppressed, Lemma writes that trans people have attempted to shut down voices like hers, when all she wants to do is "reflect" (p. 1092), "think" (p. 1097), understand "the meaning and function of any behavior, thought, or feeling . . . the everyday work of psychoanalysis" (p. 1104). For a clinician, questioning a subject's self-stated identity may be neutral, but for a transgender person to be told that their experience is false is lacerating.

The irony of the transgender community having the power to silence the institution of psychoanalysis ignores the regulatory function of the field, including the fact that our journals have been censoring (Saketopoulou and Pellegrini 2023), and in our forums, transgender people's fundamental right to self-determination is once again up for debate (APsA list serve, 2023). The pathologizing of homosexuality ruined countless lives—and, through "conversion therapy," ruins still more. The affective weight of those injustices remains sharp in our queer bodies and minds. The psychoanalytic innocence (Sheehi 2022) Lemma evokes contradicts her description of the way transgender experience has become a "central cultural site" (2018, 1092).

Let's back up. Does the identity of a psychoanalyst even matter? I mean, we would not want to judge a text just by the biography of the author, her politics, sexuality, or history. But because Lemma claims her gender and sexual identity, we are interested in how her specific corporeality (not her interiority or psyche per se) intrudes into the text (Grosz 1995, 13). And, again, I think Lemma asserts her cis gender and heterosexuality to gain credibility. Even when she is talking about all transgender people, not just the adolescents whom she believes aren't truly transgender, she refers to transition surgery or body modification as "the best compromise under the circumstances," a tepid endorsement of a transgender life, at best. Lemma does state that almost all research on those who have transitioned shows positive outcomes, but that fact is almost parenthetical in her paper. She never offers examples of a positive use of body modification. Or, conversely, even though she tells us that both patient and analyst need to make a sustained effort to question the signifiers that shape their relationships to their bodies, she never questions the etiology or legitimacy of being cis-gendered. Or examines identity difficulties among those who hew to the norm. Could cis-gendered heterosexuality be a "best compromise" for straights? Should we try to change them?

Even as the tendency to ask gay people to account for the etiology of their object choice has lessened, transgender subjects are now being forced to answer "the why" of their identities to people who have the power to regulate their lives. Lemma may be aiming for something more subtle, but this is the therapeutic agenda that comes through when she seeks to distinguish *real* transgender adolescents from those who are using their identity to shore up something else. This is especially true when she has evidenced no excitement or even awareness of the beauty or wonder of transgender life.

Without doubting the stated motivations of psychoanalytic authors, there is always potential conflict between how you represent your work and how a published piece lives and breathes in the world (Grosz 1995). As Lemma herself is aware, no written text is a simple communication of neutral information or ideas. "A text needs a reader, cosigner, a reception" (Derrida 1984, 52–54). In this cultural moment, where "it has become routine for conservatives to liken transgender people and their allies to pedophiles, and to equate discussion of gender identity with "grooming" children for sexual abuse" (Astor 2023)—it is crucial to think about how our work will be used.[1]

Whatever Lemma's goal, her ideas could easily be recruited (and may already have been) to prop up efforts to re-pathologize transgender experience as development gone awry. In England and the US, a trendy new (pseudo) diagnosis named rapid gender onset dysphoria (RGOD) has taken hold, with the "cure" being to stop teenagers who want to transition. ROGD grew out of a markedly unscientific survey of distressed parents (neither peer-reviewed or double-blind) on a website known for transphobia. According to the ROGD classification, "rapid onset" gender dysphoria in adolescents arises out of nowhere, doesn't last, and is fueled by peer pressure and transgender agendas, particularly via online resources and support groups. I hear echoes of the time when being gay was a "phase," or something we might catch.

Decades of careful studies, cited in the DSM-5 and other professional guidelines, do not support the conclusions drawn from the parent survey. To the contrary, it's been well established that people may become gender dysphoric and/or come out as transgender at any age; and many who come out later do not report gender issues earlier in their lives. Nor are these transgender adolescents more or less likely than others to subsequently change their minds about their gender.[2] Although the "rapid onset" phenomena has been repeatedly refuted as fake science, it's still being used by parents to reject an adolescent's gender identity, as well as to restrict young people's interactions with transgender peers and access to trans information and services. ROGD also provides political cover for those who wish to roll back transgender rights and access to medical care for transitioning.

Asking therapists or psychoanalysts to decide who is *really* transgender is asking the impossible, because it relies on a concept of identity as if there were an authentic truth. Further, such determinations suggest that we *can* objectively know a subject's unconscious fantasy or object relational history, that it's independent of the anxious work of cultural regulation (Langer 2011). When Lemma suggests that transgender people may be managing the inherent "opacity of the other that is at the core of our embodied experience" (Lemma 2018, 1101), I agree. But that the "the unfathomability or inaccessibility of the other resides under the skin, as it were" (p. 1101) is true for all of us. The work of translation of enigmatic messages (Laplanche 1987) has many outcomes across a lifetime, for the cis-gendered person as much as anyone else. We establish our subjectivity and sometimes our identities again and again.

The gender binary

As mentioned earlier, Lemma marks as a special category for consideration young people who identify as "trans" and wish to customize their bodies but don't plan to fully transition. In her normative framework, those who question the binary divide, or whose gender affiliations are fluid, are the "transient" trans; they're apt to want to abandon the identity (notwithstanding the research disproving that). Thus, Lemma only feels comfortable allowing medical intervention for transgender people who are resolutely sure about the divide between male and female. Only if the individual can be made more fully male or more fully female can their transgender identity be "real" enough to qualify for hormones or surgery. This notion aligns with standards of care for transgender folks in the late 1960s and early 1970s: the ideal outcome was for people to blend into the cisgender binary population, to successfully present as the gender they sought to be, to "pass."

However, decades of feminist and queer theory, transgender studies, and mainstream psychological research have challenged the need to function within the binary system—and correspondingly demonstrated that gender fluidity should not influence decisions to facilitate medical intervention. Gender is a complex and enigmatic series of internalizations and identifications that may "cohere" much less frequently than has been assumed. Nonconforming gender expresses neither a failure of certainty nor a statement of ambivalence, but a choice to live outside the binary. As González (2017) writes, "Both/neither' have taken center stage and bodies and their parts may be omnipotentially sexed and gendered, geared to shift, [and be] anything but static" (p. 1065).

Indeed, queer theorists argue that we've overvalued congruence and psychic equilibrium, while underexploring how gender regulation constricts gender's "wide arc" (Langer 2011) and the productive possibilities of variance. In failing to reflect this theory and research, Lemma's paper shares similarities with articles that purport to be "trans-friendly" but actually are written from a blatantly trans-antagonistic standpoint. Such pieces acknowledge that transgender people should not be persecuted, but then pivot to the possibility that some (perhaps many) adolescents who socially transition may not be "really transgender" (Whipping boy, online). For the many teenagers I have seen, this conclusion feels very painful, and paternalistic.

Choice and body modification

For a teen to "choose" an identity—one that is in Lemma's mind not long-standing or deeply rooted—"denudes identity of its essentially conflictual nature and of its intimate connection with desire and unconscious phantasy" (p. 1090). She continues:

> The body is the primary site of inscription and meaning arising from external forces as well as internal, unconscious ones. Severed from its unconscious psychic investments, and temporal links to the past, the materiality of the body has no meaning. It is only "real" as flesh and bones.
>
> (p. 1092)

How can Lemma imagine that a decision to transition is not intimately connected with desire and unconscious fantasy? Why is transitioning necessarily a severing, and why does it land with only materiality? Our understanding of the way our bodies are inscribed and marked, and our unconscious psychic investments in them—the meaning we make of them—is ever changing, never finished. To imagine any teenager would complete that work (or even that it can ever be completed) before making a physical change is to misconstrue the meaning of transitioning. The idea of performativity (Butler 1990) offered by queer theory does not imply conscious choice. Rather, it's about the way a subject is produced discursively, rather than emerging from the essence internal to the individual (Butler 1990). As Barden (2011) suggests, think of gender as a verb, not a noun or place.

Still Lemma is troubled by a culture that increasingly valorizes individual freedom of choice and the right to self-realization, which she believes finds ultimate expression in customizing one's body (2010, 2013). People who medically or digitally alter their bodies to match their subjective experience of gender are caught up in this consumer-choice model of liberalism, Lemma believes, adding that we should beware of basing identity on "acquisitive imitations where imitation trumps identification" (2018, 1090). This invites the question of what might count as a *legitimate* transgender identification for her.

But putting that aside for now, body modifications motivated by the desire to belong to a group or signal status are ubiquitous, as Lemma herself observed in her earlier work (2010). It is profoundly ahistorical to lay the phenomenon at the feet of transgender people. Circumcising, excising, piercing, binding, and remaking parts of the body by surgical means have taken place across time and cultures as a way of marking social location and position (Grosz 1995, 34). In (particularly white) Western culture, the medicalization of the body *is* staggering. We have breast reduction and amplification; cosmetic injection of the neuromuscular poison botox; the surgical removal of fat. Dieting, exercise, movement, and what we eat are also imbued with values, norms, and ideals, Grosz writes. Think of thinness to mark class status; tanning to mark affluence and leisure. The body is a sign to be read. How is any of this ever just individual choice? How is it feasible to be outside of social values, fantasy, and desire?

As Grosz (1993) also notes, inscriptions on/of the body not only reflect an interior subjectivity, they also generate it. "What happens on the surface body forms libidinal flows, sensations, and experiences, into needs, wants, and commodified desires and constructs depth" (Grosz 1993, 199). We inscribe meaning in the materiality of bodies, produce meaning through our body's actions—and we link up with other bodies. Inner and outer amplifying and making each other. This is not transgender bodies. This is all bodies. Bodies are and have always been the threshold between psyche and materiality (Grosz 1993).

And there is no putting the genie back in the bottle. "Bodies can be altered, adjusted—parts removed or replaced—and, as a result, they're increasingly regarded as assemblies of parts that are capable of mechanical cybernetic duplication and 'pliable to power'" (Grosz 1993, 199). Reproduction has been uncoupled from biology, no longer requiring the binary coupling. Yet, unlike Lemma, Grosz believes that if "bodies are traversed and infiltrated by knowledges, meanings, and power, they can also become sites of struggle and resistance" (Grosz 1993, 199).

Certainly, a practice that threatens the gender binary is a site of such resistance. In fact, social uprisings (and many people think we're in the middle of a gender revolution) are inextricably entwined with the formation of new knowledges and changing technologies. In the technological advances that belie the dominance of biology and reveal the body as cultural site, there is the possibility of expanding the story of who is human.

The figure of the child

I am a parent of young adults and have worked with parents for many years in the psychiatry department of a large children's hospital. I know how unnerving adolescents' sense of urgency can be, and how hard it is to accept their forceful assertions of will when we oppose them. I understand the anxiety of parents who want what's best for their offspring, especially when an adolescent wants to make life-altering physical changes. Still, I think we need to rethink our very idea of *the child*. Something ideological, not just developmental, is at stake. As Stockton (2009) notes, though children live inside their own bodies, adults want them to live instead inside the figure of what we call "the child." The child is innocent and good and needs to be protected from sexuality. But this ignores children's real and alive sexuality, which, of course, was a fundamental discovery of Freud (1905). Yet, at times, psychoanalysts still take pains to differentiate childhood sexuality from the "real" version. As Bruhm and Hurley (2004) write, the child cannot be queer because to be queer is to be sexual, and to be sexual is deemed to be adult. Young sexual and gender outliers are especially likely to be denied their freedoms (Rubin 2011) because we don't like their choices. We believe 18-year-olds can vote, go to prison, die in war, and bear children. But when it comes to defining their own sexuality and gender, it's our responsibility to put the brakes on.

To Stockton, the efforts to delay young people from making this "adult" decision are rooted in shaky soil. She questions the normative theory of *gradual* growth, that the child slowly unfolds into a full (and sexual) subject capable of marriage, work, reproduction. Instead, or additionally, she offers the metaphor of sideways growth, congruent with recent cognitive science showing that while the brain develops most rapidly in early childhood, the capacity to make new neural networks is lifelong. Growing sideways, Stockton notes, suggests that the breadth of a person's experience or ideas, their motives and actions, may be meaningful at any age, bringing adults and children into lateral contact of surprising sorts. In part, she writes, children grow sideways because our concepts of childhood constrain how far "up" they can go. They cannot advance to adulthood until we say it is time (Stockton 2009).

If the concept of RODC is fueled by parental anxiety, is something greater than protecting the "child" at issue here? Protection of children often becomes the sight of moral panic regarding sex. (Recall Anita Bryant's crusade of the 1970s.) It also can function as political camouflage for the same prejudices that find more cultural resonance when focused on "the child."

Lemma is upset about body modification because she believes, among other things, that extensive changes disrupt the temporal link (Lemma 2016). What she calls the "given body," referring to both the sexed body we are born into and the body "given" to us de facto by our parents, connects us indelibly to older generations. When we change our body, we potentially sever ourselves from the continuity among different representations of the self over time (Grinberg and Grinberg 1981), and from what came before us. But changing bodies does not erase history or ancestors, and many people who transition feel in relation to who they used to be. And for those who don't, is continuity all it's cracked up to be? As Edelman notes, "the figure of the child is always bound up in a kind of frightening and (hermetically sealed) reproductive futurism" in which one's offspring "spawn delusional visions . . . of the seamless reproduction of oneself" (2005, 13).

Moreover, the whole model of passing down knowledge from parent to child is quite clearly invested in white-gendered heteronormativity. As Eng and Han (2016) write, "We inherit a means by which violence and hate are preserved indefinitely in the service of continuous psychic and political consolidation . . . embedded in a long history of colonial relations" (p. 11). For many queer children, generational inheritance means a history of being hated. The disruption of a temporal link, if there even is one, may allow the deconstruction of the subject affording new play and possibilities, (as we will see in the next chapter). What about ways we can create both past and future connectivity that don't depend merely on generational inheritance? Our narratives are rooted not just by lineage but by affect. When we shift from discovering our origins, or the etiology of our identities, something is opened up by our always-present, right from the start, involvement with the other. Affective exchange between people, between Lemma and Jane, may introduce unexpected and unknown experiences that rewrite the psychic system—and play an important role in subject formation.

Etiology

In seeking to dismantle Jane's idea of transgender, Lemma looks for etiology. Calling it an important breakthrough, Lemma recounts how Jane, who was adopted, volunteers a year into therapy that she was born into a culture that doesn't value girls. Lemma reports that Jane wonders if her birth mother would have kept her had she been a boy, and subsequently informs us of the "weakness" of Jane's adoptive mother and the rejection of Jane by boys her age. These three pieces of information become the therapist's "reasons" for Jane's desire to switch genders, the raw material that Lemma can interpret to help free her patient to remain in her female body, or so it's implied. Yet traumas inform all our subjectivities and identities. Many girls grow up where women are second-class citizens, mothers are disempowered, and, at 18, romance is scant, but they do not become transgender. Lemma's discovery of these "facts" is part of a search for what Stockton calls a "backward birthing mechanism," where "the hunt for the roots of transgender identity is a search for what led to the death of a straight life" (Stockton 2009, 7). Facts, like norms, are an expression of context, point of view, and politics. Seeking causality necessarily reduces the lived intersubjective complexity in which identity is formed, continuously, into the present.

Treatment

And what of the treatment? Is it insight that will cure? Won't Jane and Lemma need to live something out together? Although Jane's parents force her to see Lemma prior to any decisions about hormones or surgery, the therapist dismisses the power of her gatekeeper role and its impact on their interaction, even as Jane says that she's just "going through the motions" to satisfy her parents (p. 1096). When a patient needs a clinician to obtain access to gender-altering technologies, there can be, as Prosser writes in his book *Second Skin* (1988), a careful movement between, on the one hand, telling medical authorities what they want to hear, and on the other, giving authentic coherence to one's own life as lived and personally signified. That Jane cannot open up about the complexity of her gendered experience may be part and parcel of Lemma's suspicious listening. Jane tells her, "I don't expect you to understand me" (p. 1096).

Lemma downplays the role of transference in the case as well. She imagines her bias won't derail the treatment because she makes her own position, sometimes at odds with Jane's, part of their dialogue. She tells us this was her only technical choice because Jane got mad when Lemma seemed to have her own point of view. Yet how could the therapist's repeatedly articulated mistrust of Jane's feelings not have a corrosive effect on Jane's experience of herself? Or Jane's ability to surrender to the work with Lemma? Lemma knows that she's making Jane angry by doubting her motivations, but that does not stop her from pressing her patient, and us, to see that Jane's transgender identity is a product of something other than what Jane thinks it is. Lemma writes, sounding a bit frustrated:

> No sooner had she [Jane] allowed us both to take an excursion away from the "I am trans and I need to take hormones" track and to think more generally about what it felt like to be in her girl self and body, she had done a U-turn back into certainty about "really being a boy."
>
> (p. 1097)

But could Jane's resistance be provoked by the felt experience of Lemma's certainty and sovereignty, by the sense that her therapist is more knowing than curious? That she is not *being with* Jane who is also Jake, her male avatar? What does it mean when our patients don't feel our susceptibility to them, when they can't tell that they move and affect us? That we act and are acted on by them?

Lemma writes that questioning from a position of equidistant curiosity and suspicion is not about coercing someone to follow a pre-determined "healthy" path but helping them consider underlying meaning and conflicts. Leaving aside the clinical usefulness of skeptical listening, I would argue that as long as psychoanalytic clinicians *believe* that living in one's natal body is always preferable, this cannot be an open inquiry. What Lemma considers a reflective and psychoanalytic point of view may be an example of what Ahmed calls the work of repetition: repeating and enforcing established norms, which involves the concealment of labor under the sign of nature. Bodies take the shape of norms that are repeated over time and with force (Ahmed 2004).

For instance, when Jane is asked to respond to (or defend herself) against Lemma's idea that she has "decided" to be a boy, Jane angrily asserts, "I have not decided to become a boy. I am becoming who I should always have been, that's quite different" (p. 1096). Responding to Lemma's proposition that discovering gender dysphoria as a teenager makes it less true, Jane elaborates and says she has always hated her body and that she never told anybody because she did not think she would be taken seriously. And Jane is not alone in this. As touched on earlier, we know that children who feel queer, out of synch, attracted to same-sex peers can't always name what's going on until later. Their difference is often first internally grasped by exposure to others (Butler 1993). "Linguistic markers for queerness arrive only after one exits childhood—after (the child) is shown *not* to be straight" (Stockton 2009, 6). In other words, feeling different can precede conversations that could describe what that difference is about.

From this perspective, Lemma's insistence that Jane's current understanding of her gender is valid only if she was *always* aware of it is specious.

We can't know what would have been possible for Jane had Lemma been able to join in the joy of play with Jake as a participant. Jane might have been more alive to her own experiences. Lemma reports that when she imparts to Jane that she understands how Jake made her feel more powerful than her real-life body, "as if her actual body was more substantial," Jane relaxes and says more. Jane tells Lemma that the fantasied online figure and dressing in a more masculine style increase her comfort level and interest in "going out and being with others," and not just online but "in real life" (p. 1096). When she is Jake, she says she can get in touch with a new, embodied experience of her own desire; Jake is who she should have always been.

Jane seems to be trying to live in the possibility of a different world, imagining a different future. What does it mean for us as analysts to squash or temper the feeling of wonder that comes for Jane when she makes her online avatar male? Jane is not just talking about body. She is talking about psych-soma, where in the transitional space of Jake, she is feeling the ability to come imaginatively alive (Ogden 2023).

While Lemma does not doubt Jane's feelings of being wrong, or what Jake brings her in terms of "room to breathe" (p. 1095), the therapist thinks Jane is misinterpreting the situation. She wonders, as she has from their very first session, whether Jane is feeling trapped in the wrong body or, in fact, is experiencing herself as lacking strength or substance, which she confuses with being female. Given Jane's history of boys not liking her, was she someone who failed to make an impression on another, like her mother did? Lemma asks. Her conclusion is that Jane plays with "reality" (p. 1095) to find an embodied form that might guarantee what she feels she lacked.

We don't know if this interpretation is true, or truer than anything else. We are in the realm of logic where narration "involves selection and rejection. . . . Its relation to the past is not that of truth but desire" (Grosz, p. 144). We do know that many analysts have judged gendered behaviors and fantasies as true or false (in accord with the binary), rather than examining their embodied style, patients' imaginations or histories. As Langer (2011) writes:

> If one follows basic psychoanalytic presuppositions as to the ways in which fantasy is inter-implicated with embodiment, and if it is also accepted that genders evolve and become embodied in a relational world, then one would have to be open to considering the ways in which embodiment and gendered states are open to a range of fantastic expressions and relational dynamics. And one would need to consider the ways in gender is always performed with affect, tempered by defense, knit by history, done and undone through the relational excess of human life.
>
> (p. 465)

Identity and desire are lived out in their particularity, in their dynamic force, and sometimes with another. Every identity is answering to our own unconscious forces in we ways do and don't know. If Lemma is helping Jane feel more vital, and more of themselves, we don't hear it from Jane herself. Lemma gives words to Jane when the two disagree, but Jane does not speak about her perspective regarding her reported reversion to a female identity.

I want to clarify that I don't necessarily think Lemma must accept Jane's point of view. I agree with her, as I have just discussed in Chapter 8, that using empathy and identification to help someone feel understood can sometimes perpetuate nonunderstanding. And while I am sympathetic to Lemma's stance that it can be important *not* to join in on what feel like frozen repetitive narratives in our patients, I have a different idea of what is called for when that is the case. For me, finding my own place of genuine not knowing—rather than entering with certainty or even theory—can open possibilities for patients to feel more deeply understood and, importantly, alive.

Jane seems to be in a process of unbecoming. As Butler writes,

> At moments of significant shift or rupture, we may not know precisely who we are or even what we mean by "I" when we say it. If the I is separated from the you or indeed the they, that is from those without whom the I has been unthinkable, then there is doubtless a rather severe disorientation that follows.
>
> (Butler 2015, 8)

Jane might need Lemma inside her disorientation, not locked in an opposing understanding. But rather than immerse herself in the patient's *experience* of "creatively discovering meaning for himself, and in that state of being, becoming more fully alive" (Ogden 2019, 661), Lemma remains wedded to an object-relations view in which there is cause and effect.

As I have written in other chapters, when patients are facing the profound and sometimes catastrophic anxiety of not being—in Jane's case, not being a girl at least—what may be needed is less leading from our abilities to think and analyze and interpret, and more from our capacities to be with the other in a less represented state, one where our certainty and sovereignty make no sense. When we undergo a situation with our patients and enter as human beings with our own confusion, and if that is genuine, not technique, something transformative may occur. Here I am talking about listening with negativity capability, not with preformed desire.

What in Jane's existential crisis might move Lemma to her own version of primal anxiety? Before Jane can understand herself, she might need to *feel* Lemma in her dilemma, and what that engenders—not just for Jane but for Lemma as well. Jane might need a different kind of sensing and being sensed, a different kind of entanglement where affective interplay between subjects holds the potential for new experiences.

What bestows value?

If we think with Berlant and Edelman (2014), as we did in the Ferrante novels, about the way "a story implies a direction . . . a movement that leads to some payoff or profit, some comprehension or closure, however open-ended," what might that suggest about the case history of Jane? Or how might we comprehend her story if we applied Edelman's observation that "any leading toward necessarily entails a correlated leading from" (p. 3)? The way Lemma has shaped Jane's case, I experience being led from queerness toward heteronormativity. At the beginning, Jane is a queer child—that is, a child who "doesn't quite conform to the wished-for way children are supposed to be in relation to gender and sexual roles" (Bruhm and Hurley 2004, x). She is born in a female body, feels herself to be a boy and likes girls, but then, after working with the analyst, she remains in her female body. We are told that while she still has a girlfriend at story's end, there is a potential for heterosexuality in her future.

We hear in Lemma's storytelling a seeking for what went wrong in Jane's childhood: how this child came to be a queer one. This child can be transgender as long as we understand the queerness as a series of mistakes or misplaced desires that we can correct (Bruhm and Hurley 2004, xx). In this case, you can see the psychoanalytic story "in which the becoming normal of the sexual body, the straightening of its perverse possibilities, entails the theoretical superimposition of one version of a Freudian developmental narrative," in which "the perversions are the unproductive detours passed through and left behind en route to the final destination of heterosexual reproductive life" (Kelleher 2004, 155). There is indeed pressure on the narrative to produce a proper ending, that is, a projected cis, heterosexual end. And one that conforms to the theory we were meant to see.

We might say Lemma is inventing a utopian future for Jane. According to Lemma, Jane is now a bearer of strong womanhood and the chance of heterosexuality. Ideology has been rendered invisible, but as Edelman tells us, the child is a product of physical *and* cultural reproduction. "Both the utopianism and the nostalgia invoked by the figure of the child are in turn, the preferred form of the future. . . This child of the future—anti queer—innocent is a symbol of family values" (Edelman 2005, 13). The telos of projecting the child into heteronormativity also establishes heterosexuality and the invention of humanity (Bruhm and Hurley 2004). In other words, in Lemma's story of Jane's misgendered self, set against the goodness of a cis-heteronormative bourgeois alternative, there is an unarticulated discursive truth that remains unquestioned.

If we believe with Edelman that the story Lemma writes—which leads from Jane's "refusal of story" (to live a normative life)—will "always enact the story of its refusal" (Berlant and Edelman 2014, 3), what is the story Lemma is refusing to see? Jane's disappearance as transgender male may be more Lemma's story than Jane's. What would Jane's own story of hope and disappointment, attachment and rupture, accommodation and liberation be? I thought Jane was trying to tell us. Doesn't Jane's life, like Lila's in Ferrante's novels, offer a critique of the suffocating conventions she has been subject to? If she had been supported in discovering her self-defined subjectivity, perhaps a very different tale might have emerged.

Because of expanding choices, Jane lives in a world where she can imagine other ways to live. There is emergence and potentiality in the body (Massumi 1995) and in the way it connects with other bodies. As Ahmed (2004) writes, when queer pleasures put bodies into contact that have been kept apart by compulsory heterosexuality, worlds open. My gender queer patients want a different thinkable "I." They don't want a better origin story, and they don't want to understand etiology. They need my psychic, not just professional, involvement.

The possibility of breaking certain norms as they "exercise the power to craft us" (Butler 2015, 9) happens when countervailing norms intervene. Like the rest of us, transgender people long to be accepted, wanted, eroticized (Sedgwick 2011)—loved. We psychoanalysts have the opportunity to give the recognizing look found in the eye of the other. "To give this look," Barden writes, "as obvious as it sounds, you have to meet some(one) who you recognize. When we recognize a (patient), it is meaningful because we create a connection through which they can see, through us, in themselves, something they knew or hoped was there" (Barden 2012, 284). Jane does not find ready home in her parents' or Lemma's minds (Spezzano 2007).

Trans as trendy and softball

Returning to Lemma's contention that "trans" has become trendy—a "central cultural site" (p. 1089) rather than an index of marginality—how does this square with the fact that more than half of transgender people consider suicide by their 24th birthdays, and 19 percent actually attempt it? In 2022, dozens of trans or nonconforming gender people, predominantly Black and Latinx, were murdered in the U.S., and hundreds were killed worldwide. Many transgender people receive death threats and harassment; and suicidal thoughts and actions are often driven by bullying and isolation.

At the same time, research shows that transgender children whose parents reject them or try to "fix" them are especially vulnerable to suicide[3] and depression, as well as the inverse: the incidence of depression among adolescents whose gender identity is well supported in their social environments is similar to that of cis gender controls. Likewise, several studies demonstrate that adolescents with gender dysphoria who are given gender-affirming treatment in a comprehensive gender-care center grow into well-functioning adults.[4]

Curiously, while Lemma notes statistics that show children denied access to treatment become desperate and suicidal, she still suggests that Jane's "frantic" efforts to find out about transitioning—and to connect with people who help her feel visible and intelligible—is problematic. But support groups and information-sharing are how transgender and non-binary people offer each other holding environments. Women did the same in the 1970s, when they sought mutual recognition of their own subjectivities in consciousness-raising spaces, away from male definitions of gender and sexuality. Broadly speaking, seeking others for support or to build self-awareness is a life-affirming, even lifesaving, task of adolescent identity formation. And marginalized populations, including queer young people, have long relied on community to counter the regulatory power of dominant ideology and their parents.

I understand why Lemma, or anyone, might think young people would be drawn to the heady work of identity and group formation. Many transgender young people experience incredible joy in who they are and are becoming. But I think one can only call transgender "trendy" if one is outside the very real sources of pain and discrimination that cause kids, or anyone relegated to the culture's edges, to band together.

Which brings me to the transgender people with whom I came to play softball. There is great value in clinicians spending social time with people similar to those they treat. It makes it much harder for us to "other" our patients when they sit across from us, or to make skewed determinations about what might be "real" or "wrong" with them. While structural and legal discrimination based on sexual orientation was largely eradicated after decades of activism, changing the hearts and minds of straight allies often came only after they got to know us as real people—both different and like them.

About two decades ago, some friends asked if my partner and I would be interested in helping form a gender-inclusive softball team. I hadn't been on a softball field since my twenties, but we were in. About 20 people signed up—a few lesbians like us, some transgender folks who had transitioned, and others who were just beginning the process. My partner and I were much older than most of our teammates, who were roughly the same age as the people Lemma writes about, but we were happy to be with the group. First, though, we needed a league to play in.

The women's league, primarily lesbians, wouldn't have us. Too many of our players no longer defined themselves as women. Similarly, the gay league rejected us because not everyone on our team considered themselves gay (only two people on each team could be straight-defining). Finally, we joined a coed league of teams largely comprised of cis-gendered men. Not just any men. These men were so into the sport that, in addition to playing in a single-sex league, they formed coed teams (by recruiting two wives or girlfriends) to get in extra games. Even the D-league, the bottom rung of competitiveness, was packed with serious players. Meanwhile, on our team, a couple of butch dykes were the only ones who'd ever really played before. The wages of gender displacement meant we looked about as good as a new T-ball team.

One of the unofficial rules of the league was that the fielders moved in when women were batting, and out when men were at the plate. Because so many of our players looked gender-indeterminate, the umpire instructed our batters to announce themselves as woman or man. Many of those announcing "man" were at the beginning of their gender transitions and looked feminine. They endured wave after wave of mocking laughter as the infield moved back to where our balls never landed; that is, when one of us even managed to make contact in the first place. Batter after batter struck out, until the slaughter rule was called.

More than once, our opponents approached us after the games, swinging bats and proposing a round of beers. We always declined, out of fear; we didn't think the invitations were friendly. But we stayed in that league for a whole year, determined to play ball. Over that time, we also organized and agitated, and the next season, the gay league agreed to take us because transgender politics had begun to shift. We were crushed there, too, but the atmosphere was much friendlier. The gay teams also had physically imposing men, but those of us who *were* men could play without fear. We lost, over and over. The league and the teams came to know us, and many ignored us, but some championed us, offering us tips. Eventually, we won some games, but more importantly, we won a space for our team to exist. And we spawned another team that joined the gay league.

Belonging was arduous, hard-fought, and partial. We won entry, but not just because the league had to take us. Movement-building had laid the groundwork, and we capitalized on it. Organizing with other ball players—game by game, beer by beer—we chipped away at the rationale for excluding us as misfits, for virtually making us homeless.

I tell this story for a few reasons. While I count many transgender people in my social world now, at the time that wasn't the case. The softball team gave me a very human, and delightful, view into a community of young transgender people. Which is something I think Lemma seems to be missing. Her adherence to a psychoanalytic theory of gender development reads as incompatible with an *appreciation* of transgender life: the struggle *and* the creativity and excitement that can be found there.

On the grimmer side of things, the softball team offered me the briefest glimpse of what transgender people are up against every day, not just in conservative quarters but in purportedly progressive women's and queer contexts—and in a city that was the first in the nation to pass transgender non-discrimination laws. The overt transphobia we encountered continues, of course, and it has very real consequences: in housing, employment, and, yes, recreation. At best, trans people face constant, insidious ignorance; at worst they're insulted, humiliated, and physically attacked or killed. To be transgender is to be perpetually vigilant: Is that stranger I just met friendly or menacing? If the latter, am I at risk of violence, even murder? Knowing all this, it would be hard for me to ever believe that transgender is trendy. Risky, yes.

At its worst, psychoanalysis operates through conditions of diagnosis and practice that not only govern gender's intelligibility but also direct our ways of knowing and speaking, forcibly circumscribing what counts as truth and what is defined as real (Langer 2019). At its best, psychoanalysis can open worlds and possibilities.

Notes

1 Conservative anti-gay groups like Alliance Defending Freedom, the Family Policy Alliance, the Heritage Foundation and the American Principles Project have funded and fueled the activism, according to Astor, Dec 10, 2022). An exposé of the funding and pseudo-science behind the think tank, The Society for Evidence-Based Gender Medicine, being cited in numerous legislative proposals is frightening (Leveille 2023).

2 See Serano (2018) for summary article. For instance, in the current WPATH Standards of Care (published in 2011), the section entitled "Phenomenology in Adolescents" explicitly states: *"many adolescents and adults presenting with gender dysphoria do not report a history of childhood gender-nonconforming behaviors (Docter 1988; Landén, Wålinder, and Lundström 1998). Therefore, it may come as a surprise to others (parents, other family members, friends, and community members) when a youth's gender dysphoria first becomes evident in adolescence."* Serano notes, as from Zinnia Jones, that the *DSM-5* diagnosis for gender dysphoria (published in 2013) contains similar language: Late-onset gender dysphoria occurs around puberty or much later in life. Some of these individuals report having had a desire to be of the other gender in childhood that was not expressed verbally to others. Others do not recall any signs of childhood gender dysphoria.

3 Research Examines Parental Acceptance of Transgender Kids; www.goodther apy.org

4 Health Disparities Facing Transgender and Gender Nonconforming Youth Are Not Inevitable, Daniel Shumer, MD, MPH

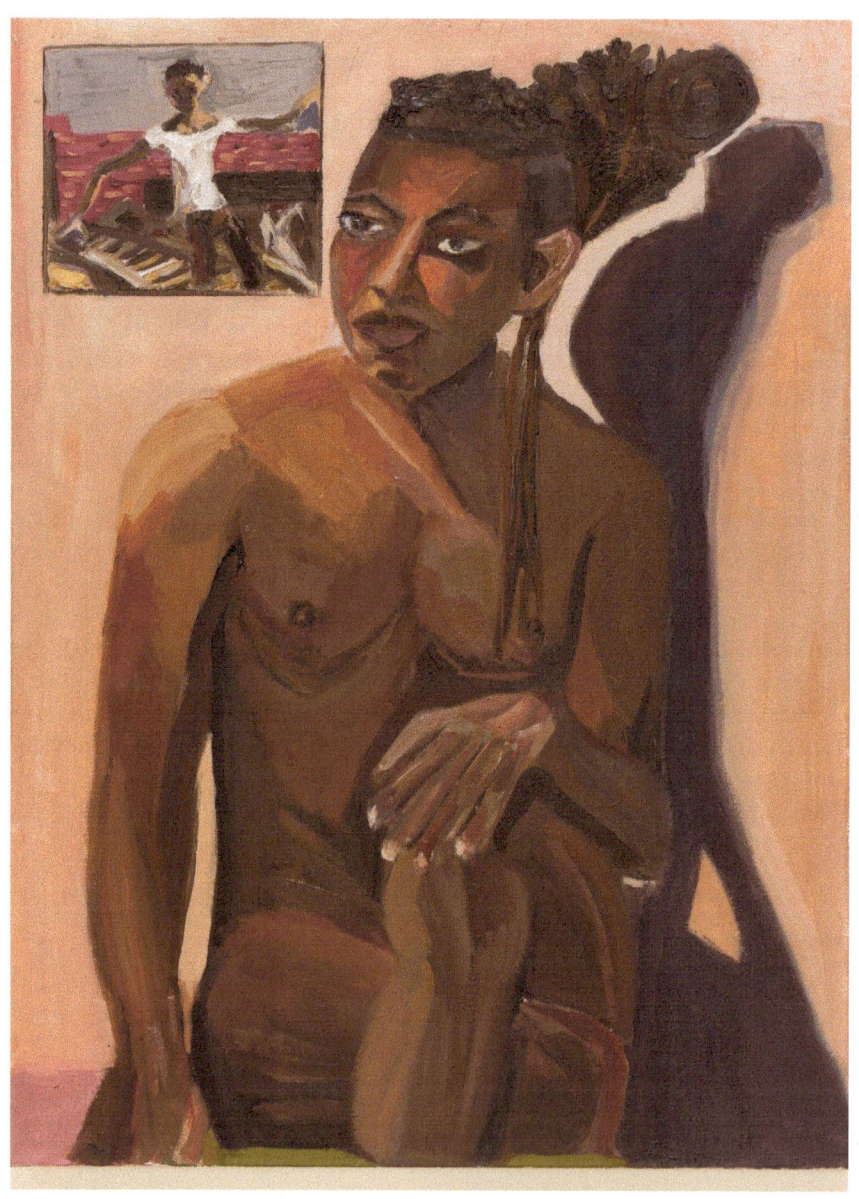

Figures 12.1 and *12.2: Dreaming Hughie Lee Smith/Dreaming a pink chair.*
Oil. 24x18. McGleughlin

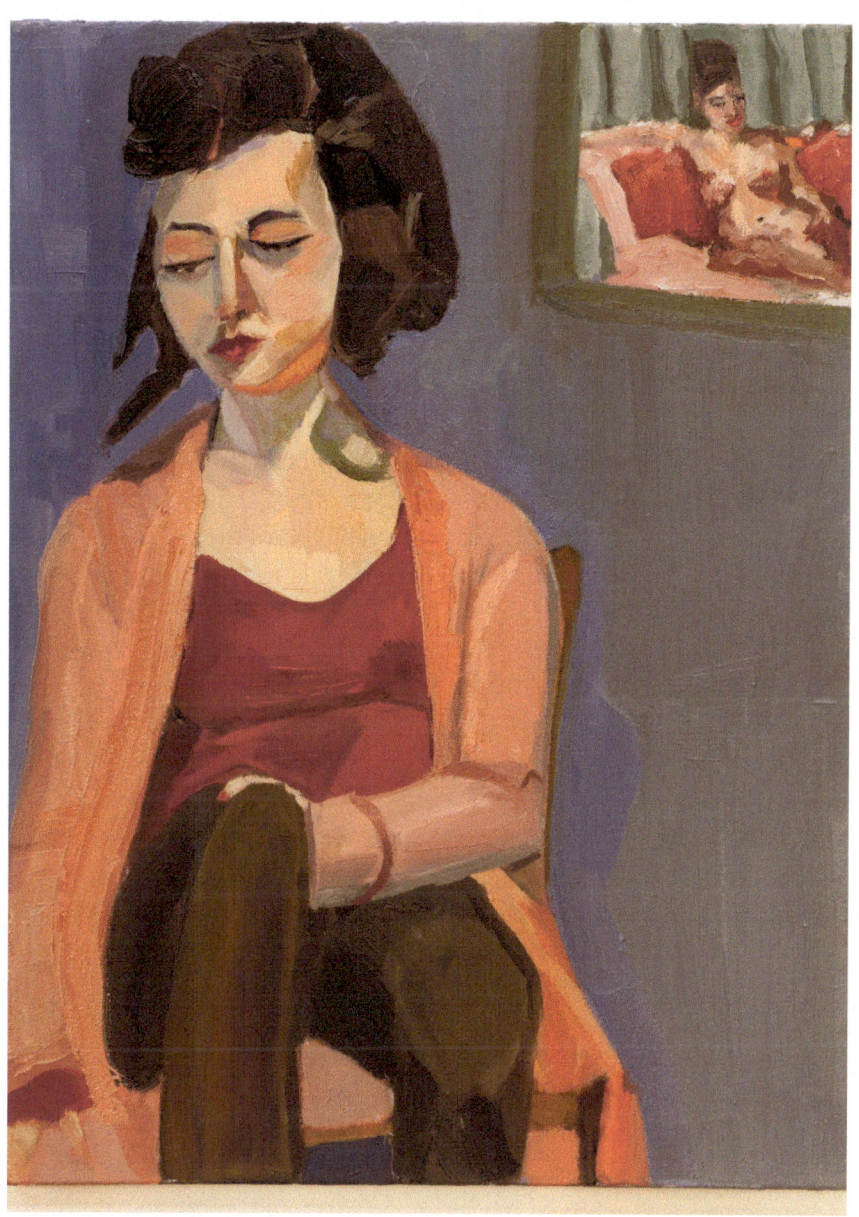

Figures 12.1 and 12.2: (Continued)

Chapter 13

Thinking outside the Oedipus box (2021)

In a paper I discussed for *Psychoanalytic Dialogues*, psychologist Shelly Nathans begins with a story of her 4-year-old daughter, who sees in a set of dolls a family that her mother does not see. "Where is the daddy?" my colleague reflexively asks, only to be reminded (incredulously but gently by her daughter) that it's a lesbian family, of course! The incident prompts my colleague to reflect on the difficulty of changing her unconscious bias despite her real comfort with the varieties of modern family life. She is grateful that the incident reveals her "confining myopia" (Nathans 2021, 312).

I was reminded of a similar story with my own daughter. On a crowded airplane, not quite 3-year-old Jesse was sitting with her two mothers and infant brother and noisily engaging with the people in the row ahead of us, one of whom asked which woman was her Mommy. "Both," my daughter answered. "But no, which is your *real* Mommy?" the woman asked again. Jesse replied in a way that was as incredulous as my colleague's daughter's response: "Do you believe in ghosts?"

The two anecdotes echo each other, but Jesse's story also contains something more troubling. Jesse is exposed, then and often, to a not-so-subtle idea that something in her family of two lesbian mothers, two gay fathers, and several equally important aunties (*not* the nuclear family of biological reproduction) is off. Maybe, in fact, not even "real." The unconscious bias that likely kept the woman from "seeing" Jesse's family is girded and rearticulated by the culture and state through normative family ideology and policy. These powerful doctrines shape and impinge on a child's experience of her psychic and material world—they affect and infect her. While my colleague's daughter happily corrects her mother, and her mother is happy to be corrected, the (not so) enigmatic message passed to Jesse requires

DOI: 10.4324/9781032670348-17

translation, and it conjures ghosts; it imposes a liminal state on her. We cannot account for the ways negation's haunting will get animated, vitalized, and transformed across the après coup of development.

My colleague is aware of the ghosts, but her solution is to generate a more inclusive theory for families. Anchoring her paper with Oedipus, whose blindness to reality handicaps him, she seeks to correct the blindness of analysts who ignore unconscious biases in clinical theory and rely on normative frameworks (Nathans 2021). She challenges the assumption that non-heteronormative families are different from traditional ones, that they're any less healthy (or sick). While she underscores the dangers of assuming universal structures of development or equating alternative families to heterosexual ones, she believes it is possible to separate Oedipus from its harmful history and enfold those cast out of its realm.

Many progressive thinkers—those whose models of sex and gender incorporate variety, fluidity, and multiplicity—hold the same view as Nathan. And when psychoanalysis "offers" queers like me a chance to be part of "normal," a wrong seems righted after decades of movement-building. The longing to be included in a society that is organized primarily by institutions like the family (even as we critique them) is powerful. Why wouldn't we want to feel such a cosmic connectedness across generations and cultures, to have a place of meaning in the world that will outlast our lives? I want to align myself with any clinician who argues with clarity and fair-mindedness that LGBTQ+ and single-parent families are as healthy as heterosexual ones.

Yet such parallelism, as political theorist Margaret Cerullo (1987) writes, reveals

> our continued alienation, our yearning for what never was: a moment in which gay people are not only accepted or tolerated, but normative, in which we are the definers of the streets and the bedrooms, . . . where night vision emerges on the daytime streets.

In other words, recognition resurfaces how family ideology has banished and punished us, and how we've been shaped by our nonbelonging in ways we embrace.

While I agree that imagining ways we are the same can be useful, especially for clinicians who might otherwise stigmatize marginal families,

I prefer to advance another, equally true idea: that by disregarding substantial differences between queer and heteronormative families—like the gap between my daughter's experience and Nathan's—we seek a sanitized, overly simplified notion of LGBTQ+ sexuality and family. The Oedipal tent of "normal" might be another comforting illusion "render[ing] us less able to navigate our way in the world" (Nathans, p. 312). I argue that continuing to use Oedipus, even altered and repurposed, deadens our imaginations and leaves us relying on theory that constrains us. Noting the perils of universal developmental stories but continuing to promote them falls short.

The problem with the idea of *all families*

Analytic thinking is that all children, including those not living within heteronormative structures, must come to terms with the anxieties and demands of the Oedipal situation. In fact, many psychoanalysts continue to assert that the successful negotiation of Oedipal issues *creates* psychological health. The notion of "all children or families" makes me nervous, especially when psychoanalysis omits so many from the story of "normal" and showcases a developmental theory constructed in another time and place. Psychoanalytic origin stories have too long been modeled on the western family and reify it as universal.

Black scholars and analysts have noted the same, illustrating how monolithic stories of being "human" have excluded Black people (Leary 1997; Wynter 2015). Freud's theory of Oedipus, developed shortly after the end of legal slavery in the U.S., is a story of a (white) God-like father in triad with a pure (white) mother and son, mirrored symbolically and materially (Nast 2000). During and after slavery, Black families were unrecognized and often forbidden or destroyed. With enslaved children routinely separated from their parents, "the only sure inheritance passed from one generation to the next was this loss, and it defined the tribe . . . an identity produced by negation" (Hartman 2008, 103). This negation, rather than resolution of an Oedipus negotiated or denied, remains formidable today, as structural racism denies access to the family constellations that we psychoanalysts cling to. As Halberstam (2011) writes, "The model of passing down knowledge from parent to child is quite clearly invested in white, gendered heteronormativity; indeed, the system inevitably stalls in the face of scenes of difference" (p. 124).

The current racial reckoning, and in particular the articulations of Black Lives Matter, give existential reply to the history of negation. When we consider the negotiation of the Oedipus as an inevitable universal or as a psychological necessity for health, we deny the complexity of how development occurs. Development is a melding of culture, body, and mind; intersubjective, fractal, idiosyncratic. I think Nathans believes this too, but her push for universal models undercuts other cherished ideas that we both hold: ideas of multiplicity and gender's "soft assembly" (Harris 2008). When psychoanalytic theory fails to grapple with the myriad ways people construct families, whether from choice or necessity, we repeat a colonialist project.

We are situated in conditions of life that differ radically across race, economics, and kinship. With varying access to power, we are always creating and being created by its dynamic (Combahee River Collective (1983) and our resistance to it. All these distinctions shape our development, identities (Crenshaw 1991), and psychic structures. How we think shapes what is being thought. Our perspectives on development or clinical work will depend on our model of the mind and our understanding of culture. For instance, the Oedipal idea that "frustration, loss, and relinquishment of the phantasy of omnipotent control" (Nathans 2021, 312) are inevitably part of a child's experience means very different things depending on the child's circumstances. We need to focus on the manifold degrees of loss, frustration, and powerlessness, and at whose hands.

Developmental stories

Comparative psychoanalysis has helped us understand that each theory determines our ideas of development, and that therapeutic action and definitions of health and pathology shift accordingly. We have multiple theories of how subjectivity occurs and even what it is. But developmental stories have been unitary and unchanging, despite the dissemination of new theories based on complexity, variety, fluidity, and multiplicity. While feminist and queer theorists have devised models of development that complicate typical gender formation and sexual object choice—from Oedipal "ice-cream cones" (Seidal 2019) to "multiple circulating narratives" (Corbett 2001)—they don't seem to take hold. The Oedipal narrative remains formidable. And it relies on unquestioned mechanisms embedded within normative white developmental theory: the primacy of "the family," the child internalizing the parental couple, and the couple performing a containing, limiting, and reflective function.

Drawn from Klein, this model emphasizes that the resolution of Oedipal conflicts is *the* path to achievement of the depressive position, subjectivity, and capacity for intimacy. While some argue that one can move through Oedipal conflicts *without* a specifically gendered set of relations, the internal "parental couple" is always foregrounded. The Oedipal negotiation, we are told, strongly influences the capacity "to form a creative couple relationship, maintain loyalty to it, and refrain from enacting unresolved Oedipal dynamics through infidelity or other boundary violations" (Nathans, p 318). But who *is* the ideal couple described in Oedipal theory?

LGTBQ people have long written about the failures of desire that mark heterosexuality, and about the culture of respectability that cloaks its fragility (McGleughlin 2008). As young queers, we knew to suspect the rhetoric of "upright" straight people. We took note of the preachers and politicians who had a secret life. And we knew the neighbors, ladies next door, and married men and women who sought solace in our arms and our bedrooms. With plenty of reason to distrust the idealized internal parental couple, we recognized that even as it was seen as a lynchpin of development, it was a fantasy.

Intrapsychic development that returns to the primacy of the child internalizing the parental couple—and of the couple performing a containing, limiting, and reflective function—cannot escape the constraints of white heterosexism. That conception seems to ignore that subject formation is also the "*social* formation of the interior mind" (Dimen 2011), thus disregarding the omnipotence of "a white imaginary that has held unwarranted sway over the unruly complexities of subject formation" (Swartz 2019, 168). Heterosexual outcome is considered "mature." I don't know how many times I've heard the terms "immature" and "arrested development" used to describe LGBTQ+ people, which to me echoes how often Black families are referred to as "broken" or "dysfunctional." Heterosexism, racism, and normative developmental theory sneak in the back door.

We are left to wonder about the internalizations of the other family configurations. What does it look like if a child has four parents, or six? What happens if she has a primary secure attachment to multiple generations, or lives under many roofs, or receives primary care at school, in communal childcare, or a place of worship? Or, if a child has parents who do not believe in the model of a parental couple that excludes a child but instead think children "grow sideways," bringing adults and their offspring into lateral contact of surprising sorts, as Stockton writes (2009)? What of a child who is separated from a mother or father because of incarceration or immigration or placement in foster care? Is such a child never able to achieve "maturity"? Or do we stretch theory to come up with a new "internal parental couple"?

Also entrenched within the Oedipal story are notions about the power of the phallus, and the centrality of castration anxiety to master relinquishing the phantasy of omnipotent control and facing reality. Yet, when we remove gender and sexual orientation from the mix in an attempt to cleanse the concept of its sexist and racist history, what are we left with? When the threatening phallic power of the father (which drive the fears of castration) is invisible, the route to these Oedipal achievements goes unexplained. Separating this theory from its basic features gives us a neutered Oedipal, one without a vital theory of sexuality. If we imagine that Oedipus can bypass racial exclusion and the historic pathologizing of gender and sexuality, aren't triangles (lacking any explicit basis for desire) and patterned relating all that remains? Why call it Oedipal? Alternatively, if we hold on to the Oedipus as a milestone on the road to achieving maturity, are we not back at problematic heteronormative and racist theorizing?

Clinical choices

Some progressive psychoanalysts sidestep the landmines of gender identification and sexual orientation intrinsic to the critique of Oedipal theorizing by putting aside the psychosocial sexual development of children. Instead, they keep their focus on clinical issues that arise in couples and adults related to what are considered unresolved Oedipal dynamics. This often involves pointing to dilemmas over triadic relating in alternative families and showing how skilled attention to hidden Oedipal knots loosens them. Many couples, including queer ones, do of course have trouble with feelings of inclusion and exclusion, jealousy, rivalry, boundary violations, and defensive triangulations that Oedipal configurations are used to describe. But I am not convinced that attention to triangular relating and dynamics *requires* the association to an Oedipal model. As the story of Nathans and her 4-year-old suggests, if you think only triangles, triangles are what you see.

For example, in Nathan's paper she attributes the decline in sexual contact in a lesbian couple she treats to difficulty maintaining psychic separateness. Accordingly, when the couple's sex life wanes and one woman starts an affair, defensive triangulation is postulated, suggesting that the threat of merger wasn't solved during an earlier Oedipal developmental phase. This hypothesis harkens back to a project I did in the mid-1980s called "The Freedom to Want Passionately: A Theoretical Exploration of Women's Desire." I explored how sexuality and desire had been consistently constructed as male, and the obstacles that created for understanding sexuality among lesbians. The few authors who examined the sexual (rather than emotional) component of lesbian relationships at the time were preoccupied with the infrequency of genital contact between long-term partners. The cause of this so-called "bed death" (McGleughlin 1987), they suggested, was that lesbians get caught in a never-ending Möbius strip of too close/too much alike (Gagnon and Simon 1973; Jay and Young 1979; Peplau and Amaro 1982; Vetere 1983).

Though theoretically disparate, these merger authors all used a heterosexual, gender-biased model and, like Nathans, proposed that lesbians need better boundaries and greater individual autonomy. This "solution" failed to grapple with studies that consistently showed that coupled heterosexual women frequently reported low desire, even those with regular sexual contact with a partner (Blumstein and Schwartz 1983). The women told researchers that they often felt they had to adapt to male sexuality (focused on genital contact), when what they wanted was a feeling of closeness better expressed in cuddling or foreplay. Also, when it was up to women to take the sexual initiative, satisfaction did not improve (Blumstein and Schwartz 1983). This data raised fundamental questions about women's desire in the absence of male power. It also challenged the conventional wisdom as applied to lesbians: If heterosexual women's lack of desire wasn't due to fusion, (though differentiation is *presumed*, not studied, between heterosexuals), why should it be the key factor for lesbians? The fusion/merger authors confuse what Jessica Benjamin (1988) calls "alienated desire" with sexual subjectivity for women, and they disregard the problem of desire for women.

My point is, in the case of the lesbian couple dealing with an affair, why are we using defensive triangulation at the expense of other ways of thinking about sexual subjectivity and desire? How are we back to focusing on the importance of an internalized parental couple to create adequate boundaries?

A new generation of queers is exploring ways to be in sexual relationships that treat the unruliness of desire as normative, as well as challenge the primacy and pleasure of long-term monogamy. But absent new developmental stories to draw from, and with clinicians regularly looking to psychoanalytic theory to understand subject formation, normative family romance (Corbett 2001) strikes again, and again. Just as psychoanalysis has been forced to unhitch gender and sexuality from the normative Oedipal, so, too, the family as ideological hotspot needs to be considered anew. After all, feminist psychoanalysts have been refiguring Oedipal dynamics for over 40 years.

Feminist psychoanalysts refigure the Oedipal

By now we are long familiar with the work of Nancy Chodorow (1978), who moved away from Oedipal theorizing and reimagined the preoedipal period as crucial for both men's and women's development, with the mother at the center. Turning the norms of health and pathology on their heads, Chodorow redeemed what had been diminished in women's domain: qualities of relatedness, connection, and attachment. Ultimately, however, she argued that the girls' identification with their mothers meant that women's relational needs may not be met by heterosexuality; and to compensate for what they couldn't get from men, they turned to mothering. The result, though, was that we were left without a model of how a girl might develop sexual agency.

Feminist psychoanalyst Jessica Benjamin first made note of this missing piece. In her groundbreaking book *Bonds of Love* (1988), she conceptualized that women may come to claim their desire through the then-novel idea of *intersubjectivity*. Benjamin theorized that the experience of having a sense of self, of knowing who I am, requires two steps: the Winnicottian transitional space where an infant registers its impulses and drives as real and coming from within and a subject powerful enough to recognize the child's desire as their own. Mothers, culturally disempowered and desexualized, could not take this role, while fathers—the carriers of desire, will, and engagement with the world—could. The result is that boys can discover their desire; with only access to the mother, girls have no such opportunity. (Girls *could* identify with/be recognized by the father and thus develop agency, Benjamin added, but it would mean a loss of culturally defined "secure" gender identification (1988).

Benjamin's model emphasized the real experience of interacting with another *subject* in which autonomy is rooted in relationship, and differentiation and connection are held in tension. Psychoanalysis could create such an intersubjective space: combining a safe holding environment, where desire is allowed to emerge freely, with a recognizing other (the therapist).

Both Chodorow and Benjamin retained a heterosexist bias, which I critiqued then, and neither could conceive of the impending explosion of categories of sex and gender and the potential for revolutionary change that would follow in next two decades. Many now think of gender not as a destination but as a shifting configuration of desire and identity (Halberstam 2018).

As you can hear, my own thinking was limited by binary constructions and focus on white women. In the 1987 project, I did, however, argue that collective social movements could and should be considered a third kind of intersubjective space, one beyond the analyst's office and the Oedipal crucible of the family. Melding Benjamin's ideas with earlier academic work I'd done reading hundreds of Women's, Gay, and Black liberation newspapers, I saw that the importance of the Women's Liberation Movement, in particular, went beyond the blooming of public political consciousness. Despite class-based and racial tensions (and the aforementioned heterosexist bias), it offered women a transitional space where they had the freedom to create, imagine, and discover themselves. Without men to establish the value of their work, or sexuality, women became subjects with the power to recognize one and other. Subject met subject. And with subjectivity came agency, the ability to act on erotic urges rather than submitting to an imposed ideal.

In fact, the early movement was partially a response to a crisis of sexuality among (mostly white) women, their determination to call out the oppressive institutions of the family and heterosexuality. This impulse created the opportunity for refusal, and in the fiery discussions that ensued, women generated ways to transform the intimate terrain where sexuality is lived out (Lewis and Joseph 1981). Sexual agency and satisfaction beckoned— and what happened at a deeply personal level also became part of the larger political struggles for liberation. For feminist theorists like Chodorow and

Benjamin, the early movement provided a glimpse of intersubjectivity, and a fresh context from which to challenge the norms of the culture. Meanwhile Black women's collectives like Combahee and the writers from *This Bridge Called My Back* (1981), like Moraga and Anzaldúa critiqued second-wave feminism for its failures of intersectionality, including the very different way Black women lived out gender oppression. Many collectives started their own powerful intersubjective spaces.

Coming full circle in my 1987 thesis, I applied intersubjective ideas to the lesbian fusion literature. If it is only in recognition from the other that one develops a sense of self and agency, women's problems of desire could not be solved by greater differentiation outside of relationship. Yet fusion and feminist-psychoanalytic theorists didn't think beyond the lesbian-feminist ideal of soft, diffuse, friendly, mutual, egalitarian encounters when considering sex for women. One model of subjectivity, I suggested, were mid-twentieth-century butch/femme relationships. "Old world" lesbians were sexual agents who took responsibility for their own desire prior to the second-wave feminist awakening. These relationships, Nestle wrote (1981), were not phony replicas of heterosexual couples but complex erotic statements expressed in an exclusively lesbian language of stance, dress, gesture, loving, courage, and autonomy. They were "erotic partnerships serving both as a conspicuous flag of rebellion and as an intimate exploration of women's sexuality. In the 1950s the courage to feel comfortable with arousing another woman became a political act" (p. 21).

Pre-Stonewall lesbian culture demonstrated that women do have very real sexual desire for one another. Further, it challenged the fusion literature's portrayal of lesbianism as a one-dimensional category that did not include gender differences among lesbians. Butch-femme couples dynamics could not be understood by counting how many times a week or month they had sex. And it wasn't just that butch-femme pairs were differentiated by gender. They lived in a sexual culture that created subjectivity and agency in its resistance to homophobic attack. Bar culture was sexy.

A return to Oedipal theorizing takes us away from applying the lessons of earlier lesbian life.

Writing in the second decade of the 21st century, I don't imagine the family as the only site of subject formation, nor its reformation as the site of liberation. My understanding of sexuality has been influenced by Laplanche, by queer theory, and by an abiding belief in the need to refigure our discussions of desire and health outside of an Oedipal family drama, which I think of as one of Swartz's "monuments." In her words, they're

> alive with meaning and ferociously signal not only their history but also their claims to future time. They become the setting for resisting change to historical narratives; for this reason, they also represent barriers to change in the search for new perspectives on both histories and future possibilities.
>
> (Swartz 2019, 169)

Although the Oedipal situation has been a taken-for-granted landscape—or monument—of psychoanalytic theory, "it is neither solid [and I would add, scientific] nor continuous, and is always enmeshed with the phantastic and phantomic" (Swartz 2019, 168). The dismantling of a monument "ruptures (and) shake the solidity of an imaginary" (Swartz 2019, 168). Bring on the rupture. To sever Oedipal theory from its ghosts requires a change in the symbolic. This can only happen when alternative narratives supplant traditional theorizing in our social unconscious. When other meaningful kinship networks are built, they engender other modes of being, feeling, and knowing—creating other kinds of internal constructions that also can constitute "health." Joyous subcultures are built from our marginalization; they're transformative to us and to our worlds. Other ways of living shift the meaning of the phantasy of omnipotent control—who is in or out, and what it means to be excluded or to suffer loss.

Chapter 14

Translation

An alternative developmental mother story (2020)

My own mother practiced the art of not knowing, forgetting, and lying. She wanted to break from the Judaism she feared would doom her. Because she wouldn't be Jewish, she couldn't interact with her family. So she broke from them. Her father, dead when she was 17, disappeared from stories; she voluntarily lost her sexless mother. Without contact with her family, she felt free to create other narratives. In the habit of not knowing, forgetting, and lying, she persisted. She lied about my own father's death: he, too, disappeared from our narrative. She was denying *origin*, hers and ours.

Because I am her daughter, loss and not knowing are my inheritance. Of course, there are many other inheritances. These are internal, unconscious, drive-inflected experiences, as well as relational and intersubjective knowings. But here I want to focus on sexuality. The biggest shame I felt in the private girls' school I attended on full scholarship was not being less privileged or fatherless, but having—not once or twice, but three times—a different last name than my mother. Everyone could see it on the class list. Marriage shame. I was humiliated by her wrongness made public, exemplified not only by her being a failed woman, a divorcée, but also by the obviousness of her sexual life. She must have been having sex. A lot of it. Her low-cut clothes, big breasts, and bad rental address coded us being from the "the wrong side of the tracks," the opposite of Upper East Side WASPs, even as her own aspirations had everything to do with feigning respectability. She structured her life around a series of "omissions" that would help her belong, and yet she remained an outlier. No matter how many times she married, how relentless or performative her effort, the family form failed her, and she failed the family. And no matter the failures, she clung to normative family ideology.

DOI: 10.4324/9781032670348-18

The struggle with the complexity of who she was—the feeling of ver-boten behavior, our (my mother's and mine) unconscious identifications—meant that I sought out the only other "wrong" girls in the school: two Jews, one Catholic, one African American, one Puerto Rican, and one West Side bohemian. Later, I lived queer lives with girls like them. In her appall, and my abjection, I had to lose my mother before I could take her back. That, too, is my inheritance.

I didn't lose my mother's lessons about sexuality and identity, however. I learned the lies behind "right living," the failures of desire, the fragility of heterosexuality and respectability. But that's not all. In the break from Oedipal rivalries (to remain within a psychoanalytic frame), my mother was my lover, though I was not hers. She didn't like women—certainly not as lovers, even friends. She was a man's man. But my mother had real sexual subjectivity. And her desire couldn't be policed. This marked her as gender nonconforming and family-busting. Hungry for her own pleas-ure, embodied, she was the first powerful woman with a desire of her own whom I ever loved, jazzy with sexual subjectivity. I'll call that mixture of sexual power and gender wrongness "butch" for now. So, to her implied butch, I became her declared femme. And I have done what femmes do: try to make the wrongness of the other right. I thought, before I came out, *I will never be like my mother. No bad men for me.* But I wanted nothing more than her happiness. I wanted her to fit. My mother named my queer-ness defiance, but it might have been about achieving respectability for her (the worst kind of substitution). I wouldn't do it with a man exactly, but I did manage three things my mother yearned for but didn't have: a lifelong partner, a "real" job, and a mortgage. All the things she and I were ashamed of—her not choosing between a sexual life and motherhood, her matriar-chal insistence that her children were hers and that men were peripheral, her hidden ethnicity—I claim them. I queered the family, but I am still my mother's daughter. And she is still not performing "mother."

Halberstam (2011) tells us that women are often the repository for the "generational logics of being and becoming" and transmit that logic to the next generation (p. 70). Who was my mother becoming when she sought a place unfettered by memory, tradition, or a usable past? Forgoing a mother, she did not receive the logics of her becoming.

Psychoanalysis frowns on severing the temporal link, disrupting the con-tinuity of what has come before (Lemma 2013). Our bodies link us indel-ibly to our parents, theory tells us, and if we detach ourselves from what came before, we are at grave risk, masochistic. Instead, psychoanalysis offers us mourning—remembering, repeating, working through. In my own psychoanalysis, I dutifully reach for her pathology, her badness, and I dwell in what it means to be without a family, history, religion, or culture. I know intimately what it means to form around another; I know the disorientation of not knowing who you are when you break from those who form you (Butler 2005).

Is my mother's choice to cut herself off from history and origin masochistic? Or does the effort to live in some other way interrupt a familiar Oedipal story that is bound to reproduce exactly what has come before? Bersani (1986) names masochism as the counternarrative of sexuality that undergirds the propulsive linear maturational story installed by psychoanalysis; he suggests that the heroic organizing narrative defines sexuality as an exchange of intensities between individuals. But the masochistic version he tells constitutes a "condition of broken negotiations with the world, a condition in which others merely set off the self-shattering masochism of jouissance" (p. 41). If my mother's masochism, in his language, constitutes a "condition of broken negotiations with the world," then her "self-shattering masochism of jouissance" opens possibility. In this broken line of unbeing, my mother is forging a way out of an endlessly repeating story. She is rejecting generational inheritance. She is refusing to merely transmit a set idea of who a woman can become.

Stockton (2009), employing Edelman (2005), writes,

> The figure of the child as the emblem of parents (impossible) continuity spawns delusional visions . . . of the seamless reproduction of oneself whose future is always represented by (one's) children. Thus, the future and our children are bound together in a kind of frightening and (hermetically sealed) reproductive futurism.
>
> (p. 13)

For Edelman, like Bersani, the death drive, "its energetic jouissance," is an "open-eyed denial of a person's continuance" (2005, 12). My mother's choice to cut herself off from connections might be seen as a self-preservative death drive—an unconscious choice to live in the break, to move toward pleasure albeit with unbearable pain.

The idea of the break (Moten 2003) is made infamous in the wake of slavery when children were routinely separated from their families (Halberstam

2011). Halberstam reads Saidiya Hartman (2008), who writes that "the only sure inheritance passed from one generation to the next was this loss and it defined the tribe . . . an identity produced by negation" (p. 103). Hartman's book *Lose Your Mother* indicates a loss that has always already happened for African Americans. Using her text, Halberstam argues against a simple genealogical account of history that stretches back in time through the family line. It is the colonized mind, he argues, that is passed down Oedipally from generation to generation (p. 132).

Halberstam asks, are there other models of generation, temporality, and politics available to world-making? He urges us to think "in terms of the negation of the subject rather than formation, the disruption of lineage rather than its continuation, the undoing of self rather than its activation" (p. 126). Losing one's mother, Halberstam suggests, frees us from the Oedipal model and allows us other models of time, space, place, and connection.

What I have been naming as my mother's unknowing, forgetting, and lying, in Halberstam's hands, is not pathology but radical edge; a potent intervention. Of course, my mother didn't "choose" as I imply here. And this re-visioning story leaves out her suffering and mine. As kids we wanted to be "normal," and we wanted her to be normal, too. But I don't mean this story as a true object-relational version of anything like what really happened. I don't want to draw any linear connections about my mother and a theory of agency, identification, or subjectivity. I cannot know what enigmatic messages she passed on to me or what kind of libidinized object I was for her, or how my efforts to translate her messages reflect their potential meaning. And, again, I don't imagine the family as the only site of subject formation, nor its reformation as the site of liberation. Both ignore the social as it is lodged in our unconscious and lived out in our material lives. But in this inflected translation, my mother is forging a way out of the reproduction of mothering, of the generational transmission of who she can become.

Women and queers, Halberstam says, *should* forget, *should* lose our mothers: "Delinking the process of generational inheritance from the force of historical progress is a queer project" (p. 70). In fact, if the queer project seeks to uncouple becoming from the supposedly organic and immutable forms of family identity and inheritance (Halberstam 2011), we might say my mother was the first queer I ever knew. Her own break from stultifying forms of family life came not from mourning but from refusal. She uncoupled motherhood from right living, wedging open space for new forms of kinship, maybe creating room for my queerness to grow.

Without my mother's welcome, without a history or culture, my own opening to women—to "our sharp jester's tongues, our cartwheels of pleasure, the queen's own pearl at our fingertips"—was everything (Broumas 1977, 47). I found home in other queer minds and theirs in mine, the basis of one psychoanalytic story of subjectivity. Coming into lesbian identity, finding community with other women, living collectively, being recognized and wanted, being eroticized (Sedgwick 1990), saved me. It was about pleasure, and it was about survival, and it was about developing agency. And, of course, it was about critique.

And so we raised our children queerly with other families where queer has meant not just the consolidation of normative identity with two same gendered people but an effort to live alternatively. We belonged to a tribe. We tried for loose collectivity, for no nuclear, no simple two. And so we rub up against and disrupt the symbolic order. And sometimes we fall into queer heteronormativity. The struggle for recognition as queer families can manifest in the language of legal rights and recognition—"Our relationships are just like yours"—but those claims are often covers for a deeper set of longings: to be seen as whole, as full citizens (McGleughlin 2008). The urge to be included in a society that is organized not just by one's origin story but by a place in its primary institutions—like family, even if we critique them—is powerful. The underbelly of this, of course, is the way we remain psychologically tied to *belonging* in the very culture we forswear. The psychic reproduction of certain desires is not a matter of individual wish or personal alienation but is inculcated into our hearts and minds and lives in the symbolic realm. This is how ideology is replicated. It hails us to become a particular kind of subject (McGleughlin 2008). Still, we risk. Like my mother, but with intention. The kinship we make is buzzing. The view from the margins is keen.

Our adult kids are actively living other forms of world-making. They are not spared the hunger to belong, nor do they escape the symbolic meanings of mother or father or origin, despite having a very different "nuclear family" and forms of kinship. But being queer is also a difference that matters. And they wouldn't give up our queer world, for anything. They are shaped by queer pleasures.

Max, our now-grown son, is rethinking origins. As the child of more than a few queers, Oedipal narratives fail him. He writes that while origins have, by their nature, a singular starting point, for him, origin scenes, such as the primal scene in his dreams and the scene of physical conception, invariably raise questions that cannot be satisfied by a singular symbol that marks a first point of becoming. He writes,

> These two scenes must be held in tension. . . . Without a marking point for my beginning, a congruency between my mothers' creative act and biological reproduction, and in the absence of a knowable legacy, projected into the future, I began my translation [of origin] empathetically, focusing on those messages contained in affect, in the unseen, with little regard for the visually discernable origin of a birth father or the physical reality of a family history, about which I knew little.
>
> (M. McGleughlin 2017)

Origin is rooted in affect, in longing. "[History is] a thing which is not yet there," Munoz (2010) says.

We rework origin, make new models, disrupt. But Max and his sister are his mother's son and daughter. The enigmatic messages we pass to the children, like the ones our mothers passed to us, seek new translation (Laplanche 1987). Certain recurring aspects of ourselves return again and again, and no narrative can contain them. Because we cannot interpret these messages, they remain as the unconscious core of our subjectivity, signifying something important but unknowable and eroticized, disrupting psychological life. Subjectivity—interiority and unconscious fantasy—are built from the labor of translation, but they alert us to the implantation of the other, the inevitable mystery of the other inside us. The repetitive presence of these messages breaches our continuity of being (already a fantasy) and suggests the nonsovereignty of the self (McGleughlin 2020). Identity is always disrupted, nonsovereign, fractal.

And identity matters. Some of my queer patients come because they need my susceptibility. They feel crushed by norms that produce a them that feels strange to themselves. They are trying to make a break—as I had to—with an atmosphere, an expectation, an insistence on a way to be, to be able to create something else. They want me to "wander away from pre-fab ways of understanding . . . (to know) the unlabeled bed, the off-site Eden, a preference for the uncategorizable" (Koestenbaum 1978, xii, xiii). Sometimes they want a mother, like my mother, cut off from the weight of history without being cut off from desire. They don't want to be their mother; they don't want *me* to be their mother. (If I am the same mother, only better, than the mother they already have, the affective future cannot be very different.) Their health does not necessarily require an internalized parental couple, when so often that image rejects their queerness in subtle and not-so-subtle ways. They want other ways to live and love that they can and can't imagine. They think I might belong to the same tribe that they do, that we might share, in Eyal Rozmarin's words (2019), a notion of an unconscious that is not *within* subjects but *between* them. With Butler (2005), they might believe, "I am not formed once and definitively, but continuously or repeatedly. I am still being formed as I form myself in the here and now" as I form myself (queerly) with you. In such explorations outside the norms, we open up an imagined future.

My mother lived in an imagined future in which emotions circulate between bodies (Ahmed 2004), and there is emergence and potentiality in relation to the body and to the way it links with other bodies (Massumi 1995). There is the push to collectives and the pull to their undoing. There is affect, and desire, and it connects us. It is the animating condition of our lives.

Part 4

The negative

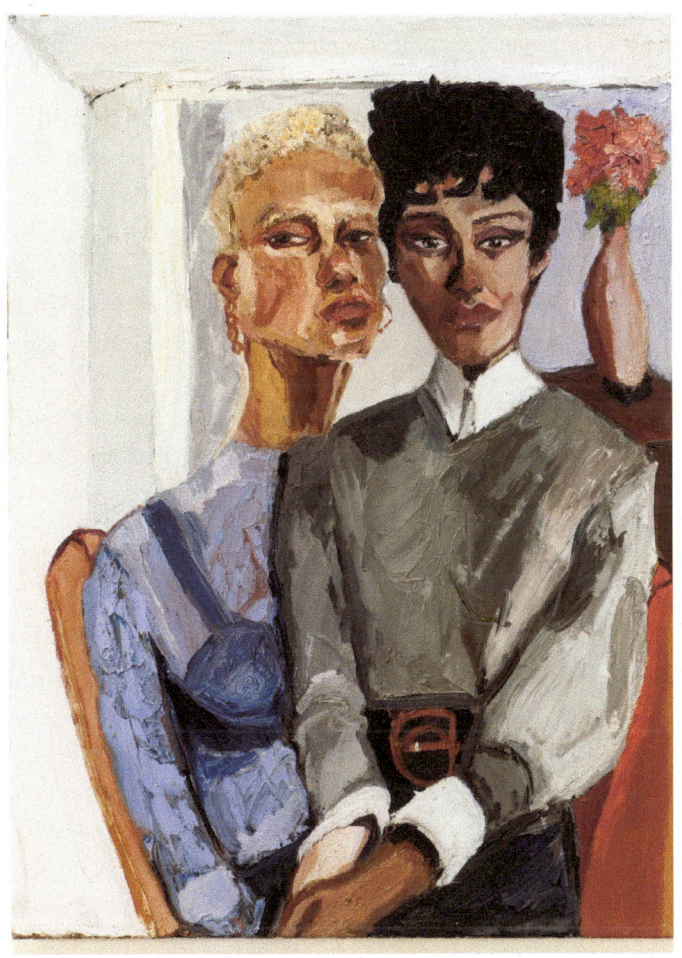

Figure PIV.1 *She knows/she doesn't know.* **24x18. McGleughlin**

DOI: 10.4324/9781032670348-19

Introduction: where we are heading: blurring boundaries and reaching from within and without

When Marlene Dumas (2008) writes,

> There is a crisis with regard to representation. They are looking for Meaning as if it was a Thing. As if it was a girl, required to take her panty off. As if she would want to do so, as soon as the true Interpreter comes along. As if there was something to take off,

(p. 63)

I resonate. Like Dumas, I want to stop looking for meaning as if it is a thing waiting for its interpreter.

Part 4 continues the work of my own clinical writing in the enactive mode (Naiburg 2015) through an even more radical experiment than that attempted earlier. The main clinical paper, "The Analyst's Necessary Non-sovereignty and the Generative Power of the Negative," returns to my core themes but is not structured linearly. Instead, I envisioned its three main parts as lying alongside each other, to offer alternative ways of understanding the negative: through thinking, perceiving and bewilderment. Like the dialogue in Lauren Berlant and Lee Edelman's *Sex, or the Unbearable* (2014) that inspires me, this paper is not meant to be read forward toward a decisive conclusion. My hope is that the blank spots and gaps created in my encounter with Berlant and Edelman—and in my dialogue with you—will destabilize and open space for creativity, even if missed connections and dissonance remain. Like Marlene Dumas, I want to stop looking for meaning as if it is a thing waiting for its interpreter.

To be specific, in the section of "The Analyst's Necessary Sovereignty" that focuses on understanding through thinking and reason, I briefly introduce the idea of the field. Field theory has radically altered psychoanalysis and stands, along with the idea of the third, as a major advance in our thinking. Since Baranger, Baranger, and Mom (1983) brought the concept into psychoanalysis 40 years ago, theorists have been drawing on it to consider how the analytic situation is forged between patient and analyst in unconscious and bidirectional ways. The field is now "the name we give to the emotional dimension created by the unconscious affective interaction and interactivity of the patient and analyst" (Levine 2022, 7). It *is* the narrative action of the session as it "reflect(s) the emotional disturbances caused by the presence, actions, and interventions of the analyst," and it "offers an unconscious running commentary on the quality and condition of the analytic relationship and process" (Levine, p. 8). But if the field is also "the patient's experience of the degree of accessibility and availability of the analyst's mind" (Levine, p. 8), who is its reader?

There is significant divergence between field theorists (see Stern 2013) over whether the analyst can, in fact, read the field. Here, I critique Bionian field theorists for their implicit sovereignty: the claim to having a greater capacity than our patients to know, read, or service the field (Civitarese 2019). This stance not only obscures the unconscious symmetry between patient and analyst but it also strengthens the belief in a knowing self, separate from other selves.

In the next section of the paper, inspired by the psychologically savvy *Sex or The Unbearable*, I center perceiving and attempt to have a dialogue with you, the reader. I contemplate the problem of transforming core psychic fantasy, and the limits to doing so. Employing Berlant and Edelman's language, I produce a "phantasmatic staging" of their ideas through a constructed clinical case presentation. This staging of the telling of the case (and every telling of every case) puts into play "reaction, accommodation, transference, exchange, and the articulation of narratives" (Berlant and Edelman 2014, viii). My hope is that it disrupts your sense of what is true.

I also play with how roles imperceptibly determine meaning. As the analyst/writer, I perform as the patient and make indistinguishable whose history and experience are being narrated. This ushers in a different kind of nonsovereignty of the self. While Part 2's "Do We Lose or Find Ourselves in the Negative" blurred the lines between patient and analyst by covering the patient's history with my own, here I use the first person to invite the reader to imagine the story as all mine. There is no longer a patient and an analyst but one merged figure, problematizing the relationship between looker and looked at, self and other, patient and analyst. This fogging of distinction and origin suggests the existence of an unstable nonunitary self. That is to say, we are always ourselves and the other, not just contiguous but maybe continuous.

Yet this experiment is chancier than earlier ones. If what I create is taken as my actual history rather than the fiction that it is, I risk intruding on my patients, supervisees, family, and others: veiling or obliterating the self that they might need me to be. And yet, I mean to upend certainty about who I am, or who anyone is. In confessing the unreliability of my tale, I alert the reader to the disappearance of the patient as narrativized subject.

Motivated by the idea that aesthetic experience can make it easier to access the creativity and power of the negative, the final section of the paper explores bewilderment and the art of Agnes Martin. Martin's paintings and the words she wrote about them contain the spirit of the negative that I am trying to bring to our work as analysts. It is the force of the negative—her helplessness, nonsovereignty, and vulnerability, sometimes even entropy, regression, repetition, and defeat—that allows Martin her generativity. In her work, and sometimes in ours as analysts, we enter chaos, vibrate with the unknowable, and let the field run through us (Blanchfield 2016). Perhaps you and I can create a reader/writer field that might enact themes from the case itself.

Beyond the hope of bringing the reader into the experience of the clinical encounter, I want something else. If, as I believe, psychoanalytic writing is the analyst's story and not a representation of the real, or patient's story, how might we tell this story that shifts our gaze and implicates ourselves? Might there be a narrative strategy for clinical storytelling that does not just survey the patient as object but requires the writer to be vulnerable, sparking us all, including the reader, to interrogate ourselves and each other?

The book's last chapter, "The Impossibility of Meaning: Joining and Rejoining," emerged in dialogue about the ideas I developed in "The Analyst's Necessary Nonsovereignty." That paper was first published in *Psychoanalytic Dialogues*, in 2020, and the same issue featured the generous, thought-provoking discussions of Donnel B. Stern, Antonio Ferro, and Amy Schwartz Cooney. Their comments and questions helped me deepen my own thinking. Here I bring their voices forward to set the stage for my responses.

I clarify issues of subjectivity and nonsovereignty and suggest that sovereignty always rests upon the idea of a unitary knowable subject, a concept I interrogate. I am asking readers to consider how our subjectivities oscillate between more sovereign and nonsovereign poles. Our nonsovereign pole puts us in touch with aspects of human experience that *cannot be represented*, which I refer to as the negative, but can still meaningfully register in us. By underscoring this dialectic, I'm seeking to turn readers' attention to the moments when an analyst is broken in on (not necessarily consciously), allowing access to something that is more in line with an area of nonsovereignty in ourselves (in order to help our patients access their own). This move challenges identity and necessarily summons our vulnerability.

Working from our nonsovereignty then shifts our analytic stance, as I try to demonstrate both in my discussion of the limits of field theory and in an expanded clinical section. Through the narrative experiment in the presentation of a clinical case, I ask the reader to imagine a figure that emerges rather than one that originates from the position of a reified self that exists prior to an encounter with another. In merging the figures of self and other, I offer a fictionalized (yet in another sense real, as well) means of perceiving the "you" as inseparable from the "I." This blending offers an ontological challenge to the notion of a discrete self that is in the position to know highlighting how the asymmetrical nature of a psychoanalytic frame can bypass the deeper *symmetry* between the unconscious of the analyst and patient. I return to the art of Agnes Martin and the philosophy of Elizabeth Grosz to refocus on the importance of bewilderment.

Without focusing on the unknowableness of what lies outside symbolic representation, we can omit an undertheorized dimension of the theory: the generative force and intrinsic relationality in what will never be formulated but is between us.

Chapter 15

The analyst's necessary nonsovereignty and the generative power of the negative (2019)

One life to live, to live again. Singularity recast as multiple. That is, one subjectivity run through by a performance not one's own. Here at the authorless site of my thrill, producing a replacement time in place of time . . . something expresses in me, the way ground water is said to express intermittently as a spring. . . . A sense of it having run under all along.

—Brian Blanchfield, *Proxies*, 2016

Psychoanalysis traditionally values articulating what is hidden, replacing symptoms with narratives, making the unconscious conscious. With the increasing recognition, across many schools of psychoanalysis, of the importance not only of what is hidden but also what might never have been represented, the field has been intent on finding ways to symbolize. A growing body of work, including my own (Director 2016; Grossmark 2018; Levine, Reed, and Scarfone 2013; McGleughlin 2001, 2011, 2015a, 2015b), addresses our engagement with unrepresented states in which symbolic representation has been foreclosed, as it is in massive psychic trauma or primitive mental states. (See Levine 2012 for a discussion of the nuances of registration and representation.) This scrutiny of what remains unregistered, unsymbolized, and unknowable has usually focused on its power to disrupt, prevent integration, or limit thinking. The fundamental assumption remains that what is unrepresented needs to find ground for representation; what is unsymbolized needs marks. We work to discover what additional technique may be required of the analyst in order for psychic representation to occur prior to symbolization. Yet what is not represented may also be nonpathological, ubiquitous, and generative. It may even be the creative pulse of being human.

DOI: 10.4324/9781032670348-20

Our most obvious encounter with the unrepresented comes when we face experiences that defy linguistic description. In my own work, feelings of wordless chaos and vertigo engulfed me as I sat with one particular patient's prolonged silences and pull towards death. That treatment (with Sarah, whom I introduced in Part 1) was the most dramatic of my career, in part because of what the agitated months of silence unleashed in me. As I struggled to hold onto meaning, that treatment compelled me to approach an objectless existence, corresponding to my patient's experience—a terrifying absence at the center where I endured forceful sensory states outside the limits of representation.[1]

In this paper, I approach the unrepresented not as void to be filled but as a creative force, what I will be calling the negative, that expands beyond ordinary unconsciousness.[2] Efforts to know the enigmatic elude our grasp, but the effort to translate enigma is unremitting and generative. I want us to value aspects of subjectivity and identity that are not representable (Phelan 1994, 1). This is not "calling for greater visibility of the hitherto unseen," as in symbolizing the unsymbolized (an operation that marks the hierarchical gaze of the symbolizing analyst upon the non-symbolizing patient), but examining how we honor the enigmatic, the "power of the unmarked," in our clinical work and writing. I am interested in a way of analytic being that does not take surveillance of the other as an aim (Phelan 1994, 1–2).

Grappling with the negative

Unrepresented experience is often linked with the negative. The negative has a complex history, starting with Freud's important negation paper (1925) and continuing in the wondrous work of Andre Green (1999). I use "the negative" here in two interrelated ways. The first draws attention "to a state of things which, contrary to appearances, continues to exist even when the sense cannot perceive it, not only in the external world, but in the internal world consciousness" (Green 1999, 16). The second refers to a force that disrupts the positive, challenging our sense of the way things are. I use both meanings to engage negativity's potential to transform our clinical work and psychoanalytic writing.

The negative runs through all life and connects the living to the non-organic forces and qualities of the material world (Grosz 2008). As a force inherent in being, its valence is neither positive nor negative in a value sense, neither creative nor destructive. Generations "of vibratory waves and rhythms traverse the body and make of the body a link with forces it cannot otherwise perceive and act on" (p. 23). It cannot be symbolically represented in human language because it is beyond representation. This is not the negative as necessarily traumatic or unbearable, but something that cannot be symbolized while at the same time binding us to all things. It is an impossibility that returns again and again like "a force that runs through us" (Blanchfield 2016, 127) and between us.

We might sense the force of the negative as disrupter when trauma splits us open, dispersing and casting us into an unbearable sensory experience, as it did with the silent patient Sarah referenced earlier. Such inchoate sensory states are usually outside of perception because they are overwhelming. When these "shards" land and are slowed in time and space, they affect our bodies and potentially frame something new. Despite the terrifying silence and "necessary vertigo" I experienced (McGleughlin 2011), the inexplicable connection I felt to my silent patient alerted me to a powerful pull: the vibrations, networks, and fields that can link us to each other and the universe and that have the power to transform (Grosz 2008).

These terrifying and transformative aspects of the negative co-exist. We might also be alerted to the negative when something unseen and powerful interrupts an idea of ourselves or our world, as when we are unmade and strange to ourselves.[3] Or we might become aware of the negative in moments of awe, as when we blur with another in spiritual communion. Or in sex. Or in an analytic session in which boundaries dissolve and something that was contained in separate bodies or temporal registers flows in from outside, revealing an unlivable chaotic force (Grosz 2008). Or we might know it when we feel affective power stir in us, as when we respond to nonrepresentational artists, such as Agnes Martin or Mark Rothko, who frame and unframe our universe, attuning us to something greater than our individual subjectivity. When I saw Martin's work in the spiral of New York's Guggenheim Museum and attuned with my fellow museum goers to the collective state of immanence that permeated the exhibit, I experienced how the unrepresentable takes us out of our perceptual range and alerts us to what is unbounded in space and time, connecting us to each other.

These examples share ways the negative refuses our coherence, our sense of discreet separate subjectivity. Queer theorists Berlant and Edelman, in *Sex or the Unbearable* (2014), refer to negativity as "the psychic and social incoherencies and divisions, conscious and unconscious alike, that trouble any totality or fixity of identity. It denotes . . . the relentless force that unsettles the fantasy of sovereignty" (2014, vii). That relentless force may be close to Lacan's concept of the real: that which cannot be symbolized or even imagined, a recurrent impossibility that returns again and again and is present for all subjects.

When Berlant and Edelman deemphasize self-knowledge, authority, and self-control to emphasize our misrecognitions of ourselves, they undo the organizing principle that we call identity and pose a relational alternative to identificatory processes. The negative draws our attention to the limits of individual subjectivity to contain or explain what runs between us. We don't make sense to ourselves, and we can't, yet our connection to others lies in that "can't." In the acknowledgment of the limit, we confront our own unknowableness and *need* for the other. This is the negative at work. Preferring their use of "sovereignty" and "nonsovereignty" to the more familiar psychoanalytic term *subjectivity*, I focus on how we cannot ever know ourselves. Encountering ourselves as non-sovereign is to encounter relationality itself.

Inspired by both the form and content of Berlant and Edelman's book (2014), this paper is an engagement with and loose application of ideas that emerge from their dialogue, where they enter the negative through an "encounter with the estrangement and intimacy of being in relation" (p. viii) in order to imagine new ways of world-making. Following on their use of dialogue, highlighting inevitable gaps, risks, lack of control, and failures in communication, I stage a dialogue with you, my imagined reader. In the encounter with another's ideas, blank spots and caesuras become available in missed connection and dissonance as much as in synchrony. Those gaps in understanding that we often patch over in everyday analytic life create disequilibrium, breaks that can open space for creativity even if they remain unmarked. I want this paper to do the same. I invite disequilibrium, in an effort to enact a critique of psychoanalytic valuing of logic over affect, symbols over sensations, knowledge over uncertainty, analyst over patient. I'll write in three discrete sections, laying each section side by side to offer different ways of understanding the possibilities and limits of the negative. Like their dialogue, this paper is not meant to be read forward toward a putative end.

In the first section, I critique post-Bionian work on the analytic field where unrepresented experience is valued and may become manifest: this theory makes room for the analyst's nonsovereignty while simultaneously portraying the analyst as acting in sovereign ways. I suggest that this sovereignty is a necessary consequence of the pressure to make and represent meaning. In the second section, I experiment with how our clinical writing might reflect nonsovereignty; I write with the performative "I," combining my story with a patient's as if we were one person, introducing the unpredictable with you, the reader. Finally, in Section 3, I turn to the abstract paintings of Agnes Martin, whose art highlights work in the negative that is not translated, or translatable, but is felt as a persistent force through time, a source of struggle and of pleasure, too.

1. Bionian field theorists: working with the unrepresented but forgetting nonsovereignty

Influenced by Bion, a number of contemporary writers have expanded our understanding of somatic resonance (Lombardi 2005), the field's contracting the patient's illness (Ferro 2009), functional symbiosis, and other forms of mutual containment (Goldberg 2012; Ogden 2005; Civitarese 2008). They underscore that from a live sensory state, sensation can be translated to affect representation, mentalized, and ultimately fantasized. This process involves loosening or destroying old links while forging new ones. Their focus is on "reclaiming and enhancing the mind's capacity to transform . . . emotional and sensory experience not by increasing symbolic capacities alone, but by broadening domains and types of psychical experience" (Peltz and Goldberg 2013, 662). The belief in taking up negative capability is seminal and brilliant. Post-Bionian field theory, more than most theories, makes room for the power of the unmarked to influence the analytic field, thereby explicitly acknowledging the analyst's nonsovereignty. Paradoxically, the theory articulates, but does not illustrate, the unremitting power of the negative by imagining that the analyst can and should interpret the field, asserting the analyst's sovereign position before the negative and omitting the value of the analyst's vulnerability.

Making room for the unexpected

Ferro (1993) situates analyst and analysand in the field, the site where meaning is happening at this very moment. Horizontal and vertical, the field includes all sources of emotional data—the interior of a consulting room and the interior of the minds—in interaction. This loosens the grip of old narrative organizations (such as yesterday's roles in the transference) as characters are freed from the burden of representation and allowed a new fluidity (Frankel 2017). Meanings are not fixed; individual and historical realities are deferred. The analytic couple uses the characters in the field to reflect upon emotional possibilities that float freely, untethered from manifest content (Ferro 1993). A conclusive assessment of the analytic path is not required.

In this model, the analyst's narrative comment (something as accurate or opaque as "it's foggy here") is proposed not as a deep interpretation of the patient's psyche but to offer a first level of containment and transformation of the unconscious fantasy of the field. The analytical dialogue, described as "a kind of forge, where interpretations acquire form and sense thanks to hermeneutic cooperation in which the patient possesses equal, though not identical, dignity of function . . . " (Bezoari, Ferro, and Politi 1994, 38) is understood to be founded intersubjectively, through the unconscious communication of two. This idea is appreciated and documented by disparate writers in American relational and field theorists as well as by Ogden's work (1994) on the intersubjective third. The radical edge of this theory allows for nonsovereignty because subjectivity is not discrete, and play invites the unpredictable.

But how do the field theorists work clinically as they describe the shared creation within the field? The field represents an amalgam of analyst/patient contributions, yet Ferro still characterizes the analyst as the receiver and metabolizer of the patients' needs (including distortions) for object relations that have not been satisfied, "the primitive parts [of the patient] need to obtain access to symbolization there in the consulting room" (1993, 927). For the analytic couple, this involves

transforming into an object-relationship, in which separation and communication are stressed, those aspects of the relationship previously dominated by confused, manipulatory, narcissistic ways of thinking and expression. Viewed in this light, the analyst or patient's contributions, whether we call them "interpretations," "associations," "memories," or "dreams" (better "accounts of dreams") assume relatively less importance. The most important thing is the transformative function actually *performed by these parts of the dialogue, in so far as they are symbolic and conceivable.*

(Bezoari, Ferro, and Politi 1994, 39; my italics)

Telling the story together in this way, Ferro believes, contains transformative potential. Yet there is a sleight of hand. We have a function "performed by these parts of the dialogue." Which agency, which performer? Who is seen as "confused, manipulatory, narcissistic"? The couple? The field? Pronouns drop out because the characters are seen as intertwined aspects of the field. To reiterate, Ferro and his colleagues describe the analytical dialogue as "a kind of forge," in which *hermeneutic cooperation* allows the patient to possesses "dignity of function" (Bezoari, Ferro, and Politi 1994, 38).

This implies the field represents a true amalgam of bidirectional analyst/patient projective identifications, yet Ferro still concludes that the patient transfers to the psychoanalyst those needs (and distortions) for object relations that have not been satisfied. The analyst works to enable the patient to metabolize the paralyzing projective identifications: "This may be a slow, laborious and often painful task: the 'betaloma', . . .—clumps of beta elements which contrast with thought—is owned, digested, transformed and, if possible, resolved in a narration which the patient is capable of owning" (Ferro 1993, 926). But if symbolization is facilitated by a spirit of [mutually nonsovereign] play with its "accompanying suspension of reality judgments . . . " (p. 35) how does that square with the analyst's assessment of the patient's confusion, manipulation, and narcissistic needs?

There are emergent phenomena of intertwined subjectivities, a bidirectional field, even shared psychosensory experience, but it is primarily the patient's *projections* and the analyst's *capacities* that are narrated when the route towards transformation lies in the analyst's capacity for reverie, for sensing the bi-personal unconscious fantasy of the field, for the often silent metabolizing of the patient's projections. Despite the analyst's willingness to "allow himself to be involved in—one might almost say captured by—the forces of the field" (Ferro 2009), he is still able to

> reaffirm his status as a third party through interpretation and take a "second look" which makes it possible to view from a distance the process that he helps to initiate, but whose specificities he must be able to grasp and describe.
>
> (Ferro 1993, 917)

He can "wake from the dream" and interpret (Ferro 1993).[4]

Despite the field theorists' agreement that the analyst will have divisions and bastions (Baranger and Baranger 2008) and their articulation of the importance of negative capability and nonsovereignty, in practice, those

theories are obscured in this sovereign stance. Where is the analyst's (problematic, implicit, presumed, unconscious) contribution described as it is
enacted with the patient? (Stern 2013).

A self-fulfilling loop can be seen or imagined in Ferro and colleague's
portraiture. As Hartman (2015) notes, field theory's

> bracketing the patient's primitive states and the analyst's higher order
> symbolic capacity stations the analyst in the role of portrait maker and
> analysand in the role of model, roles that by definition reproduce exactly
> the images (container/contained) that their roles were functionally
> designed to produce.
>
> (p. 242)

While there may be new joint characters in the field, they are photographed
by the analyst/director's gaze and establish a field mimetic of the analyst's vision. This reproduction of the known aims to assure us of our self-
authority and presence (Phelan 1994). The concept of a joined intertwined
patient/analyst couple minimizes that the analyst is marked with capacity
and "takes she who is unmarked and re-marks her, rhetorically and imag-
istically, while he who is marked with value is left unremarked" (Phelan
1994, 5). The beauty of characters freed from representing to just presenting (Frankel 2017) is then circumscribed by a predictable set of power
relations that can limit new relational imaginations/new dreams. Despite
Ferro's acknowledgement of nonsovereignty, and faith in the deeply intersubjective and dialogic nature of the work and his belief in the necessity
of the patient's contribution for making sense of the field, his discussion
includes few signs of an inchoate, divided, vulnerable analyst. Relational
thinkers have noted that the field is limited by an Other who is absent as a
full human being (avoiding the intimacy, risk, and estrangement of mutual
relationship the field theorists deem unnecessary for psychic transformation). But I am adding there are also limits when we only illustrate the
analyst's moves towards symbolization.

The view of the analyst as reader of the field or GPS signaling device
(Levine 2013) privileges the analyst's competence—her alpha function—obscuring what can't be represented and functionally ignoring the
analyst's ontological inability to know herself, even as the theory acknowledges the same. Levine refers to the "representational imperative" (Levine 2013, 671) that assumes "the primary function of the psyche is to deal

with raw overwhelming sensation by taming beta elements . . . and creating symbols, thoughts, narratives" (p. 671). This underemphasizes the potential in raw sensory states that go untranslated (Goldberg 2012) where there is creativity born of destruction—breaking up old meanings to allow reconfiguring. When the analyst primarily demonstrates capability and does not reveal the psychic states associated with the destruction of the links of her own mind, for example, negative capability, something may be foreclosed: the possibilities that emerge from the experience of living together in a shared contained entropy (which would be unbearable alone).

I want to distinguish the critique I am making of the analyst's assumption of sovereignty from the recognition that some of our patients may require a great many things from us, including our capacity to think when they cannot and to foster representation of unrepresented experience in the sense of figurability (Botella and Botella 2005; Levine 2013). We have many roles and responsibilities towards our patients. For patients with poorly represented mental states, or what Alvarez (2012) calls the undrawn patient, our willingness to be the ground on which they might construct a self is essential. For the undrawn patient, psychic touch, our willingness to seek and engage our patients, may be necessary to catalyze growth. But we should not confuse the analyst's capacity to be helpful with sovereignty. However important it is to lend my thinking/dreaming/creating mind to my undrawn patient in a given moment, something of my *incapacity* may also be important. While reorienting from the mutuality of unconscious communication to the "asymmetry needed to treat the patient" (Ferro and Civitarese 2013, 650) is necessary, we know less about the importance of working "undone." For instance, in treating Martin with an (a), when I bore my helplessness, despair, and aloneness, and conveyed that to my patient rather than trying to contain and narrate hers, something shifted (Slavin 2011; McGleughlin 2011).[5] It was (unknowingly) living aloud (not necessarily in words) in negative capability with my patient, without the goals and methods of normative repair, that expanded the field of affective potentialities between us (Berlant and Edelman 2014). This was not technique or metaphor, but raw experience metabolized together in real time.

Perhaps the analyst's surrender to herself, in plain view, may also be required in some cases to make room for the unrepresented state of the patient. I mean more than receiving and interpreting emergent phenomena in the field, sharing countertransference or living in an enactment, but rather being willing to live in the breach of our own nonsovereignty. Ferro

(1993) acknowledges that not all experience can be represented and that as analysts we "have a responsibility not to map these still unexplored territories 'excessively'" (p. 918). But when we demonstrate that the route to transformation and growth is primarily through greater symbolization, facilitated by the alpha function of the analyst, we may do just that. The experience of dispersion or entropy, lived with another in a moment or over time, may deeply facilitate transformation. When we still mind and let the external world appear to us, letting where we are access us (Arsic 2016), we may find the world and each other.

In our overemphasis on moving from bewilderment toward symbolization and understanding, there is a fantasy of integration as cure. The oscillation promised in Bion's theory (1962) between being and knowing tilts towards analytic knowing. Post-Bionian theorization of the field champions a radical present, but at times its reparative vision of psychoanalysis is limited by a prescribed telos or cure. Perhaps this is also the limit of psychoanalysis in general. As long as "theory is the strong arm of knowing" and we resist theory's negativity (Morris 2005), we are (partially) sunk.

2. Stumbling upon performative writing

Few analysts would choose work in the negative. It chooses us. One stumbles into it unaware and never quite grasps it. I wonder whether it is possible to intentionally write about our work in the negative while asserting less sovereignty—without confirming that we "got it" either by using the right method, deploying a certain theory, or adopting a "relational" conviction that whatever it was that happened in the negative fostered some quantity of "subjectivity" or capacity. (As you will see, I, as writer, am guilty of just this! Trying to represent the negative is an oxymoron: it can't be rendered explicitly.)

Still, I want to challenge clinical writing in which we rarely acknowledge that we are inventors rather than conveyors of fact. Presented as both historical and narrative truth (Spence 1984), the accepted format of psychoanalytic case histories is influenced by a "network of constraints and censorship" (Johnson 1998, 168) that privilege in the name of clarity the objectivity and authority that can be anathema to the work.

We narrate aspects of subjectivity that can be known and described, neglecting an encounter with what is enigmatic and unsymbolized. We report affect that is stirred up in clinical encounters, but we don't inhabit it in our writing. Our neutrality can foster the impression that we knew what we were doing when we found ourselves caught in an abyss with our patients (McGleughlin 2015a) or that we *know*, now. What would it be like to write a clinical vignette in a way that dodged such certainty?

In earlier papers (2001, 2011, 2015a), to confront problems of precocious representation, I relied on enactive writing (Naiburg 2015) to communicate an unbearable experience of work in the negative. I told a story in the only way I could: by combining poetry, prose, dreams, and theory to convey gaps in subjectivity and affect states not yet symbolized. Without being fully conscious of it, I forced my readers into the same floating, rudderless experience of vertigo I had endured. By unwittingly enacting something with the reader, I discovered a way to write about the turmoil within the treatment and to convey, as Bion stressed, the emotional "truth" of the situation. I embrace this unconventional method.

Performative forms of psychoanalytic writing may address the overvaluing of the symbolized reflecting our confusion of the real with the represented. And sometimes they intensify affect. In this paper, I am asking: What would it mean to think and write without pinning things down? Without assuming our stories are "true" or relying on post-hoc temporality to shape meaning? I am trying to align with a shift in contemporary psychoanalysis away from a "neutral" observational stance of analytic knowing to one recognizing the importance of close attention to shared aliveness and uncertainty *in the field*. I believe that for deep, transformative work to happen, we need not just interpretation, in the sense of looking in from the outside, but "being at one with" our patients in the here and now, potentially ushering in unknown psychic reality that has not come into being (Slavin 2013; Ogden 2016). How can we write clinically to create such a field with the reader? Our clinical stories might not be just the application of knowledge or the satisfaction of a personal desire. Rather, they might be experiential: a two-way learning process. Yet hard as I try, it's difficult to unfold a story without a line of intention that promises progress toward meaning (Berlant and Edelman 2014) as certified by the analyst's function or theory or facility with narrative. I am hoping the three sections of this paper create such an effect, but I am alert to its failures.

In the clinical "vignette" that follows, I self-consciously combine my own story with a patient's as if we were one person. I mean to play with the usual binary between me, the writer, and you, the reader. To affect that confusion, I am self-consciously telling a story about myself and the patient as if it we were one, evoking a different kind of "we" than the Post-Bionian's. In creating a way of being at one with my patient here on the page and with you, the reader, I attempt to displace a form of telling that separates us from our patients and forces them to be an "other." Identities, meanings, and time are deliberately confused in an effort to highlight commonality rather than individual specificity; to challenge coherence and suggest the instability and timelessness of subjectivity. You may instinctively try to sort things out and ascribe (auto)biographical footprints, but I invite you to imagine us as fused, living a shared experience that belongs to both and all of us. We are chair to couch or couch to chair or just occupying a single space, but we also have (separate) bodies.

In combining patient and analyst in a single figure, "I," I am suggesting a different kind of origin where temporality flows in more than one direction and has access to the logic of dreaming and a two-way reaching (McGleughlin 2017). When boundaries are punctured and we allow chaos to accrue, the blurring of distinction and origin frees trauma from its fixity in narrative time and one-way directionality.

All experiences of the negative, of puncturing, take place in at least two registers—the one of experiencing and the one where the experience rewrites all that came before it. I wish to evoke the moment before we bracket what is outside us and deploy narrative to regain symbolic control. It's a gambit. I can't know what will happen. How will you experience the "me" that is also not me, the tangle between patient/analyst/writer/reader? Enactive writing keeps the unpredictable in play and foregrounds our uncertainty and nonsovereignty. I am trying to create an aliveness in the writer/reader field by enacting a scene with you.

Two stories as one

I dream (my patient dreams). I am with a baby who is inert, perhaps sleeping. I put homemade soft, closely knit, chunky yellow-stitched bootie socks on her, and she wakes up cooing and giggling, positively laughing with what seems at once like delight. It seems she has understood a good joke. She is staring at me with deep love and also with a wink and a nod.

In the same week, I see a local three-and-a-half hour production of the play *Amadeus*. A reviewer wrote, "Too many words that never seem to stop," and at 11:20 p.m. I agree. But as the audience sleeps for the last hour, I have been weeping. In this fictionalized story, Salieri, whose envy has caused him to starve, deprive, poison, and trick Mozart, is trying to confess to Mozart that he is responsible for the genius's demise. Nonetheless, Salieri wants Mozart to forgive him. Mozart lies on the floor alone, deranged, and impoverished, singing nursery rhymes over and over to shut Salieri out. There is not enough left of him to forgive.

I am weeping still, as I am always weeping, not for Mozart and his destruction but for my mother, because it is also too late for her. On a recent trip with her last friend, she became ill. Away in another country and unable to get home, she did what she always does—turned her pain, helplessness, and rage against those near her. Her friend called after the trip to let me know he would not be speaking to her anymore. He was done with her narcissism, negativity, and attack. Sober for many years, he took up (potentially deadly) drinking again. He couldn't stand it. In the weeks since, my mother has struggled in the most disavowed way to understand what happened, but however gentle my suggestions, whatever my attempts to help her see herself and her impact, it is too late. She is Salieri, and there will be no relief or understanding. Time is real, and she had no help against the ready-to-appear sense of absence and nothingness that undergirds human anxiety and makes her so wild with another. Her friend will not forgive her, and she will be alone.

The way the narrative helps patient/analyst

Dreaming the dream and seeing the play link up and nudge something liminal from the shadows. Watching *Amadeus*, where Mozart has been poisoned by envy, an image percolates on the heels of my mother's recent experience, her friend insinuating she poisoned him. I can begin to feel something I have *known* a lot about but couldn't bear to feel in *this* particular way: my mother has been envious and undermining of me—she is my own Salieri.

In analysis I tell that story. My mother's envy of me has lurked unawares, perhaps even more than lurked. Perhaps it was an anchoring idea inside of me all along? Seems I have always known such a mirror, seems like a fantasy at my core. An unthought known? (Bollas 1983). A structure? An aspect of my being that was never represented? Now it seems that way. An image of my mother's mirror of who I am, "too much," "too little," has registered, a deadly tincture that can't be reversed. The metaphor of poisoning lodges inside me, makes mental image, alphabetizes chaotic sensations. Builds. Takes space.

I now know her active (but not conscious) undermining of me, the way she cannot let me come into being. Watching *Amadeus* I can *feel* my utter helplessness, and for the first time my mother's intentionality, a poisoning that has no antidote. A cruelty. And I can feel what has not been possible because of it. A certain kind of disavowal is broken in on. A haze lifts and opens towards acknowledgment. I am in a kind of dreaming, what Ogden (2016) calls unconscious thinking that allows a reordering of things and creates psychological growth.

This symbolization, this transformative moment, happens against the background of a shift in atmosphere (Berlant and Edelman 2014), the analytic work. The analyst has been dreaming me up and dreaming with me, allowing the warming of my body and the bringing to life of a new capacity, symbolized by the baby's yellow booties and her delight. The laughing, chunky, yellow-footed baby kicks me, and I break open. Now I can bear this image. This dream can unfold because the analyst has been willing to be poison and to be poisoned. The analyst has been abandoning and cruel, but mostly the analyst has been the discarded, disgraced, envied, and undermined Mozart; has become the hated child's not being enough to please the mother; has allowed herself a corresponding place of smallness; has lived in that smallness; had her own inadequacy seen, sited, and underlined; has been willing to surrender to that shame, to have us find that strand of trauma in her (maybe without her knowing that place before?) has lived and survived that with us out loud, in her actions, with her words—in acknowledgment.

Something is transformed. Now a reversal of fortune seems possible, a new kind of mourning that will not be too late. I am not Mozart. I am not Salieri. Things remain for me. I can change the image of the overwhelmed, vulnerable, helpless-to-be-able-to-be-a-better-mother mother to someone more lethal and can bear the site of killing, the terrifying knowledge of a mother's hatred. And in this fantasy, the transformative moment makes bearable the unbearability of the crushing encounter with love and loss (Berlant and Edelman 2014).

And new relational possibilities follow. We feel gratitude for the analyst's willingness to be poisoned first by us and for us so we can know this poisoning. We can see her help now, and we can tell her of our gratitude. Something else has become possible: we will give up some lingering fantasy of self-sufficiency, of being everything to ourselves (Bollas 1987). It is she, the analyst, who must have knit the dream booties, weaving warp and woof.

This is what we aim for as psychoanalysts. Transformation, not just insight. Transformation begets the possibility of new psychic structure and with it new meaning and new relational possibilities. We (the analyst) feel the dream baby's adoring look, see the coo, hear the warmth of the booties. Creativity takes hold. We (the patient) can move with what has been the most painful reality of a life—a mother's hatred. We (both) can use this story now, we and my patient who we are, too. A feeling of bone beneath the skin (Davis 2009), marbles in our pockets forms. Solid. Something else becomes possible. And with that new sense of bigness, of goodness, we want to make the translation to you the reader, who is also part of our we. We reach out, tell our story. In doing so, in trying to use this place of pain creatively, we assert mastery over our wild nonsovereignty, the unknowable otherness of a mother, ourselves. The story imposes time, linear narration, a kind of coherence. Checks the pain, makes it bearable in time and rhythm, seduces us, maybe you.

Narrative's underside: the return of the enigmatic message: the analyst speaks

In discussing our "story" later, I bring to bear the debate between Berlant and Edelman (2014) and use their ideas to play with how representation can and cannot transform.[6] On one hand, the quest to establish a narrative worked. Something in the experience of the characters in the field—the baby and her yellow booties, Mozart, Salieri, the poisoner, the mother, etc., and the play with them—allowed a metaphor about an emotional truth (that of being hated and envied, and of having been poisoned by this) that we (patient and analyst) could digest in a transformative way. But in the move toward symbolic representation, as writer and constructor of this "combined story," something gets filled in, covered over, and lost. The narrative transformation fails to hold. The feeling of hope and creativity collapses, and we are scared; the narrative is a conceit. As unconscious content, fantasy is timeless, both persistent and outside of narrative structure, hard to dislodge.

As we, the patient/analyst/writer, go to reconstruct the story for you, the reader, in the "uncuratedness of conversation," to surrender "to the inevitably of non-sovereign relationality," we feel endangered, as though you are our mother. Something gets repeated (we are still poisoned), and our mother's idea of who we are (too little/too much) carries forward, and you, the reader, become her. Now it seems we are "forcing our internal state on to you," and we don't know what we are revealing, enacting (Berlant and Edelman 2014, 94). We don't know who you are, what you will think, and we can't control you and your otherness. We feel exposed. Ready to be misunderstood, maybe even hated. Our mother's idea of who we are carries forward, and you become her.

Not just because we have been disloyal, made the story one directional, vilified our mother, made ourselves a victim. Or because the story leaves out ways we might have seduced, invited this kind of interaction, and actively sought this persecution, been not enough and too much. Not just because we have allowed even a momentary forgetting of her exquisite vulnerability, our identification with her, our merged selves, exposed her, perhaps become Salieri ourselves, poisoning her with this paper.

But because even though I, the writer, have changed the setting to us, writer and reader, and addressed you now from my role as the analyst, there is something immutable about the fantasy. Even if you, the reader, are drawn into the narrative and undergo the situation with us, feel the joy of the baby's warming, the ironic wink to symbolism's saturated booties, the deadliness of envy's destruction, the requiem for a kind of coming into being that might not ever happen, or the too-lateness of the situation, I, the writer, don't know if we are experiencing something together. You are too far away, "a largely silent listener," and our fantasy follows us forward. We may have changed the narrative device but without affecting the psychic structure lodged inside of us.

We can't help ourselves. As soon as we allow you to have a response that we cannot control, we are up against the enduring quality of (an old) us. Repetition is inevitable. We replay our past scene with our mother onto the present stage not just because it was unconscious (it isn't now) or unanalyzed but also "because self-identity needs to be continually reproduced and reassured precisely because it fails to secure belief" (Phelan 1994, 4). Any new representation of myself needs shoring up, bolstering, but can never erase the original fantasy, nor the unsayable, unseeable, unrepresentable, and therefore immutable nonsovereign (the mother's message inside of us). We are (now me, again—or me and you?) almost just back to where we started.

In this sense, then, the mother is also a fantasy, a skeleton, a placeholder (exchangeable for others), used to mark that with which we cannot be in relation (Berlant and Edelman 2014).

Our hope of something different in each encounter with our mother (looking so much like you now) involves a return to a site of fantasy that enables us to believe that nearness to mother—the very pleasure of being inside a relation with her—is sustaining regardless of the content of the encounters. We are bound to a position of threat that is highly confirming (Berlant and Edelman, p. 2). Something inside us, reader, writer, patient, analyst, irreducible and strange, seeks something in repetition, libidinally, repetitively, with you or elsewhere. This, after Laplanche, is ". . . the unstated erotic pleasure that places us in relation not only to what we have been casting as the subject's unbearable access to his own radical unrepresentability, but also to the sensual pleasures of relationality itself" (Berlant and Edelman 2014, 90).

The pleasure or force or drive or fantasy that keeps us wanting to be "in the neighborhood of the object," our mother, is also "overwhelming insofar as it reveals the necessity of relationality itself" (Berlant and Edelman 2014, 91). Berlant and Edelman call this being

> unmastered by need that one senses but does not know, in the terms of knowledge as mastery; a sense clustered with the sense of a need for the objects or scenes that hold up the world and pleasure in that need . . . the form of enduring repetition itself.
>
> (p. 91)

We see that our return to the fantasy, the placeholder of our mother, is not just organized by the movement between acknowledgement and the disavowal of that negativity (she is poisonous, she is vulnerable)

> but also by negativity that is sensed inarticulately as a condition of being in the world—a certain way that is as a feeling of displacement that is inevitable, non-sovereign, and at the same time a pressure to which the subject remains attached.
>
> (pp. 90–91)

In psychoanalysis, we talk of our attachment to bad objects, the difficulty of wanting to stay the same while changing, the libidinalization of pain, or the repetition compulsion, but none of these quite carries the force of the irreducibility, the inescapable human reality that immutable fantasies are a condition for being in the world. We live in cycles of disavowal, acknowledgment, repetition.

But repetition is not futile. The inescapability of nonsovereignty is related to Laplanche's (1987) enigmatic message, which is still and always seeking translation while remaining beyond translation, signified now by our too muchness. The enigmatic messages in our body (writer, reader, patient/ analyst), some important aspects of our sensibility, does not, cannot yield. Something runs through us, is us, but is strange.

The fantasy cannot be dislodged because it is a work of registration and translation outside or beyond the symbolic. The confrontation with the other, the enigmatic message installed in our child body from our mother's own unconscious sexuality can never be represented veridically and is always in excess of understanding. Because we cannot process these messages, they remain as the unconscious core of our subjectivity, disrupting psychological life, signifying something important but enigmatic and eroticized. Subjectivity—interiority and unconscious fantasy–is built from such labors and alerts us to the implantation of the other, installing in us the nonsovereignty of the self. The repetitive presence of these messages breaches the continuity of being (already a fantasy) and suggests a loss—the inevitable unknowableness of the other inside us.

The excess living in us is a form of both resisting and claiming our mother, declaring the boundary where we diverge and merge with her (and you). "In that declaration of identity and identification, there is always loss, the loss of not being the other and yet, remaining dependent on the other for self-seeing, self-being" (Phelan 1994, 13). The wish to tell our story, to represent it, is about an impulse to use you as a mirror to see our self. (We'll be probing to see if it can be different this time.) How much can we risk? How much can we change?

What of this enduring repetition? Certainly, what patient/analyst have built together, the yellow booties and what they symbolize over long years of living side by side, creates the possibility for transformation. Ferro would argue that telling this story together contains the transformative potential, and that it is the dialogue that matters. And it does. But in the story that I, the writer, have narrated, it was also patient and analyst being together facing the negative, each at risk, that (in my fantasy) fostered transformation: acceptance of a mother's hatred and the capacity to use that knowledge to break through old defenses and allow new relational possibilities. It was the willingness of my (my patient's) analyst to be poisoned—to find in herself a corresponding place of badness, that ultimately made it possible to transform experience. The analyst's reliance on the patient to know some enigmatic part of herself (Hoffman 1983), to live that badness out loud with the patient without technique or goal, never having quite known or been able to bear that place before, allowed something unlivable for the patient to become bearable in both (McGleughlin 2011, 2015a). Central to this was the analyst's vulnerability. There was two-way reaching.

When my patient and I lived in a state of defeat individually and together, without knowing, enduring our poisoning, going on that way, repeating over and over, the negative created an opening. This is the encounter with the negative where being in relation with another risks rupture and also may allow repair.

Now if I tell a story to you, the reader, "who has barely consented to be there," "giving my story over consciously or not," I open "the possibility of its crumbling in front of another . . . in the expansive, uncuratedness of conversation, a scene inevitably of nonsovereign relationality as such" (Berlant and Edelman 2014, 94)—again. This is the estrangement and intimacy of relationality. Without the risk of being in fuller relation, we may limit connectivity and our possibility to access another way to perceive the forces running through us and between us. An invitation to live in entropy, together, to allow "negativity's multiplicity" without achieving story, Berlant suggests, offers its own potentialities. Berlant believes we do this not just intrapsychically but in our multiple investments with others, our work, our political commitments, our collaborations. What *I*, writing, am saying to you, reading, is that we may have to live something with our patients, side by side, in our unconscious fantasy and aloud, facing the void at the center of the edifice so that the enigmatic may thrive and the negative may do its work. When my patient and I lived in a state of defeat individually and together—without knowing, enduring our poisoning, repeating over and over, misunderstanding, helpless—the negative created an opening. That field without narrative meaning allowed us to bracket the mother's enigmatic message and find something generative, something unknown but there all along.

3. Agnes Martin—negativity's potential power and art as the negative

To think about how we might surrender to the negative's generative force and our ineluctable nonsovereignty, I turn to art. Recently I saw the paintings of Agnes Martin. There, in the perfect spiral of the Guggenheim as

I ascended ever higher into abstraction, I wept, upended. It is hard to know quite what prompted these affective stirrings. I felt an almost indescribable set of chaotic feelings looking at art devoid of representation. I believe Martin brings us into contact with the creative force of the negative; something that has run under all along, creating excess, potential and creativity, some other agent "continually keeping its time" (Blanchfield 2016, 126) even as it remains unmarked, unseen.

Martin created art from the late 1940s until 2004, when she died at 92. She destroyed many of her paintings but left hundreds of 72-inch square canvases filled with rows, columns, and stripes of varying widths and hues. They remain, 15 years after her death, truly astonishing (Als 2016). Martin's paintings pull the viewer in, exerting a kind of force felt in the body that is close to what Grosz (2008) describes: art is where intensities proliferate, forces are expressed for their own sake, sensation lives. Martin wanted her work to be emptied of referential meaning to allow something unknown to enter. She pays attention to the dynamic forces of the field as she empties her mind and awaits inspiration, what she calls the courting of something that surprises.

Although her inspirations came in images the size of postage stamps, voices commanded her to produce large canvases. She appreciated these voices as forces of joy that coursed through her and connected her to the world. She wanted her work to make us feel our own inner states, suggesting how we could empty our minds of something like memory. She suggested we crawl into the box in her grids, look out from the inside, and wait (Glimcher 2012). We might then be surprised by the ineffable. This she called perceiving, which she said, "is the same as receiving and it is the same as responding. Thinking, on the other hand, leads to pride, identification, confusion, and fear" (Glimcher 2012, 145). And indeed, Martin's work can't be thought.

Martin rejected any purposeful, mimetic goal for art. Goals, she thought, directed us to pre-experienced sensations guaranteed to affect in particular ways. Critiquing the impulse to produce what we already know, to assure ourselves, she discouraged reproduction of "self-image within the representational frame" (Phelan 1994). She sought to detach herself from her work. She said in 1981, "To live truly and effectively, the idea of achievement must be given up" (Als 2016). With Grosz she would believe that "art proper emerges when sensation can detach itself and gain an autonomy from its creator and its perceiver, when something of the chaos from which it is drawn can breathe and have a life of its own" (Grosz 2008, 7). This is the work of the negative. Listen to her words:

> Suffering is necessary for freedom from suffering . . . the wiggle of a worm is as important as the assassination of a President . . . our work is very important but . . . we are not . . . a sense of disappointment and defeat are an essential state of mind for creative work. . . . Defeat means we cannot move . . . but still we go on, without hope, without desire, and without dreams, then it is not I, then it is not us, then it is not conditioned response . . . going on without hope and desire is discipline,. . . defeated you rise to your feet like dry bones,. . . undefeated you will only say what has already been said. . . . We feel cast into outer darkness as though some fatal error has been made . . . feelings of loss and catastrophe cover everything and we tremble with fear and dread but when fear and dread have passed as all passions do, we realize that helplessness is the most important state of mind.
>
> (As recorded by Jill Johnston in 1970 interview)

Martin endured schizophrenia. After her first psychotic break, in the 1960s, she left New York and a community of artists there to live alone in an adobe house in New Mexico. Her work was widely sought after and considered "among the most disciplined and rigorously programmatic work in the history of modern art" (Als 2016). In Martin's paintings, finely drawn lines (often in grids) appear at first as uninterrupted color fields. Hilton Als (2016) believed Martin used the grid as "a form for belief—a space where the viewer as well as the artist could contemplate the hand making the thing being observed." Martin herself said the grids came from thinking about the innocence of trees (Morris and Bell 2015). When you see her grids, it's hard not to think of Bion's grids and his sensibility. Statements like "one who becomes all eyes does not see" and "to try to understand is to court misunderstanding" pepper her writing.

Some critics believed that "by converting her personal and plaguing disconnection from space and time into a structural mapping of the most elegant and minimally contained mannerist art likely ever produced," (Denson 2016) she labored her way to sanity. To look at Martin's vast body of paintings with their obsessive tiny lines repeated in infinite variation, a corpus whose creation consumed her almost every waking hour for over 50 years, it's easy to imagine someone trying to impose order on chaos.

Beta to Alpha. But it's hard to imagine Martin thinking of her art as something done for the sake of something else, even sanity: she insisted that schizophrenia had no effect on her life.

Martin would have us believe that she tried to convey the vibratory infinite waves that connect us to the world, to the negative. I believe her. Think O (Bion 1962). I see her pursuing what Grosz (2008) cast as a wish to explore the peculiar relations that art establishes between the living body, the forces of the universe, and the creation of the future, where "generations of vibratory waves, and rhythms traverse through us and link the body to forces it cannot otherwise perceive" (Grosz 2008, 23). Maybe she wanted to attend to the most abstract questions, which, Grosz says, if abstract enough, provide us with renewed understanding of the concrete and the lived. For Martin, sensations of renewal emerge from attuning to some other agent "playing the thinking thing" while something continual is "keeping its time in the plain continuousness of her own lived span, and while the meadow runs through her" (Blanchfield 2016, 126).

Martin's paintings and her descriptions of them contain the spirit and force of the negative that Berlant and Edelman (2014) describe and that I hope to bring to our work as analysts. In her work and ours, we enter chaos, vibrate with the unknowable, and let the field run through us possibly encountering the sublime. Generativity requires the force of the negative—helplessness and vulnerability and the ability to live in sensory affective states without symbolization, despite entropy, regression, repetition and defeat. Even more, art is "among the most forceful ways in which culture generate[s] a small space of chaos" (Grosz 2008, 23). Art "makes mystery into a solid object" (Als 2016). With Martin, I think of psychoanalysis as generating spaces where chaos "can be elaborated, felt, and thought" (Grosz 2008, 23). At its best, psychoanalysis, like art, "through [the] plane of composition it throws over chaos, gives life to sensation that, disconnected from its origins or any destination or reception, maintains its connections with the infinite it expresses and from which it is drawn" (Grosz 2008, 8). This is transformation.

Addendum

I want to close with a story. Sarah, the silent patient I begin this book with, left treatment in the early 2000's. We had a very deep connection that could not be continued. She was a patient who functioned professionally at a very high level but had few social connections in the world. The patient felt my proximity was too much. She was unsettled by the idea that the breath I breathed out, she had to breathe in. While this patient has not been in treatment for 14 years, I call her once a year on her birthday, a call that is short but that we each very much look forward to.

So present was she as I traveled through the Martin exhibit that I decided to contact her outside of our never-violated and very reliable frame. I felt I needed her to know and see this exhibit. There were obvious similarities, both artist's and patient's minimalism, their disconnection from the world, their brilliance, the way potentially steadfast obsessional work held something much more chaotic. So it is not strange that she came to mind. But it was strange that I contacted her. I texted, forgetting, of course, that she has no cell phone, and the text was returned to me. Later my phone pocket-dialed her. I saw it and hung up immediately, not wanting the call to be intrusive, although it was her work phone, in the evening and on the day after Christmas. She called a few hours later, no ID, but I picked up. She said hello and I explained what had happened—the returned text, the pocket dial, my keen feeling of the importance of telling her about the exhibit. As I was talking, I suddenly knew. Her mother was dying. I asked and she confirmed this. Maybe in hours, she thought, her mother would be dead. She was exceedingly grateful that I knew and for the call, and we hung up. As Fanny Howe says, "Chance often feels like a channel to a knowledge held together by invisible spirits. A knowledge that precedes and follows us, then vanishes" (Howe n.d.). This to me is a story not just of the uncanny or the serendipitous but also of the power and creativity of the negative—the forces that run in us and between us.

Notes

1 This work felt like being in the center of a void in Green's sense (1999), where primitive states of mind reject whatever is intolerable to the ego and point to the destructiveness of the death drive. Still, I think it links more closely to Green's (1999) sense of an absence always in dialectical relation with presence. The presence-absence dialectic is the substrate that underlies all self-other normative development (Morris 2005).
2 Bion's "beta elements" and Stern's (1997) "unformulated experience" come to mind here, among many conceptions of unrepresentability.
3 This happened to me when, at age 53, I began to paint portraits with no artistic capacity. What emerged felt miraculous and not from a me I knew.

4 See Donnell Stern's extensive discussion and critique of the post Bionian Field theorists (Stern 2013) and Levine's (2013) rebuttal.
5 In newer writing, Civitarese (2015) has emphasized the analyst's need to find the corresponding hallucinosis of his patient, bringing him closer to many relational thinkers' belief that we must live at the level of the chaos our patient is living, though he does not do that aloud.
6 See Chapter 3 of Berlant and Edelman (2014) for their rich and complex dialogue. All unattributed quotes come from that discussion.

Chapter 16

The impossibility of meaning (2019)

The negative, unrepresented mental states and their importance

Now that you have read "The Analyst's Necessary Nonsovereignty and the Generative Force of the Negative," I want to return to its epigraph, from the poet Brian Blanchfield (2016), to situate us outside of how we usually perceive reality. I am drawn to the imagistic and almost numinous way Blanchfield captures the potential of nonsovereignty and the power of the negative—in our body, between our bodies, in the field and in the world:

> One life to live, to live again. Singularity recast as multiple. That is, one subjectivity run through by a performance not one's own. Here at the authorless site of my thrill, producing a replacement time in place of time . . . something expresses in me, the way ground water is said to express intermittently as a spring. . . . A sense of it having run under all along.
>
> (Blanchfield 2016, 126)

Blanchfield calls this field running through him something "close to a higher power . . . something like the field instantiating fieldness, the welling of confluent creativity." These sensations of renewal, he adds, are "for attuning your own instrumentality, where some other agent [is] playing the thinking thing, something continual keeping its time" (p. 127).

As it was for my patient/me in "The Analyst's Necessary Nonsovereignty," Blanchfield signals cycles of change, even transformation, yet they will need to be repeated over and over. And, like the painter with whom I close the paper, Agnes Martin, for whom some other agent is keeping time, Blanchfield alerts us to how the *unrepresentable*—there all along, creating chaos and excess, potential and creativity—is unbounded in space and time and, importantly, connects us to each other.

DOI: 10.4324/9781032670348-21

This final chapter builds upon a published paper I wrote in response to the respective discussions of Donnel B. Stern, Antonio Ferro, and Amy Schwartz Cooney about the ideas explored in "The Analyst's Necessary Nonsovereignty." While their papers aren't printed here, I hope that my inclusion of their voices in this chapter will make them useful interlocuters. Stern, Ferro, and Cooney were each uniquely suited to think and feel their way to understanding: Stern, with his work with unformulated experience; Ferro, with his Bionian belief in the power of what cannot be represented; and Cooney, with her eye on vitality.

The choice to include the discussants isn't just about my need for a conversational partner. The heart of the idea for "The Analyst's Necessary Nonsovereignty" came from the dialogue between Lauren Berlant and Lee Edelman in *Sex or the Unbearable* (2014). I draw on the content of their book, as well as the form. The questions they asked each other—"how to live relationally, how to confront our self-division, how to experience the unbearable undoing of the logic that binds us to the world"—are the same ones that we psychoanalysts ask in a different vernacular.

What was so extraordinary for me was how seldom I felt the tiny tears of misrecognition in my discussants' responses. Ironically, while I call on Berlant and Edelman's (2014) dialogue to bring out the usefulness and creativity in disjunction, I experienced a feeling of grace from the gentle, generous accompaniment of my three colleagues. It was the kind of surprising zinger (Sedgwick 2011) that the negative can so often invite, and it was especially welcome in this case: when we set out to tell the story, my patient and I were gripped with fear because our own enactment pivoted around imagining that the reader would be like the mother reflecting back the too little/too muchness of us. But not only did the discussants disconfirm my old fears, they also created "a replacement time in place of time, . . . (where) something expresses in me, the way ground water is said to express intermittently as a spring. . . . A sense of it having run under all along" (Blanchfield 2016, 127).

Subjectivity and sovereignty

To challenge psychoanalysis' stabilizing framework and logic of coherence (Berlant and Edelman 2014), I avoided pinning down meaning in "The Analyst's Necessary Nonsovereignty," but my respondents made it apparent that the terms "subjectivity" and "nonsovereignty" can be confusing. The words' meanings depend on their location, whether in philosophy, political theory, or psychoanalysis. As for my use of nonsovereignty, it follows Berlant and Edelman, as well as Laplanche; I understand people to be nonsovereign beings who are forever trying to translate enigmatic messages transmitted at our formation as subjects, confronting the limits of knowing oneself.

But Cooney reads my definition of sovereignty as an objective positivistic stance, implying a "belief in knowledge and certainty that can enable the wielding of oppressive power through tyrannizing social norms, rigidities and categorizations" (p. 141). This is problematic for her, as well as for Stern, as neither see sovereignty as necessarily authoritarian. While I agree with Cooney that sovereignty need not imply a totalizing definition that is oppressive, always signifying a unitary knowable subject, I am asking readers to consider that our subjectivities may encompass a dialectical oscillation between more sovereign and nonsovereign poles.

I also, of course, acknowledge unconscious subjectivity, including the ways we are strange to ourselves by virtue of unconsciousness. But at the same time, I want to point to a strand of subjectivity that is undertheorized: aspects of human experience that *cannot be represented* and still meaningfully impact us. Contact with the negative can both disrupt and foster connection to another, and as I move toward a more ontological psychoanalysis, these experiences haven been critical for me. A belief in sovereignty as simply another word for subjectivity may keep us from opening ourselves to the important work the negative may perform in and through us.

In shifting from psychoanalytic language of subjectivity to the more philosophical language of sovereignty/nonsovereignty, I am trying to disturb the notion of a unified subject. There are already more mixed-up notions of self and other in psychoanalytic theorizing, yet they stop short of what I am suggesting. For instance, Bollas postulated as early as 1983 that the feelings of the analyst are thought to be those of the patient's objects (Bollas 1983). He argued that the analyst would have to take himself as the object of interest, insight, and, quite possibly, cure to reach the patient's cure. Yet Bollas was focused on the significant individuals *in the patient's life* that might be found within him. In other words, his inward look was about his being used by the patient as *an object*, rather than as a subject intermixing with another subject.

In contrast, Relational analysts have long taken up the analyst as subject and critiqued as overly unidimensional the notion of an action that starts with a patient (transference) and is responded to by an analyst (counter-transference). These theorists have developed an extensive body of thought centered on what patient and analyst create together (often unconsciously) from their separate subjectivities, as in the now ubiquitous notions of the "third" and formulations of mutual enactment. Emphasizing the bidirectionality of the analytic pair (as do many other kinds of field theories), Relationalists have pointed us toward the importance of the space shared *between* analyst and patient.

While I recognize the worth of this "betweenness," the very concept suggests a separateness that I'm trying to trouble by merging therapist and patient in my paper. I am suggesting that we are always both ourselves and the other, an unstable, nonunitary self. Like Butler, I do not entirely believe in the distinctness between the "I" who utters an address and the "you" to whom the address is uttered (Butler 2015, 9). Rather I am suggesting that "the you" is at once an externalized version of the "I" and an ambiguous part of the "I" (p. 9). In collapsing the figures, I offer a fictionalized (yet real in another sense) means of perceiving the "you" as inseparable from the "I." We have a paucity of language to flesh out this idea.

Through the narrative experiment in the clinical case, I ask readers to imagine a figure that emerges through "circulation, engagement, and assemblage" (Lara et al. 2017, 34), rather than from the position of a reified self who exists prior to an encounter with another. This offers an ontological challenge to the notion of a sovereign discrete subject. Stern joins me in this effort, noting that

> McGleughlin not only doesn't interpret; she doesn't even try to create intersubjectivity . . . she ceases trying to inhabit her own subjectivity . . . but nonetheless the analyst's vulnerability—that is the analyst's ongoing personal participation in the field—comes across.
>
> (Stern 2020, 153)

Ferro, too, recognizes my desire for a project that refuses our *individual illusions* of subjectivity and sovereignty. He expresses appreciation for "how [I combine] the story taking shape in the consulting room with [my] own personal story, . . . show[ing] us the fertility of immersing ourselves in confusion" (Ferro 2020, 148).

To Cooney's question of whether I seek to "abrogate[e] subjectivity" (2020, 141), I don't think so, nor could this be a goal. However, we can *occasionally* make contact with something that interferes with our sense of our isolated self. Cooney wonders if I believe in *any* "subjectness," which she defines as "the individual's unique (non-objective) sensibility: her ways of feeling, fantasizing, and experiencing the world" (p. 140). Yes, but also no, at least based on Cooney's definition, which considers arenas of subjectivity that uniquely belong to a "me," not those that are fractal, incoherent, unpredictable, and sometimes even unrecognizable as me. I emphasize a less coherent subject.

I hope the narrative device of combining figures will draw attention to the limits of subjectivity to contain or explain what runs inside us or between us. Relatedness, I think, comes not only in the construction of a self but in the deconstruction of one. Disrupting our sense of ourselves as discrete individuals, we challenge the totality or fixity of identity (Berlant and Edelman 2014) and, in so doing, become more vulnerable subjects.

Unrepresented mental states and the generative work of the negative

Much has been written about how unrepresented states can impede growth, but this neglects the powerful non-pathological forces that are part of the negative. Non-representable states co-exist with those that can become represented. They subtly impact perceptions and experience and, on rare occasions, can be directly sensed. As Stern writes, the negative doesn't "give shape to experience that can be known or interpreted: it washes over you, or surrounds you—or better, it suffuses you" (Stern 2020, 151). This is the *generative* potential of the negative, if we can be open to it.

Cooney's questions about the negative give me the opportunity to clarify what I mean by it, though I will also note that it is oxymoronic to narrate what is inchoate on the level of symbolic meaning. Even as I experiment with ideas of the negative—by narratively combining two figures as one—I recognize that the effort is paradoxical, since the negative can't really be courted. That said, certain forms of sex or play may be the best places to intentionally loosen our sense of sovereignty (Saketopoulous 2022b), which might allow the eruption to the negative. To reconfigure our sense of ourselves as continuous with each other is to open the possibility for different kinds of relating. These ideas feel to me deeply congruent with Bionian field theory, which rests upon the proposition that truths are not found in the singular mind but in a "primordial human unity" that Bion calls *at-one-ment* (Steinberg 2019, 419). I would add that this at-one-ment exists in the negative, the shaping force moving through all things.

Cooney (2020) wonders if I see the negative as a transitional space or analytic endpoint. In my view the negative is always present, a force that occasionally interrupts and may create or destroy; it's definitely not an endpoint or place of transcendence. For something that is ever with us, I don't think the language of transitional space is helpful. Perhaps it is in the idea of the "use" of the negative that the muddle occurs. The negative may or may not expand a "sense of vitality and meaning," as Cooney suggests (2020, 141). I want to accentuate my belief in its intrinsic value, as a force that is not in itself instrumental. I am trying to describe moments of simply *being* when we attune to something outside language. Here we might grasp our connection to all things, even those without consciousness.

Ferro and Stern also believe in the power of the unrepresented. Ferro (2020) says so directly, agreeing with me "that the utmost importance should be attached not only to what is hidden but also, and especially, to what has never been represented" (p. 147). But while he credits the creative potential in the unknown, Ferro retains an emphasis on its symbolization. Likening the unrepresented to an oil well, "a rich resource . . . to be protected and tolerated as unknown," he describes it as something to draw on in "the process of refining alphabetization" (p. 147)—a Bionian idea where the unconscious is continually constructed out of what is not even minimally represented via alpha functions.

Stern, too, maintains that unformulated states "quite naturally become actualized, or formulated, whenever it becomes relevant to matters at hand" (p. 157). When dissociation melts, he writes that "what McGleughlin describes as 'sovereignty,' actually expands" (p. 157). I think he means that dissociation, which relies on splitting, cuts us off from aspects of ourselves that may become available when we can bear more internal conflict; contact with these states creates a fuller sense of our subjectivity. I'm with Stern here, but I still would like to stress that some unformulated experience can never be represented *at all* but nonetheless stimulate growth. Stern ends his discussion acknowledging he will likely modify his theory of unformulated experience (Stern 1997, 2018) to accommodate the negative: "[W]e do not have to choose between portraying unrepresented states as potentially meaningful, on one hand, or the impossibility of meaning, on the other" (2020, 157)—an idea that is central to my project.

While I join a growing group of analysts who are thinking about unrepresented mental states, my contribution is to bring attention to the *generative force and intrinsic relationality* in what will never be formulated but is between us. To do otherwise is to put our weight on the side of knowing, and potentially screen out other forms of sensing, perceiving, and being with the other.[1]

Technique

Our understanding of therapeutic action has increasingly—and, for many analysts, decisively—moved away from emphasizing the analyst's superior understanding as conveyed to the patient through interpretations. Instead, contemporary field and relational theorists believe that mutative action also depends on a shared living through. As one example, Civitarese (2015) has recently written about the analyst's need to find the corresponding hallucinosis of his patient, a belief similar to my own about living at the level of chaos our patient is inhabiting (Slavin 2013; McGleughlin 2001, 2011, 2015a; Lombardi 2005).

I think all three discussants, and I believe in creating alive experience in the here and now as opposed to only processing early familial or developmental interactions and interpreting transference. And Relational theorists have been narrating problems with the analyst's authority for decades (Hoffman 1983; Aron 1999; Stern 1997); the technical issue is how to exist in the field as nonsovereign, participating subjects without neglecting the needs of the treatment and the patient. Rather than sidestepping our analytic authority, Cooney suggests that claiming it helps us to be more accountable to the power we hold (Cooney 2020). I agree. As I argue in "The Analyst's Necessary Nonsovereignty," we unavoidably shape the field as analysts, even when we're characters in it, even when we work in less symbolic regions. So I take seriously Cooney's cautionary note, especially as it pertains to frame. But while the four of us may now recognize "sovereignty" (as I am using this term) as a constant risk, we diverge at other points, particularly around the use of the analyst's vulnerability.

Though Cooney champions openness to the unknown and freeing oneself from pre-existing concepts, she asserts the importance of interpretation that emerges from the analyst's subjectivity. The analytic relationship has an inherent asymmetry because the patient's experience is the focal point, she argues, and surveilling is a necessary tool for seeking generative connections. While surveilling can be subjugating, it isn't always, Cooney says, pointing to witnessing, recognizing, understanding, and empathizing. Yet as I understand it, surveillance—to observe the activities of a person or group closely, to keep watch over or, more ominously, to monitor, supervise, or regulate—implies that we observe *for* something from the outside, rather than actively participate in and shape all aspects of an analysis.

As I tried to show in the "*Hiroshima mon amour*" and "white empathy" chapters, standard analytic ideas like empathy or recognition can rely on what we already know and potentially eclipse the other. The "getting-to-know-you" process of treatment is inescapably influenced by the analyst's specific means of perceiving and organizing the patient's experience. Each analyst sees a different patient. If we rely primarily on observing, we are employing our way of seeing to know, which is always mimetic of our self-image—we see what we know (Phelan 1994). Moreover, we use our profession's schemas as filters, reproducing a psychoanalytic logic of the real. (One example is through meta-psychological stories such as the Oedipus complex, stories that are bound up in white patriarchal biases; see "Thinking Outside the Oedipus Box.") This real promotes its own representation as if it were true, limiting possibilities. Further, what we see is never totalizing, so representation leaves ruptures—it fails to produce the real exactly.

In contrast, I am interested in allowing what's in the gaps of our seeing to come forward. The excess meanings that we pick up can *become supplements that make possible multiple and resistant readings of what is also true.* As Butler argues, "the real is positioned both before and after its representation; and so representation becomes only a moment of the consolidation of the real" (Phelan 1994, 2), one of many. Understanding only by observing our patients may limit culturally different, nonverbal, or nonsymbolic ways of perceiving.

Similarly to Cooney, Ferro notes the benefits of "looking" to read the feedback from the characters in the field and the effect of the narration on the emotions in play. But like me, he leans away from theorizing that values knowing even as he acknowledges that the analyst's vulnerability to the emotions of the field carries the risk of unconscious sovereignty and clinical practice has not always caught up with the idea of a nonsovereign analyst and a truly bidirectional field. In fact, many Bionian field theorists have been instrumental (in the best sense of the word) in formulating the limits of interpretations as insight, saturated as they are by metapsychology. Instead, these theorists value Bion's K, the transformational dreaming process where patient and analyst are freed from the burden of representation, and the field has an ambiguous power of its own.

Welcoming some "bewilderment," Ferro wonders if "psychoanalysis might be a *not* always definable or classifiable art form" (Ferro 2020, 148). We share the idea that bewilderment potentially paves the way to something unknown for both patient and analyst, and Stern points out that psychic destabilization has long been considered useful in psychoanalysis. Virtually all schools view therapeutic action as the breaking up of "overly rigid and tendentious psychic structures . . . or rigid repetitive processes in the service of allowing more flexible ways of living to emerge" (p. 154). Stern writes, "for McGleughlin, destabilization—that is, living with the negative—is valued for its own sake" rather than to yield new symbolization or psychic structures. This perspective emphasizes the relational cast when "it is not only the patient who experiences the negative, but the analyst, as well" (Stern 2020, 154).

Still, what the analyst can "see" and "know" is an area of some confusion. Ferro argues that my concern about the analyst interpreting the field and assuming sovereignty, which he shares, would not be as great had I considered the latest developments in our field rather than rely on older papers. He points to how theory has evolved away from the Barangers' concept of containing and interpreting the field (Baranger and Baranger 2008). Instead, he writes,

> The analyst loses his role, however minimal, of director in order to be captured as one of the characters in the analytic scene. The interpretative game (played by all the characters, who are a sort of de-concretising diffraction of the real people) takes the place of saturated interpretations and the transference.
>
> (Ferro 2020, 147)

I assume he means that this de-concretizing makes the analyst less the sovereign authority/reader of the field and more just another character in it.

Further, "the analyst should not have an interpretative project," Ferro states, "but a readiness for narrative play in the session which does not require or anticipate any of the possible developments. It is as if the field were an interpreting context in which interpretation has, however, been replaced by narrative" (p. 148). But I wonder if narrating the field *can* actually bypass an interpreting analyst?

Field theory is indeed changing, as Ferro suggests, but, reflecting on his 2020 discussion in tandem with some of his earlier work, I am genuinely confused about whether he believes that this new approach has eliminated the problem of sovereignty. As recently as 2016, he argued that projective identifications should go in one direction only—from patient to analyst. "When the analyst strays temporarily from this, becomes unconsciously personally involved (in a reversal of the flow of projective identifications)," he wrote, "it must be corrected as quickly as possible to restore the analyst's treatment function" (Ferro and Civitarese 2016, 145). I am not sure how Ferro could consider this a non-interpretive stance, though he may no longer endorse this 2016 idea. In 2020, he writes that there are clumps with asymmetrical features that carry the risk of sovereignty, but apart from transforming all communications into a dream, he is not sure what to do about them. Nor am I but I suggest that the analyst's vulnerability may be a route to minimizing our sovereignty.

In slightly different language, Civitarese (2019) also seems to be tacking away from notions of the analyst's sovereignty by shifting from language of interpreting to language of narrating or "*servicing*" the analytic field (to keep the theatre of analysis open and functioning). My easiest route into an emotional understanding of servicing the field is the play therapy I did for many years starting in the mid-1980s. Down on the floor in play, a child and I would jointly invent characters and scenarios. One might say we created an analytic field together through our intense unconscious communication. But it would be wrong to imagine that there was not a leader and a follower. Consciously, I went where the child led, but when the play became too much—for me, the setting, or the child—or when it provoked what Civitarese refers to as violent emotions that obscure truth, I offered something from my mind as a therapist. In Civitarese's language (2019), I serviced the therapeutic field. While the content was ours, it was mine to manage *and* influence, in what I emphasized or brought out in the play. Relational analysts have shown us (Renik 1993) that no matter how much we follow or only narrate, in every word we utter, question we ask, character we create, silence we allow (or endure), we are unknowingly *shaping* the field from our own psychology. In this situation, naming the therapist narrator instead of interpreter seems like a sleight of hand that hides sovereignty.

I am not advocating that we abandon the asymmetrical psychoanalytic frame or eschew our own capacities. Or even that we not read or service the field. We do and must. We use our capacities to find the other. I am saying that our *unconscious* participation may be quite symmetrical with our patients'—a deeper *symmetry* of the unknowableness of analyst, patient, and what lives outside symbolic representation. As Civitarese writes, "to postulate asymmetry at the level of joint unconscious creation would be problematic, asymmetry is restored at the level of conscious interpretation" (Civitarese 2019, 432).

Asymmetry is a frame issue and a manner of formalizing difference in power, as much as capacity. When we are within experiences that lie outside representation, the negative is informal and not subject to interpretation the way the frame is. This suggests that when, within that asymmetry, the analyst senses something out of usual perceptual range, when negative capability is operative, when our deep unknowing of ourselves is made apparent, the analyst is *not* the arbiter of meaning. If anything, it is the holes in meaning that might come to the fore, challenging the realm of representation itself. Here it is not reading, narrating, or the action-oriented idea of servicing we are after, but something closer to *being with the other*. As Stern writes,

> If we are receptive, we create in the field that comes about between us and the patient, or us and the work, something powerful that cannot be described as a meaning. It is not only that the meaning of the images is impenetrable . . . the direct affective and sensory impact of these images *is* their meaning.

> (2020, 152)

Despite my critique of the technique that Ferro considers nonsovereign, Ferro demonstrates in his stance as discussant, his capacity for being with the other. I sense his openness to entering my dilemma as our joint dilemma, generously looking out at the problem with me, demonstrating in "our field" that he shares my curiosity about an analytic approach that is not sovereign and does not aim at surveillance of the other. Still, I am not sure he, or other Bionian field theorists, would invite a more transparently *vulnerable* use of themselves.

Ferro, Stern, and I each agree that living in negative capacity can be terrifying. It may have a very high cost for us as analysts and make us leery of moving further (within the transitional space of the field) into difficult states. Ferro explains that what we share most with patients is *avoidance* of mental pain. Drawing on Bion, he writes, "We are entitled to remain alive (as Winnicott reminds us) and cannot, therefore, always and in whatever circumstances, be required to cross certain boundaries of destructuring, anxiety, and risk (sometimes including physical risk)" (1993, 918). Stern underscores not only the predicament of experiencing the confusion and chaos of the negative but also the steep challenge of allowing ourselves to become vulnerable to it in the first place. The impulse to avoid suffering stokes the all-too-human propensity to see what is known, and to exploit narrative as a defense against the terror of what is not. "The impossibility of meaning," Stern (2020) writes, "causes us to retreat to a defensive posture, often in the form of forcing strangeness into recognizable forms or believing that comprehensible meanings lie behind the strangeness" (p. 152). Ferro insists on the analyst's "responsibility not to map these still unexplored territories 'excessively' with false charts" (1993, 918).

Can a technical stance that includes the analyst's vulnerability be a new, important means to disrupt our knowingness and facilitate growth? I believe that when we don't allow our vulnerability into the mix-up of our joint worlds, something of our humanness is lost. I don't mean that we should share our histories necessarily, but within the treatment's transitional space, we might recognize that the field may be servicing us as much as we are servicing the field. For me, and I think for Stern, the analyst's retreat to knowing is not limited to a saturated interpretation or an occasional shying away in the face of vulnerability, as the Bionian field theorists might believe. Rather, it is built into the newest notion of servicing the field, where the technique seems to understate issues of power, human relatedness, and intimacy (at least as articulated). As Stern and other relational thinkers have taught us, without the "estrangement and intimacy of being in relation," (Berlant and Edelman 2014) where shared *risk* may be required, the field is not truly bidirectional. We need to welcome the gaps in our understanding, and even our *solidity*, to allow something different to emerge.

Risk and repair: A new kind of dialogue in the clinical story

We psychoanalysts generally believe in the power of narrative—or dialogue, in Ferro's terms—within an analytic couple to transform.

When I write my clinical story in "The Analyst's Necessary Nonsovereignty," I am wrapping affect in a story, also hoping the imagined dialogue between writer and reader will open something up. But the story I tell reveals a problem within our belief in transformation. If subjectivity forms in the translation of another's message inside of us that we are influenced by but cannot know (Laplanche), the very possibility for repair of those early messages comes into question. Can we repair? Is this a goal? Thinking with Ferro (1993), and Berlant and Edelman (2014), I want to consider the transformational possibility I narrated in my story, but also its limits.

Ferro's ideas are consistent with my experience as "the patient" (patient and analyst are a single merged figure in "The Analyst's Necessary Nonsovereignty"). Something in the play with the characters in the field—the baby and her yellow booties, Mozart, Salieri, the poisoner, etc.—allowed me to understand and digest an emotional truth in a new way. Certainly, the metaphor of the yellow booties, their construction over long years of patient and analyst living side by side, created the felt possibility for transformation. I could sense that something changed when, entangled with one another, an unbearable real, a mother's hatred, (and the mother's translated enigmatic message of my being too much/too little), became thinkable in bearable terms. For both Ferro and Berlant, narrative play potentially allows fantasy a different arc and reach.

But did I really move, and how far? Indeed, as soon as I tell you, the reader, my new metaphoric understanding, I am reliving my too muchness/too littleness. I am fearing your reaction in my projection of how you will feel, imagining you as like my mother, and failing to fell the fantasy of my too muchness that I thought had just softened. In fact, even the requirements of narration—that a story moves from here to there, has some coherence—erases something important about the incoherence and nonsovereignty of the story itself. In writing the story, my affect re-presented itself here with you, the reader, in what I think Edelman would consider a predictable way. The scene changes from mother/daughter to analyst/patient to now reader/writer, but the structure of the fantasy persists. I brought to you (and have not dismantled) both my previous object relations and the enigmatic message lodged inside me seeking translation. There is something here outside of my control, formative, early, and maybe immutably beyond symbolization, or new metaphors—further indication of my nonsovereignty. Edelman argues that our stories keep us from encountering what is truly unbearable, the lack at the center (the gap of primal negation). The resistance to symbolization of this lack lends the real its traumatic character. This is trauma that cannot be repaired.

On the other hand, Berlant, a cultural and political theorist, thinks like a relational analyst. She believes that the prospect of movement does come from unbearable encounters with others that reveal, break down, and then acknowledge the structuring fantasy of the subject—what both Berlant and Edelman consider to be the existential gap or lack we live with. Because of our desire not to be defeated by life, she writes that "we enter the scene of relationality that is also and ultimately a demand for collaboration: relationality disturbs fantasy enough that it is open . . . . to absorbing and generating new social relations" (pp. 109–10). Acknowledgement (in this case, of the mother's hatred), she argues, shifts negativity's hold on us, making possible an escape from disavowal as a defense against reality. To concretize and simplify her idea, because I work with the analyst/because the patient works with me, we no longer must deny a mother's hatred. As a result, who we are and how we understand ourselves expands. Patient/analyst are no longer *just* too little/too much. Berlant asks, "If not repair what? If not world building what? When we move forward together new world making becomes possible" (p. 110).

Ferro also tells us that the transformative function is actually *performed by the dialogue,* "in so far as it's symbolic and conceivable" (Bezoari, Ferro, and Politi 1994, 39). Symbolization, while sometimes impossible, is nevertheless held out as a goal. The recognition of impossibility does not alter the analyst's push to represent. This is the paradoxical limit of knowledge noted by Edelman: To his surprise, we keep going for it, even in the face of impossibility. In contrast to Ferro and Berlant, Edelman argues that acknowledging a psychic fantasy, creating symbolization—as my patient and I did—does *not* necessarily release us from the hold of a structuring fantasy.

Edelman does not think consciousness can dislodge metaphors (like the enigmatic message of the mother), particularly those that are "largely unconscious" (p. 86). He contends that Berlant grants cognition a truly striking degree of power over affect, defined as "at once the somatic manifestation of psychic activity and the subject's relation to bodily action" (p. 95). This concept of moving differently with affect (and our bodies) raises the question for Edelman of just what agency would generate such movement. Logically, he says,

> it can't be affect itself, but [affect] isn't the subject of cognition either. . . . A belief in the power of knowledge to operate on what knowledge doesn't govern in the first place . . . may disavow the insistence of the unconscious and the real.
>
> (p. 86)

Our conscious knowing suggests a sovereign mastered self, but Edelman suggests that to hold this understanding of ourselves is to "keep company with a distinctive version of fetishistic disavowal . . . the disavowal precisely of *the limits of knowledge*" (p. 84, italics added). As Edelman continues, "We can fantasize, as fetishism demonstrates, that we know our relation to fantasy but the image of the fantasy we believe we know differs from that of the fantasy we enact in believing that we know it" (Edelman, p. 94). The fantasizer knows that they have fetishized, let's say a boot, as a substitute for the mother's phallic power, now lost, but knowing that does not change their love of the boot.

In psychoanalytic language, Edelman's ideas might be about the inefficacy of insight to produce deep affective transformation, because the formation of our being inscribes in us an unknowable otherness not subject to change. Said more simply, we may disrupt old fantasies, break down structure, and create new symbols, as my patient and I did. Yet while this may lessen our feelings of displacement and nonsovereignty, it won't rid us of them. These feelings come from being a person in the world.

In my view, moments of disavowal and acknowledgment oscillate (Morris 2012, personal communication). We do and undo. Know and unknow. Our efforts to make meaning through knowledge, while necessary to go forward, are what Edelman calls "an illusory binding of contradictory pressures, possibilities and investments to defend the subject against the lack with which it can have no relation" (p. 97). In "The Analyst's Necessary Nonsovereignty," irreducible otherness, the lack or negativity that persists in me, is re-presented in the image of the poisoning mother—a placeholder who fills or covers the gap, or lack (Berlant and Edelman 2014). We need representation to contain chaos and terror, but it also papers over the emptiness, the negative, the nonsovereignty that I am trying to illustrate in the disagreement between Berlant and Edelman.

While it is true that the mother's enigmatic message reinvigorated itself when I narrativized my experience, I do believe, in contrast to Edelman, that "acknowledging nonsovereignty . . . does significantly transform my affective encounter with the ontological disorganization of the world" (p. 90). It is not simply knowledge or acknowledgment but more the experience of entanglement with another that Berlant claims as world building. She argues that by knowing about negativity's power to disrupt, by owning our nonsovereignty, by breaking down our fantasies, *in the intimacy and estrangement of relationship*, we become able to lay other fantasies next to the structuring one. And that can shift how we live in the world. I agree. The analyst/patient's years of living side by side with new fantasies about who the patient is have diminished the *power* of the mother's message. Berlant's theorizing here resonates with the contemporary psychoanalytic idea that *the presence of an intersubjective system* allows affects to register and become translated, contained, and transformed. New living, often unlived life, becomes possible.

But I think Berlant would also have some quarrel with Ferro, as I do. While Ferro argues that telling the story together contains the transformative potential to move with affect in new ways, this is not a dialogue with shared risk. I believe the work requires the mutual entanglement and vulnerability that Berlant suggests and that the field theorists intimate is necessary but do not welcome, at least not in their writing.

The willingness to live in our nonsovereignty, sometimes in states of destructuring anxiety, may be necessary with some patients. As I wrote in "Do We Lose or Find Ourselves in the Negative?" (2015a), for patients whose very sense of being is in question, a different kind of access to and delivery of our own states of nonbeing may be required. Because our own truths continually escape us (and neither patient nor analyst possesses the knowledge of trauma that has gone unsymbolized), it is only in the mutual engagement that our unmentalized experience becomes constituted (McGleughlin 2015a). And often action precedes symbolization. We may need to speak and listen from the site of our own trauma, relying paradoxically on what we *don't* know of our own traumatic pasts and states of nonbeing (Caruth 1996; McGleughlin 2011, 2015a). By trauma, I also mean the existential trauma that lies at the heart of our humanness, the void at the center. In the "Analyst's Necessary Nonsovereignty," it was my unknowingly living out loud (only sometimes in words) in negative capability with my patient, without the goals and methods of normative repair, that expanded the affective potentialities between us (Berlant and Edelman 2014). This was not technique or metaphor, but raw experience metabolized together in real time.

Reader/writer engagement

It is very hard to free oneself from the internal demands of our own knowing. And it is difficult to tell a story without progress toward meaning (Berlant and Edelman 2014). In reading about a treatment, we generally presume the analyst-author possesses a line of intention, often supported by the analyst's facility with narrative. While I strove to disrupt my such factors, I found myself within a paradox: my aim of troubling the analyst's sovereignty (in theory, clinical practice, and writing) has an intentionality of its own. In spite of this "caughtness," I tried to engage what it means to think and write without pinning things down or assuming our stories are "true"—and without relying on post-hoc temporality to establish meaning.

The experimental writing of this piece was arduous and humbling. Because of a limited word count and the need for clarity for the reader, I took out several cycles of confusion that had put more of my own skin in the game, so to speak. For instance, where I originally referred to our joint person as "I," increasing my own risk and vulnerability, I opted for "we" in the published version. That decision, as far as I understand it, was based on my anxiety. Given that the paper would be available on the internet, I wanted to reduce the chances of being misunderstood as revealing my history or that of "the mother." But having changed to "we," I no longer felt the discomfort of being the sole subject under scrutiny, and I wasn't sure the reader would understand my pedagogical intention. So in this book I switch back to the first person, and then again to "we."

This narrative strategy worked to create an experience of the patient's vulnerability inside of me. I felt the fear of exposure from seemingly detailing my own inner world in ways I can only partially know or control. Enactive writing kept the unpredictable in play for me, as I had hoped, and brought out my uncertainty and nonsovereignty. But I am not sure that I created an aliveness in the writer/reader field that truly enacted a scene with you. How can we invite clinician, writer, *and* reader vulnerability?

By weaving the dense ideas of Berlant and Edelman into the clinical story, I sought to stage a dialogue in the gaps of our understanding about the treatment. By encouraging you, the reader, to interrogate yourself in some of the ways I interrogated myself, could I create a textual position in which I would feel vulnerable as a writer and you would experience your own nonsovereignty? Might we both be subject to pain and the possibilities that come from opening ourselves to these psychic fissures? As the reader, you don't get to speak back, at least not directly, but I would like to believe that "thinking with" and "speaking back" nevertheless might have taken place on a different plane. Perhaps the discussants might, in some sense, stand in for "you" as organizing placeholders, as well as original thinkers.

While I felt seen, recognized, and helped by all three discussants, each engaged most heavily on the level of ideas rather than sense, perception, or bewilderment. Stern (2020), for instance, used his precise, calibrating mind to find me, and he does. He simplifies my jargon and unbraids complicated thoughts about the negative. He offers his own similar experiences, and he teaches us. I am fuller for what I learned from him. However, I was equally trying to enact being with the other (my patient, my discussants, and you) in our shared nonsovereignty.

This was, at best, a partial success. Ferro noted that "the experience in the session with the patient is paralleled by the reader's experience with a text which leaves its spaces open, revealing its ambiguities and gaps in understanding" (2020, 148). This was gratifying, as was Cooney's *suggesting her own sensing* when she resonates with the importance of uncertainty, negative capability, and the shared surrender that I illustrate. But a more experienced writer might have been able to call forth the reader's experience of being broken in on or discombobulated, awash in something akin to sensation. This is something that Toni Morrison does so masterfully with her non-narrative style in novels such as *Sula*, where she rips readers out of time and space as they know it. She shows us we are not only readers but we are also being read.

How could I have invited the readers' nonsovereignty more effectively? As Goldberg (2012) writes of clinical technique (but we might also consider this for our writing),

> at the level of sensory symbiosis, [it] eschews the search for symbolic meaning and self-reflectivity in favor of experiencing the contours, movement, and impact of objects in and of themselves. It is a psychic domain where what matters is what we do rather than what we think, imagine, or say.

(p. 802)

I don't think I managed to turn us toward "an inductive dimension of technique . . . that operates as a counterpoint to the receptive/interpretive/symbolizing dimension" (Goldberg 2012, 801). To do so, my writing would have had to allow more affect and sensation to enter and circulate among us rather than be projected onto you in my fantasy. The questions of interpretation, narration, the field's interpreting itself, and asymmetry all remain squarely within a frame of representation. As do uncertainty and even negative capability. Seeing/not seeing, knowing/not knowing are questions rooted in representation. No discussant could seek out, exactly, a sensory level of symbiosis with me, the writer. But is there value in the struggle? Through play or performance? Risk? Shared vulnerability?

I used Agnes Martin to help us understand something else that I couldn't quite convey in my enactive writing: the limits of representation and the potential of perceiving outside of it. Martin draws our attention to non-conscious events that occur in what critical theorist Ali Lara calls

> "diffraction in the mind," or the sudden appearance of space–time–matter relations that are apparently not part of the what's going on, but that are perceived by virtue of our organic engagement with matter, expanding or contracting lapses of time, and even more, bringing physical qualities from somewhere else to the present event.
>
> (Lara et al. 2017, 34)

Political scientist Davide Panagia also imagines a "politics of sensation," which involves rupturing "the sensible domain of the human body through aesthetic experience" (Lara et al. 2017), a version of what I tried to do in breaking my bounded presentation of myself as analyst. He believes it is sensory experience that perturbs our perceptual givens and possibly our authority and sovereignty. In my clinical writing, I am committed to living in meaning that is emergent, enigmatic, and that preserves the uncertainty in the analytic process. I am imagining an analyst, and writer, who is groping toward the other whom she cannot quite know, only sense and feel (Stern 2020), in an effort to *be with* the other. The project of the book has been to discover and create some of that unsettled unknown experience, where meaning is not owned by the analyst or theorist or discrete subject, and theory is more generative of uncertainty.

The capacity to be connected in a non-symbolic register highlights the way the force of the negative runs through all life and connects the living to the non-organic forces and qualities of the material world (Grosz 2008), beyond and despite our individual identities. I want us to think that committing to the idea of nonsovereignty is allowing negativity to do its positive work. In a certain sense, this is writing on behalf of excess, not the kind that has to be translated or narrated, but that is felt as a constant source of struggle, and pleasure.

In conclusion

I will end by taking us back to art and its ability to intensify meaning without narrative, pairing Agnes Martin with the philosopher Elizabeth Grosz. In each of the short paragraphs later, the first lines, in italics, are Grosz, in conversation with fellow philosopher Gilles Deleuze. The second lines, in a plain font, combine Martin's writings and my thoughts on psychoanalysis from this paper.

Grosz (2008): *Art begins from the experience of chaos, the whirling unpredictable movement of forces . . . where intensities proliferate, forces are expressed for their own sake, where sensation lives.*

Think immersion in the field, raw sensation, what shapes the world. Think without memory or desire.

. . . Life can only exist and perpetuate itself to the extent that it . . . can somehow bracket out or cast into shadow the profusion of forces that engulf and surround it so that it may incorporate what it needs.

We frame to bracket chaos, to make a space where chaos can be explored. Think grid.

Elementary life can only evolve, develop, and elaborate itself to the extent that there is something fundamentally unstable about both its milieu and its organic constitution.

Think nonlinear dynamic systems; the unpredictability of change; the problems of reifying psychic structure, making it a thing, refusing metaphor.

Art is the art of affect more than representation, a system of dynamized and impacting forces rather than a system of unique images that function under the regime of sign (Deleuze). . .where the future is affectively and perceptually anticipated, [it] takes on the task of . . . summoning sensations to come.

Think an aesthetic approach where shared sensory experience takes precedence over intersubjective object-relational dynamics. Think affect and sensation over symbols; think the real.

There is much art in the natural world, from the haunting beauty of bird song to the erotic display in primates . . . which affirm[s] the excessiveness of the body and the natural order, their capacity to bring out in each other what surprises, what is of no use, but nevertheless attracts and appeals . . . .

Think the sensory for its own sake. Think excess. Think intensification, not containment.

Sensations, affects, and intensities, while not readily identifiable, are clearly closely connected with forces, and particularly bodily forces, and their qualitative transformations.

Think of O, the ineffable, what can't be known but runs through us.

Note

1 Like Green's concept of absence, which is always in dialectical relation with presence, absence is also generative—the presence-absence dialectic is the substrate that underlies all self-other normative development (Morris 2005). I add, so too the negative.

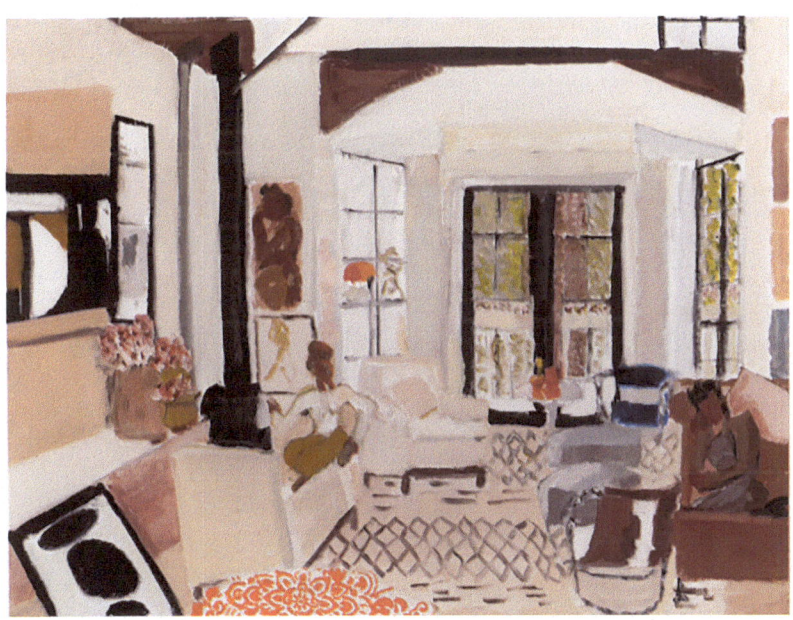

Figure 16.1 Room 1. 24x18. Oil on board, McGleughlin

Bibliography

Abelin, G. E. 1993. "Book Review. *Perdre De Vue: By J.B. Pontalis*. Paris: Gallimard, 1988, 307 pp., Fr 115." *Journal of the American Psychoanalytic Association* 41: 897–99.

Abraham, N., and M. Torok. 1994. *The Shell and the Kernel, Volume I*. Chicago, IL and London, England: The University of Chicago Press.

Aeroplane. 2010. *Without Lies [Recorded by Aeroplane and Sky Ferreira]. On We Can't Fly*. New York, NY: Ultra Records.

Ahmed, S. 2004. *The Cultural Politics of Emotion*. New York and Oxfordshire: Routledge Courtesy Edinburgh University Press.

Ahmed, S. 2017. *Living a Feminist Life*. Durham and London: Duke University Press.

Ahmed, S. 2019. *What's the Use*. Durham and London: Duke University Press.

Als, H. 2016. *The Heroic Art of Agnes Martin*. New York, NY: Review of Books. July 14

Alvarez, A. 1992. *Live Company: Psychoanalytic Psychotherapy with Autistic, Borderline, Deprived and Abused Children*. New York and London: Routledge.

Alvarez, A. 2012. *The Thinking Heart; Three Levels of Psychoanalytic Therapy with Disturbedchildren*. London, UK: Routledge.

Ammons, A. R. 1986. *The Selected Poems*. New York and London: W.W. Norton and Company.

Anzaldúa, G. 1987. *Borderlands: The New Mestiza= La Frontera*. San Francisco: Spinsters/Aunt Lute.

Aron, L. 1999. "The Patient's Experience of the Analyst's Subjectivity." In *Relational Psychoanalysis, Volume 1 The Emergence of a Tradition*, edited by S. Mitchell and L. Aron. New York and London: Routledge.

Aron, L., and A. Harris, eds. 1993. *The Legacy of Sandor Ferenczi*. Hillsdale, NJ: The Analytic Press

Aron, L., and K. Starr. 2012. *A Psychotherapy for the People: Toward a Progressive Psychoanalysis*. London, UK: Routledge.

Arsic, B. 2016. *Bird Relics*. Cambridge, MA: Harvard University Press.

Astor, M. 2022. "Transgender Americans Feel Under Siege as Political Vitriol Rises." *New York Times*, December 11, 2022.

Astor, M. 2023. "G. O. P. State Lawmakers Push a Growing Wave of Anti-Transgender Bills." *New York Times*, January 25.

Atlas, G., and L. Aron. 2018. *Dramatic Dialogue: Contemporary Clinical Practice*. London and New York: Routledge.

Baker, G., A. Daly, N. Davenport, L. Larson, and M. Sundell. 2003. "Francesca Woodman Reconsidered: A Conversation with George Baker, Ann Daly, Nancy Davenport, Laura Larson and Margaret Sundell." *Art Journal* 62 (2) (Summer): 52–67.

Bambara, T. C. 1980. *The Salt Eaters*. New York, NY: Random House.

Barad, K. 2012. "Interview with Karen Barad." In *New Materialism: Interviews and Cartographies*, edited by R. Dolphijn and I. van der Tuin. London: Open Humanities Press.

Baranger, M., W. Baranger, and J. Mom. 1983. "Process and Non-Process in Analytic Work." *International Journal of Psychoanalysis* 64:1–15.

Baranger, M., and W. Baranger. 2008. "The Analytic Situation as a Dynamic Field." *International Journal of Psychoanalysis* 89 (4): 795–826. https://doi.org/10.1111/j.1745-8315.2008.00074.x.

Barden, N. 2011. "Disrupting Oedipus: The Legacy of the Sphinx." *Psychoanalytic Psychotherapy* 25: 324–45.

Barden, N. 2012. "Response to: Research off the Couch: Re-visiting the Transsexual Conundrum." *Psychoanalytic Psychotherapy* 26: 282–89.

Barthes, R. 1967. "The Death of the Author." *Aspen: The Magazine in a Box*. 5+6. As presented at Ubu Web: http://www.ubu.com/aspen/aspen5and6/index.html

Barthes, R. 1980. *Camera Lucida: Reflections on Photography*. New York, NY: Hill and Wang, A Division of Farrar, Straus, and Giroux.

Benjamin, J. 1988. *The Bonds of Love*. New York and Toronto: Pantheon Press.

Benjamin, J. 1995. "Recognition and Destruction: An Outline of Intersubjectivity." In *Like Subjects, Love Objects: Essays on Recognition and Sexual Difference*, 27–48. New Haven, CT: Yale University Press.

Benjamin, J. 1998. "The Primal Leap of Psychoanalysis, from Body to Speech." In *The Shadow of the Other: Intersubjectivity and Gender in Psychoanalysis*. New York and London: Routledge.

Benjamin, J. 2004. "Beyond Doer and Done to: An Intersubjective View of Thirdness." *Psychoanalytic Quarterly* 73: 5–46.

Benjamin, W. 1935/2008. "The Work of Art in the Age of Its Technological Reproducibility." In *The Work of Art in the Age of Its Technological Reproducibility and Other Writings on Media,* edited by M. Jennings, B. Doherty and T. Levin. Cambridge, MA and London, England: The Belknap Press of Harvard University Press.

Benjamin, W. 2006. *Berlin Childhood around 1900*. Cambridge, MA and London, England: The Belknap Press of Harvard University Press.

Berlant, L. 2011. *Cruel Optimism*. Durham and London: Duke University Press.

Berlant, L., and L. Edelman. 2014. *Sex, or the Unbearable*. Durham and London: Duke University Press.

Bersani, L. 1986. *The Freudian Body: Psychoanalysis and Art*. New York: Columbia University Press.

Bezoari, M., A. Ferro, and P. Politi. 1994. "Listening, Interpreting and Psychic Change in the Analytic Dialogue." *International Forum of Psychoanalysis* 3: 35–41. https://doi.org/10.1080/08037069408411005.

Bianco, M. 2014. Online. March 2014. Lambda Literary.org publication.

Bion, W. R. 1959. "Attacks on Linking." *International Journal of Psychoanalysis* 40: 308–15.

Bion, W. R. 1962. *Learning from Experience*. London, UK: Heinemann.

Bion, W. R. 1967/2013. "Notes on Memory and Desire." In *Wilfred Bion: Los Angeles Seminars and Supervision*, edited by J. Aguayo and B. Malin, 136–38. London: Karnac.

Bion, W. R. 1970. *Attention and Interpretation*. London: Library/Karnac.

Blanchfield, B. 2016. *Proxies: Essays Near Knowing*. New York, NY: Nightboat Books.

Blechner, M. J. 2001. *The Dream Frontier*. London and Hillsdale, NJ: The Analytic Press.

Blessing, J., P. Phelan, and N. Trotman. 2010. *Haunted: Contemporary Photograph, Video, Performance*. New York, NY: Guggenheim Museum.

Blumstein, P., and P. Schwartz. 1983. *American Couples: Money, Work, Sex*. New York: William Morrow.

Bollas, C. 1983. "Expressive Uses of the Countertransference—Notes to the Patient from Oneself." *Contemporary Psychoanalysis* 19: 1–33.

Bollas, C. 1987. *The Shadow of the Object: Psychoanalysis of the Unthought Known*. New York, NY: Columbia University Press.

Bolognini, S. 2004. "Intrapsychic-Interpsychic." *International Journal of Psychoanalysis* 85: 337–58.

Botella, C., and S. Botella. 2005. *The Work of Psychic Figurability: Mental States Without Representation*. Translated by A. Weller and M. Zerbib. Hove and New York, NY: Brunner-Routledge.

Brickman, C. 2017. *Race in Psychoanalysis: Aboriginal Populations in the Mind. Relational Perspectives Book*. New York, NY: Routledge.

Bromberg, P. M. 1998. *Standing in the Spaces: Essays on Clinical Process, Trauma and Dissociation*. Hillsdale, NJ: The Analytic Press.

Bromberg, P. M. 2002. "'Speak to Me as to Thy Thinkings.' Commentary on 'Interpersonal Psychoanalysis' Radical Façade' by Irwin Hirsch." *Journal of the American Academy of Psychoanalysis* 30: 605–20.

Bromberg, P. M. 2006. *Awakening the Dreamer*. Mahwah, NJ: The Analytic Press.

Broumas, O. 1977. *Beginning with O*. New Haven: Yale University Press.

Bruhm, S., and N. Hurley. 2004. "Introduction." In *Curiouser: On the Queerness of Children*, edited by S. Bruhm and N. Hurley. Minneapolis and London: University of Minnesota Press.

Butler, C., R. Shiff, M. Monahan, and M. Dumas. 2008. "Painter as Witness." In *Marlene Dumas: Measuring Your Own Grave*, edited by L. G. Mark. Los Angeles: Museum of Contemporary Art.

Butler, J. 1990. *Gender Trouble: Feminism and the Subversion of Identity*. New York and London: Routledge.

Butler, J. 1993. *Bodies That Matter: On the Discursive Limits of "Sex"*. New York: Routledge.

Butler, J. 2005. *Giving an Account of One's Self*. New York: Fordham University Press.

Butler, J. 2014. "Rethinking Vulnerability and Resistance." In *Vulnerability in Resistance*, edited by J. Butler, Z. Gambetti, and L. Sabsay. Durham, NC and London: Duke University Press.

Butler, J. 2015. *Senses of the Subject*. New York: Fordham University Press.

Campt, T. 2021. *A Black Gaze: Artists Changing How We See*. Cambridge, MA and London: MIT Press.

Caper, R. 1999. *A Mind of One's Own*. London, UK: Routledge.

Caruth, C. 1995. *Trauma: Explorations in Memory*. Baltimore, MD: Johns Hopkins University Press.

Caruth, C. 1996. *Unclaimed Experience: Trauma, Narrative, and History*. Baltimore, MD and London, England: The Johns Hopkins University Press.

Cerullo, M. 1987. *Night Visions: Towards a Lesbian and Gay Politics for the Present*. Boston, MA: Radical America, 67–71.

Cho, S., K. W. Crenshaw, and L. McCall. 2013. "Toward a Field of Intersectionality Studies: Theory, Application and Praxis." *Signs* 38 (4). Chicago University Press Journals.

Chodorow, N. J. 1978. *The Reproduction of Mothering: Psychoanalysis and the Sociology of Gender*. Berkeley, CA: University of California Press.

Civitarese, G. 2008. *The Intimate Room: Theory and Technique of the Analytic Field*. London, UK: Routledge.

Civitarese, G. 2015. "Transformations in Hallucinosis and the Receptivity of the Analyst." *The International Journal of Psycho-Analysis* 96: 1091–116. https://doi.org/10.1111/1745-8315.12242.

Civitarese, G. 2019. "Reply to Goldberg and Steinberg." *Psychoanalytic Dialogues* 29: 427–34.

Coleman, E., W. Bockting, M. Botzer, P. Cohen-Kettenis, G. DeCuypere, J. Feldman, L. Fraser, J. Green, G. Knudson, W. J. Meyer, S. Monstrey, R. K. Adler, G. R. Brown, A. H. Devor, R. Ehrbar, R. Ettner, E. Eyler, R. Garofalo, D. H. Karasic,.. K. Zucker. 2012. "Standards of Care for the Health of Transsexual, Transgender, and Gender Nonconforming People, Version 7." *International Journal of Transgenderism* 13 (4): 165–232. https://doi.org/10.1080/15532739.2011.700873

Combahee River Collective. 1983. "The Combahee River Collective Statement." In *Home Girls, A Black Feminist Anthology*, edited by B. Smith. New York: Kitchen Table Women of Color Press, Inc.

Cooney, A. S. 2020. "Through a Glass Darkly: A Discussion of 'The Analyst's Necessary Non Sovereignty and the Generative Power of the Negative'." *Psychoanalytic Dialogues* 30: 139–45.

Cooper, S. 2007. "Begin the Beguine: Relational Theory and the Pluralistic Third." *Psychoanalytic Dialogues* 17: 247–71.

Cooper, S. 2014. "Clinical Theory at the Borders." *IJP- Open* 1: 1–34

Cooper, S. 2021. "Donald Winnicott and Stephen Mitchell's Developmental Tilt Hypothesis Reconsidered." *Psychoanalytic Dialogues* 31: 355–70.

Corbett, K. 2001. "Nontraditional Family Romance." *Psychoanalytic Quarterly* 70: 599–624.

Crenshaw, K. 1991. "Mapping the Margins: Intersectionality, Identity Politics, and Violence against Women of Color." *Stanford Law Review* 43 (6): 1241–299.

Davies, J. M. 2004. "Whose Bad Objects Are We Anyway? Repetition and Our Elusive Love Affair with Evil." *Psychoanalytic Dialogues* 14: 711–32.

Davis, L. 2009. *The Collected Stories of Lydia Davis: Break It Down.* New York: Farrar, Strauss and Giroux.

De Lauretis, T. 1987. *Technologies of Gender: Essays on Theory, Film and Fiction.* Bloomington and Indianapolis: Indiana University Press.

De Lauretis, T. 1999. "Letter to an Unknown Woman." In *That Obscure Subject of Desire*, edited by R. Lesser and E. Shoenberg. New York, NY: Routledge.

Denson, G. R. 2016. "On Agnes Martin and Mapping the Pathways Out of Schizophrenia and Obsession." *Huffington Post.* https://www.huffpost.com/entry/on-agnes-martin-and-mappi_b_13882410

Derrida, J. 1984. *Margins of Philosophy.* Translated by A. Bass. Chicago: University of Chicago Press.

Derrida, J. 1988. "Signature Event Context." In *Limited Inc.*, edited by J. Derrida. Evanston, IL: Northwestern University Press.

Dimen, M. 2011. *With Culture in Mind.* New York and London: Routledge.

Director, L. 2016. "The Analyst as Catalyst: Cultivating Mind in the Shadow of Neglect." *Psychoanalytic Dialogues* 26: 685–97.

Dolphin, R., and I. van der Tuin. 2012. *New Materialism: Interviews and Cartographies.* Ann Arbor, MI: Open Humanities Press.

Du Bois, W. E. B. 1920/2001. *The Comet.* Minnesota: Mint Editions.

Du Bois, W. E. B. 1935/2013. *Black Reconstruction in America.* New Brunswick, NJ and London: Transaction Publishers.

Du Bois, W. E. B. 1968. *Autobiography of W.E.B. Dubois: A Soliloquy on Viewing My Life from the Last Decade of Its First Century.* New York, NY: Intl Publishers Com, Inc.

Edelman, L. 2005. *No Future: Queer Theory and the Death Drive.* Durham, NC and London: Duke University Press.

Eliot, T. S. 1915. "The Love Song of J. Alfred Prufrock." In *T.S. Eliot: Collected Poems 1909-1962* (1991). New York: Harcourt, Brace and Company.

Eng, D., and S. Han. 2016. *Racial Melancholia, Racial Dissociation: On the Social and Psychic Lives of Asian Americans.* Durham, NC: Duke University Press.

Fanon, F. 1986/1967. *Black Skin, White Masks.* Translated by C. L. Markmann. London: Pluto Press.

Farhi, N. 2010. "The Hands of The Living God." *Psychoanalytic Dialogues* 20 (5): 478–503.

Felman, S., and D. Laub. 1992. *Testimony: Crises of Witnessing in Literature, Psychoanalysis, and History.* New York, NY and London, England: Routledge, Taylor and Francis Group.

Ferenczi, S. 1985. *The Clinical Diary of Sándor Ferenczi.* Edited by Judith Dupont. Cambridge: Harvard University Press.

Ferrante, E. 2012/2013/2015. *The Neopolitan Novels*. Translated by A. Goldstein. Book One: *My Brilliant Friend* (2011); Book Two: *The Story of a New Name* (2013); Book Three: *Those who Leave and Those Who Stay Behind* (2014); Book Four: *The Story of the Lost Child* (2015). New York, NY: Europa Editions.

Ferris, A. 2003. "The Disembodied Spirit." In *The Disembodied Spirit Exhibition Catalog*, 32–43. Brunswick, ME: Bowdoin College Museum of Art.

Ferro, A. 1993. "The Impasse Within a Theory of the Analytic Field: Possible Vertices of Observation." *The International Journal of Psychoanalysis* 74: 917–29.

Ferro, A. 2009. "Transformations in Dreaming and Characters in the Psychoanalytic Field." *The International Journal of Psychoanalysis* 90: 209–30.

Ferro, A. 2020. "A Discussion of 'The Analyst's Necessary Nonsovereignty and the Generative Power of the Negative'." *Psychoanalytic Dialogues* 30: 146–49.

Ferro, A., and G. Civitarese. 2013. "Analyst in Search of an Author: Voltaire or Artemisia Gentileshi? Commentary on 'Field Theory in Psychoanalysis, Part 2: Bionian Field Theory and Contemporary Interpersonal/Relational Psychoanalysis' by Donnel B. Stern." *Psychoanalytic Dialogues* 23 (6): 646–53.

Ferro, A., and G. Civitarese. 2016. "Confrontation in the Bionian Model of the Analytic Field." *Psychoanalytic Inquiry* 36: 307–22.

Flood, A. 2015. "U.S. Poet Defends Reading of Michael Brown Autopsy Report as a Poem." *The Guardian*, March 2015.

Foehl, J. 2017. *Introduction in Interpersonal Psychoanalysis and the Enigma of Consciousness*. New York: Routledge.

Foehl, J. C. 2008. "Follow the Fox: Edgar A. Levenson's Pursuit of Psychoanalytic Process." *Psychoanalytic Quarterly* 77: 1231–68.

Forché, C. 1981. *The Country between Us*. New York: Harper and Row.

Foucault, M. 1980. *The History of Sexuality*. New York: Vintage Books.

Fournier, L. 2021. *Autotheory as Feminist Practice in Art, Writing, and Criticism*. Cambridge, MA and London: MIT Press.

Frankel, R. 2017. "Presentation for Massachusetts Institute for Psychoanalysis." Unpublished manuscript, Cambridge, MA.

Frankenberg 1993. *White Women, Race Matters: The Social Construction of Whiteness*. Minneapolis, MN: University of Minnesota Press.

Freud, S. 1905. "Three Essays on the Theory of Sexuality (1905)." *The Standard Edition of the Complete Psychological Works of Sigmund Freud* 7: 123–246.

Freud, S. 1914. "Remembering, Repeating and Working-Through (Further Recommendations on the Technique of Psycho-Analysis II)." *The Standard Edition of the Complete Psychological Works of Sigmund Freud* 12: 145–56.

Freud, S. 1920. *Beyond the Pleasure Principle. The Standard Edition of the Complete Psychological Works of Sigmund Freud*. London, UK: Hogarth Press.

Freud, S. 1925. "Negation." In *The Standard Edition of the Complete Psychological Works of Sigmund Freud*, 235–39. London, UK: Hogarth Press.

Freud, S. 1937. "Analysis Terminable and Interminable." *International Journal of Psychoanalysis* 18: 373–405.

Friedman, L. 2005. "Psychoanalytic Treatment: Thick Soup or Thin Gruel?" *PsychoanalyticInquiry* 25: 418–39.

Fuentes, C. 2001. *The Years with Laura Díaz*. Translated by A. J. Mac Adam. San Diego, New York and London: Harvest Book.

Gabbard, G. O. 1997. "A Reconsideration of Objectivity in the Analyst." *The International Journal Psycho-Analysis* 78: 15–26

Gagnon, J., and W. Simon. 1973. *Sexual Conduct: The Social Sources of Human Sexuality*. Chicago, IL: Aldine.

Gerson, S. 2009. "When the Third is Dead: Memory, Mourning, and Witnessing in the Aftermath of the Holocaust." *The International Journal of Psychoanalysis* 90: 1341–57.

Ghent, E. 1990. "Masochism, Submission, Surrender—Masochism as a Perversion of Surrender." *Contemporary Psychoanalysis* 26: 108–36

Gilroy, P. 1993. *The Black Atlantic: Modernity and Double Consciousness*. Cambridge: Harvard University Press.

Glimcher, A. 2012. *Agnes Martin: Paintings, Writings, Remembrances*. London and New York: Phaidon Press.

Goldberg, P. 2012. "Active Perception and the Search for Sensory Symbiosis." *Journal of the American Psychoanalytic Association* 60: 791–812.

Goldberger, M. 1993. " 'Bright Spot,' a Variant of 'Blind Spot'." *Psychoanalytic Quarterly* 62: 270–73.

González, F. J. 2009. "Moving Fragments." *Studies in Gender and Sexuality* 10: 54–74

González, F. J. 2017. "The Edge is a Horizon: Commentary on Hansbury." *Journal of the American Psychoanalytic Association* 65: 1061–73

Green, A. 1972. *On Private Madness*. London, UK: Hogarth Press.

Green, A. 1975. "The Analyst, Symbolization and Absence in the Analytic Setting (On Changes in Analytic Practice and Analytic Experience)—In Memory of D. W. Winnicott." *International Journal of Psychoanalysis* 56: 1–22.

Green, A. 1998. "The Primordial Mind and the Work of the Negative." *International Journal of Psychoanalysis* 79 (4): 649.

Green, A. 1999. *The Work of the Negative*. Translated by A. Weller. London, UK: Free Association

Greenberg, J. 2001. "The Analyst's Participation: A New Look." *Journal of the American Psychoanalytic Association* 49: 359–81.

Greenberg, J. R., and S. A. Mitchell. 1983. *Object Relations in Psychoanalytic Theory*. Cambridge and London: Harvard University Press.

Gregg, M., and G. Seigworth, eds. 2010. *The Affect Theory Reader*. Durham and London: Duke University Press.

Grinberg, L., and R. Grinberg. 1981. "Modalities of Object Relationships in the Psychoanalytic Process." *Contemporary Psychoanalysis* 17: 290–320

Grossmark, R. 2018. *The Unobtrusive Relational Analyst*. New York and London: Routledge.

Grosz, E. 1993. "Bodies and Knowledges; Feminism and the Crisis of Reason." In *Feminist Epistemologies*, edited by L. Alcoff and E. Potter. New York, NY: Routledge.

Grosz, E. 1995. *Space, Time and Perversion: Essays on the Politics of Bodies*. New York: Routledge.

Grosz, E. 2008. *Chaos, Territory, Art; Deleuze and the Framing of the Earth*. New York, NY: Columbia University Press.

Halberstam, J. 2011. *The Queer Art of Failure*. Durham: Duke University Press.

Halberstam, J. 2018. *Trans**. Oakland, CA: California University Press.

Halberstam, J. 2020. *Wild Things: The Disorder of Desire*. Durham and London: Duke University Press.

Hambourg, M., and M. Fineman. 2002. "Avedon's Endgame." In Catalogue Essay from Exhibition Publication *Richard Avedon: Portraits September 26, 2002– January 5, 2003*. New York, NY: Harry N. Abrams.

Hansbury, G. 2017. "The Masculine Vaginal: Working with Queer Men's Embodiment at the Transgender Edge." *Journal of the American Psychoanalytic Association* 65: 1009–31.

Haraway, D. 1991. "A Cyborg Manifesto: Science, Technology, and Socialist-Feminism in the Late Twentieth Century." In *Simians, Cyborgs and Women: The Reinvention of Nature*, 149–81. New York: Routledge.

Harris, A. 1997. "Aggression, Envy, and Ambition: Circulating Tensions in Women's Psychic Life." *Gender and Psychoanalysis* 2: 291–325.

Harris, A. 2000. "Politicized Passions: A Discussion of Dianne Elise's Essay." *Gender and Sexuality* 1: 147–56.

Harris, A. 2008. *Gender as Soft Assembly*. New York: Routledge.

Harris, A. 2009. "You Must Remember This." *Psychoanalytic Dialogues* 19: 2–21.

Hartman, S. 1997. *Scenes of Subjection: Terror, Slavery, and Self-Making in Nineteenth-Century America*. Oxford, UK: Oxford University Press.

Hartman, S. 2008. *Lose Your Mother: A Journey Along the Atlantic Slave Route*. New York: Farrar, Straus and Giroux.

Hartman, S. 2015. "Drowning in a Sea of Love." *Psychoanalytic Dialogues* 25 (2): 237–47.

Himes, M. 2012. "The Weight of the Proper Name." *Division|Review* 4 (Spring): 15–18, American Psychological Association.

Hoffman, I. 1983. "The Patient as Interpreter of the Analyst's Experience." *Contemporary Psychoanalysis* 19: 389–422.

Holder, A. 2018. "The Afterlife of Black Citizenship." Unpublished presentation, The American Studies Association, Atlanta, GA, November 2018.

Howe, F. n.d. "Notes Following an Afternoon with Catherine Kehoe." https://catherinekehoe.com/essay-fanny-howe-

Jay, K., and A. Young. 1979. *The Gay Report: Lesbians and Gay Men Speak Out about Sexual Experiences and Lifestyles*. New York: Summit Books.

Johnson, B. 1998. *The Feminist Difference: Literature, Psychoanalysis, Race, and Gender*. Cambridge, MA: Harvard University Press.

Johnson, B. 2000. "Using People: Kant with Winnicott." In *The Turn to Ethics*, edited by M. Garber et al. New York: Routledge.

Johnson, B. 2014. "Barbara Johnson." In *The Barbara Johnson Reader: The Surprise of Otherness*, edited by M. Feurstein, B. J. Gonzalez, L. Porten, and K. Valens. Durham and London: Duke University Press.

Jones, A. L. 2020. "A Black Woman as an American Analyst: Some Observations from One Woman's Life Over Four Decades." *Studies in Gender and Sexuality* 21: 77–84.

Jones, L. 1964. *The Dead Lecturer*. New York, NY: Grove.

Jones, Z. 2017. "Fresh Trans Myths of 2017." Posted online on Gender Analysis, July 1, 2017.

Joseph, B. 1975. "The Patient Who Is Difficult to Reach." In *Melanie Klein Today, Volume 2*, edited by E. Bott-Spillius. New York and London: Routledge.

Kelleher, P. 2004. "How to Do Things with Perversion: Psychoanalysis and the Child in Danger." In: *Curiouser: On the Queerness of Children*. Minneapolis, MN and London: University of Minnesota Press.

Keller, C. 2013. *Francesca Woodman 1958–1981*. New York: San Francisco Museum of Modern Art with DAP Museum Catalogue.

Klein, M. 1948. "A Contribution to the Theory of Anxiety and Guilt." *The International Journal of Psychoanalysis* 29: 114–23.

Knoblauch, S. H. 2020. "Beyond Racial Visibility and Invisible: Reply to Hartman and Sheehi." *Psychoanalytic Dialogues* 30: 331–35

Koestenbaum, W. 1978. *Barthes: A Lover's Discourse, Fragments*. Foreword by W. Koestenbaum. New York: Hill and Wang.

Kohut, H. 1972. "Thoughts on Narcissism and Narcissistic Rage." *The Psychoanalytic Study of the Child* 27 (1): 360–400. https://doi.org/10.1080/00797308.197 2.11822721.

Kraus, R. 1986. "Problem Sets." In *Francesca Woodman: Photographic Work*, 41–51. New York, NY: Wellesley College Museum and Hunter College Art Gallery.

LaCapra, D. 2001. *Writing History, Writing Trauma*. Baltimore, MD and London, UK: The Johns Hopkins University Press.

Langer, S. J. 2011. "Gender (Dis)Agreement: A Dialogue on the Clinical Implications of Gendered Language." *Journal of Gay and Lesbian Mental Health* 15 (3): 300–7.

Langer, S. J. 2019. *Theorizing Transgender Identity for Clinical Practice: A New Model for Understanding Gender*. Philadelphia, PA: Jessica Kingsley Publishers.

Lanzoni, S. 2018. *Empathy: A History*. New Haven and London: Yale University Press.

Laplanche, J. 1987. *New Foundations for Psychoanalysis*. Translated by J. House. New York: The Unconscious in Translation.

Lara, A., A. Liu, C. P. Ashley, A. Nishida, M. B. Liebert, and M. Billies. 2017. "Affect and Subjectivity." *Subjectivity* 10: 30–43.

Laub, D. 1991. "Truth and Testimony the Process and the Struggle." *American Imago* 48: 75–91.

Layton, L. 2020. *Toward a Social Psychoanalysis: Culture, Character, and Normative Unconscious Processes*. Edited by M. Leavy-Sperounis. London and New York: Routledge.

Leary, K. 1997. "Race, Self-Disclosure, and 'Forbidden Talk': Race and Ethnicity in Contemporary Clinical Practice." *Psychoanalytic Quarterly* 66: 163–89.

Leavitt, J. 2021. "A Letter to Kathleen Del Mar Miller: Skin to Skin, Bone to Bone." *Psychoanalytic Dialogues* 31: 551–63.

Leavitt, J. 2022. "Plea for a Measure of Social Un-belonging." Paper presented at the Psychology and the Other Conference, Boston, MA, October 5, 2022.

Lemma, A. 2010. "An Order of Pure Decision: Growing up in a Virtual World and the Adolescent's Experience of Being-in-A-Body." *Journal of the American Psychoanalytic Association* 58: 691–714.

Lemma, A. 2013. "The Body One has and the Body One is: Understanding the Transsexual's Need to be Seen." *The International Journal of Psychoanalysis* 94: 277–92.

Lemma, A. 2016. "Present Without Past: The Disruption of Temporal Integration in a Case of Transsexuality." *Psychoanalytic Inquiry* 36: 360–70.

Lemma, A. 2018. "Transitory Identities: Some." *The International Journal of Psychoanalysis* 99: 1089–106.

Leveille, L. 2023. "Shadow Money Behind a Leading Anti-Trans Think Tank." Health Liberation. Now.com

Levenson, E. 1972. *The Fallacy of Understanding.* New York and London: Basic Books, Inc.

Levenson, E. 1983. *The Ambiguity of Change.* New York and London: Basic Books, Inc.

Levine, H. B. 2012. "The Colourless Canvas: Representation, Therapeutic Action and the Creation of Mind." *International Journal of Psychoanalysis* 93: 607–29.

Levine, H. B. 2013. "Comparing Field Theories." *Psychoanalytic Dialogues* 23: 667–73.

Levine, H. B. 2022. *Affect, Representation and Language: Between the Silence and the Cry (The International Psychoanalytical Association Psychoanalytic Ideas and Applications Series).* London and New York: Routledge.

Levine, H. B. 2023. "A Metapsychology of the Unrepresented." *Psychoanalytic Quarterly* 92: 11–25.

Levine, H. B., G. Reed, and D. Scarfone, eds. 2013. *Unrepresented States and the Construction of Meaning: Clinical and Theoretical Contributions.* London, UK: Karnac.

Lewis, J., and G. Joseph. 1981. *Common Differences: Conflicts in Black and White Feminist Perspectives.* Garden City, NY: Anchor Books.

Leys, R. 2000. *Trauma: A Genealogy.* Chicago, IL and London, England: The University of Chicago Press.

Likierman, M. 2006. "Unconscious Experience: Relational Perspectives." *Psychoanalytic Dialogues* 16: 365–76.

Lombardi, R. 2005. "On the Psychoanalytic Treatment of a Psychotic Breakdown." *Psychoanalytic Quarterly* 74: 1069–99.

Lombardi, R. 2010. "Flexibility of the Psychoanalytic Approach in the Treatment of a Suicidal Patient: Stubborn Silences as 'Playing Dead'." *Psychoanalytic Dialogues* 20: 269–84.

Mantel, H. 2009. *Wolf Hall*. New York, NY: Henry Holt and Company, LLC.

Maroda, K. 2022. *The Analyst's Vulnerability: Impact on Theory and Practice*. New York and London: Routledge.

Massumi, B. 1995. "The Autonomy of Affect." In *Cultural Critique*. Minneapolis: University of Minnesota Press.

McGleughlin, J. 1982. "Power, Liberation and Sexuality." Unpublished manuscript, Hampshire College.

McGleughlin, J. 1987. "The Freedom to Want Passionately: A Theoretical Exploration of Women's Desire." Thesis, Smith College School for Social Work.

McGleughlin, J. 2001. "The Demand for Intersubjectivity before the Birth of the Patient's Self and the Problems That Follow, or How Poetry Always Leads Theory." Unpublished manuscript for Completion of Psychoanalytic Training, Massachusetts Institute for Psychoanalysis, Boston, MA.

McGleughlin, J. 2008. "Can A Diamond Ever Be Gay?" *Studies in Gender and Sexuality* 9 (2): 184–205.

McGleughlin, J. 2011. "The Analyst's Necessary Vertigo." *Psychoanalytic Dialogues* 21 (5): 630–42.

McGleughlin, J. 2015a. "Do We Find or Lose Ourselves in the Negative?" *Psychoanalytic Dialogues* 25 (2): 214–36. doi:10.1080/10481885.2015.1013838.

McGleughlin, J. 2015b. "Answering Gestures." *Psychoanalytic Dialogues* 25 (2): 256–64.

McGleughlin, J. 2019. "Translation." *Studies in Gender and Sexuality* 21 (1): 53–57.

McGleughlin, J. 2020. "The Analyst's Necessary Nonsovereignty and the Generative Power of the Negative." *Psychoanalytic Dialogues* 30: 123–38.

McGleughlin, J. 2021. "Rethinking Oedipus or Not." *Psychoanalytic Dialogues* 31: 329–39.

McGleughlin, M. 2017. *Two Way Reaching: Graduation Paper*. Middletown, CT: Wesleyan University.

McKay, R. K. 2019. "Bread and Roses: Empathy and Recognition." *Psychoanalytic Dialogues* 29 (1): 75–91.

Melville, H. 1851. *Moby Dick*. New York, NY: Penguin Group; Reprint edition (1992).

Michaels, A. 1997. *Fugitive Pieces*. New York: Knopf.

Michaels, A. 2001. *Poems: The Weight of Oranges, Miner's Pond, Skin Divers*. New York: Alfred A Knopf.

Michaels, W. B. 1996. " 'You Who Never Was There': Slavery and the New Historicism, Deconstruction and the Holocaust." *Narrative* 4: 8.

Mitchell, S. 1988. *Relational Concepts in Psychoanalysis: An Integration*. Cambridge, MA and London: Harvard University Press.

Modell, A. H. 1970. "The Transitional Object and the Creative Act." *Psychoanalytic Quarterly* 39: 240–50

Moraga, C., and G. Anzaldúa. 1981. *This Bridge Called My Back*. Boston, MA: Kitchen Table—Women of Color Press.

Morris, F., and T. Bell. 2015. *Agnes Martin*. London, UK: The Tate Modern.

Morris, H. 2005. "Discussion of 'Conflict, Structure, and Absence: The Relevance of André Green's Ideas to the Treatment of Difficult Patients,' by Gail Reed and Francis Baudry." Unpublished manuscript, Boston, MA, Boston Psychoanalytic Society and Institute. September 23.

Moten, F. 2003. *In the Break: The Aesthetics of the Black Radical Tradition*. Minneapolis: University of Minnesota Press.

Munoz, J. E. 2010. *Cruising Utopia: The Then and There of Queer Futurity*. New York: New York University Press.

Naiburg, S. 2015. *Structure and Spontaneity in Clinical Prose: A Writer's Guide for Psychoanalysts and Psychotherapists*. New York and London: Routledge.

Nast, H. J. 2000. "Mapping the Unconscious." *Annals of the Association of American Geographers* 90 (2): 215–55.

Nathans, S. 2021. "Oedipus for Everyone: Revitalizing the Model for LGBTQ Couples and Single Parent Families." *International Journal of Relational Perspectives* 31 (3): 312–28.

Nestle, J. 1981. "Butch-fem Relationships: Sexual Courage in the 1950's." *Heresies* 12: 21–24.

Nguyen, L. 2012. "Psychoanalytic Activism." *Psychoanalytic Dialogues* 29 (3): 308–17.

Ogden, T. H. 1989. "On the Concept of an Autistic-Contiguous Position." *International Journal of Psycho-Analysis* 70: 127–40.

Ogden, T. H. 1997. "Reverie and Metaphor: Some Thoughts on How I Work as a Psychoanalyst." *International Journal of Psycho-Analysis* 78 (4): 719–32.

Ogden, T. H. 2005. *This Art of Psychoanalysis: Dreaming Undreamt Dreams and Interrupted Cries*. New York, NY: Routledge.

Ogden, T. H. 2012. "Psychoanalysis as a Pocket of Resistance against Inhumanity: Commentary on Paper by Rachael Peltz." *Psychoanalytic Dialogues* 22: 291–95. https://doi.org/10.1080/10481885.2012.679595.

Ogden, T. H. 2016. "Some Thoughts on Practicing Psychoanalysis." *Fort Da* 22: 21–36.

Ogden, T. H. 2019. "Ontological Psychoanalysis or 'What Do You Want to Be When You Grow Up?'." *Psychoanalytic Quarterly* 88: 661–84.

Ogden, T. H. 2023. "Like the Belly of a Bird Breathing: On Winnicott's 'Mind and Its Relation to the Psyche-Soma'". *International Journal of Psychoanalysis* 104: 7–22.

Olds, S. 2001. "The Space Heater." *The New Yorker*, January 22, 2001.

Oliver, M. 1986. "Wild Geese." In *Dream Work*. New York: The Atlantic Monthly Press.

Orange, D. M. 2008. "Recognition as: Intersubjective Vulnerability in the Psychoanalytic Dialogue." *International Journal of Psychoanalytic Self Psychology* 3: 178–94.

Orange, D. M., G. E. Atwood, and R. D. Stolorow. 1997. *Working Intersubjectively: Contextualism in Psychoanalytic Practice*. Hillsdale, NJ: The Analytic Press.

Peltz, R., and P. Goldberg. 2013. "Field Conditions: Discussion of Donnel B. Stern's Field Theory in Psychoanalysis." *Psychoanalytic Dialogues* 23: 660–66.

Peplau, L. A., and H. Amaro. 1982. "Understanding Lesbian Relationships." In *Homosexuality: Social, Psychological, and Biological Issues*, edited by W. Paul, J. D. Weinrich, J. C. Gonsiorek, and M. E. Hotvedt, 233–47. Beverly Hills, CA: Sage.

Phelan, P. 1994. *Unmarked: The Politics of Performance*. New York, NY: Routledge.

Phelan, P. 2002. "Francesca Woodman's Photography: Death and the Image One More Time." *Signs: Journal of Woman in Culture and Society* 27: 979–1004.

Phillips, A. 2006. *Side Effects*. London, UK: Harnish Hamilton.

Pizer, B. 2003. "When the Crunch is a (k)not: A Crimp in Relational Dialogue." *PsychoanalyticDialogues* 13: 171–92.

Pontalis, J. B. 1999. *Perdre De Vue*. Paris, France: Gallimard.

Powell, D. 2018. "Race African Americans and Psychoanalysis. Collective Silence in the Therapeutic Conversation." *JAPA* 66: 1021–49.

Prosser, J. 1988. *Second Skins: The Body Narratives of Transsexuality*. New York: Columbia University Press.

Racker, H. 1968. "The Meanings and Uses of Countertransference." *Transference and Countertransference* 73: 127–73.

Rankine, C. 2015. "The Condition of Black Life is Mourning." *New York Times Magazine,* Op Ed. June 22, 2015. https://www.nytimes.com/2015/06/22/magazine/the-condition-of-black-life-is-one-of-mourning.html.

Rankine, C. 2019. *The White Card: A Play in One Act*. Minneapolis, MN: Graywolf Press.

Raymond, C. 2010. *Francesca Woodman and the Kantian Sublime*. Surrey, England and Burlington, Vermont: Ashgate Publishing.

Reed, G. S. 2001. "The Disregarded Analyst and the Transgressive Process: Discontinuity, Countertransference, and the Framing of the Negative." *Journal of the American Psychoanalytic Association* 49: 909–31.

Renik, O. 1993. "Analytic Interaction: Conceptualizing Technique in Light of the Analyst's Irreducible Subjectivity." *Psychoanalytic Quarterly* 62: 553–71.

Rich, A. 1973. *Diving into the Wreck: Poems 1970–1972*. New York and London: W.W. Norton and Co.

Rich, A. 1978. *The Dream of a Common Language; Poems 1974–1977*. New York and London: W.W. Norton and Co.

Robbins, M. 1996. "The Mental Organization of Primitive Personalities and Its Treatment Implications." *Journal of the American Psychoanalytic Association* 44: 755–84.

Roberts, D. 2022. *Torn Apart: How the Child Welfare System Destroys Black Families—and How Abolition Can Build a Safer World*. New York: Basic Books.

Rothberg, M. 2019. *The Implicated Subject: Beyond Victims and Perpetrators*. Stanford, CA: Stanford University Press.

Rowling, J. K. 1997. *Harry Potter and the Sorcerer's Stone*. New York, NY: Scholastic.

Rozmarin, E. 2019. *Identity In-Formation*. London, England: Presentation for The International Psychoanalytic Association. July 2019.

Rubin, G. 2011. *Deviations: A Gayle Rubin Reader*. Durham and London: Duke University Press.

Rukeyser, M. 1976. *The Gates: Poems*. New York: McGraw Hill. ISBN: 978-0070542693.

Russell, P. 1983. "The Theory of the Crunch. (Unpublished). Published Posthumously (2006)." *Smith College Studies in Social Work* 76 (1–2): 9–21.

Russell, P. 1998. *Trauma, Repetition and Affect*. Edited by G. Teicholz and D. Kriegman. New York: The Other Press.

Saketopoulou, A. 2022a. "On Trying to Pass off Transphobia as Psychoanalysis and Cruelty as 'Clinical Logic'." *Psychoanalytic Quarterly* 91 (1): 177–90.

Saketopoulou, A. 2022b. *Sexuality Beyond Consent*. New York: New York University Press.

Saketopoulou, A., and A. Pellegrini. 2023. *Gender Without Identity*. New York: The Unconscious in Translation

Schafer, R. 1980. "Narration in the Psychoanalytic Dialogue." In *On Narrative*, edited by W. J. T. Mitchell. Chicago and London: The University of Chicago Press.

Schutz, D. 2017. *Open Casket*. New York, NY: The Whitney Museum.

Searles, H. 1965. *Collected Papers on Schizophrenia and Related Subjects*. London, UK: Hogarth Press.

Sedgwick, E. 1990. *Epistemology of the Closet*. Oakland, CA: University of California Press.

Sedgwick, E. 2011. *The Weather in Proust*. Durham and London: Duke University Press.

Seidal, R. 2019. "Queering the Psychoanalytic Family." Unpublished manuscript.

Seligman, S. 2007. "Mentalization and Metaphor, Acknowledgment and Grief: Forms of Transformation in the Reflective Space." *Psychoanalytic Dialogues* 17: 321–44.

Serano, J. 2018. "Everything You Need to Know About Rapid Onset Gender Dysphoria." *Medium (online)*

Shaw, P. 2006. *The Sublime: The New Critical Idiom*. 1st ed. New York and London: Routledge.

Sheehi, L. 2020. "The Reality Principle: Fanonian Undoing, Unlearning, and Decentering: A Discussion of 'Fanon's Vision of Embodied Racism for Psychoanalytic Theory and Practice'." *Psychoanalytic Dialogues* 30: 325–30.

Sheehi, L. 2022. "The Ideology of Apparitions: Disrupting Supremacist Temporalities of Being (White)." *Psychoanalytic Dialogues* 32: 598–609.

Shiff, R. 2008. *Doubt*. New York and London: Routledge, Taylor and Francis Group.

Slavin, M. O. 2011. "Lullaby on the Dark Side: Existential Anxiety, Making Meaning, and the Dialectics of Self and Other." In *Relational Psychoanalysis, Vol. IV*, edited by L. Aron and A. Harris. Hillsdale, NJ: The Analytic Press.

Slavin, M. O. 2013. "Meaning, Mortality, and the Search for Realness and Reciprocity: An Evolutionary/Existential Perspective on Hoffman's Dialectical Constructivism." *Psychoanalytic Dialogues* 23: 296–314.

Slavin, M. O., and D. Kriegman. 1998. "Why the Analyst Needs to Change: Toward a Theory of Conflict, Negotiation, and Mutual Influence in the Therapeutic Process." *Psychoanalytic Dialogues* 8: 247–84.

Smith, S. 1983. *Collected Poems*. New York: New Directions.

Smith, Z. 2013. "Man vs. Corpse [Online]." *New York Review of Books*, December 5, 2013.

Smith, Z. 2017. "Getting In and Out: Who Owns Black Pain?" *Harper's Magazine*, July 2017.

Spence, D. P. 1984. *Narrative Truth and Historical Truth: Meaning and Interpretation in Psychoanalysis*. New York: W.W. Norton & Company.

Spezzano, C. 2007. "A Home for the Mind." *Psychoanalytic Quarterly* 76: 1563–83.

Steinberg, B. 2019. "Civitarese on O: Bion's Pragmatic and 'Aesthetic-Intersubjective' Theory of Truth, the Growth of the Mind, and Therapeutic Action: Discussion of 'Bion's O and His Pseudo-Mystical Path'." *Psychoanalytic Dialogues* 29: 418–26.

Steiner, J. 1993. *Psychic Retreats: Pathological Organizations in Psychotic, Neurotic and Borderline Patients* (The New Library of Psychoanalysis, Vol. 19). London and New York: Routledge.

Stephens, M. 2020. "Getting Next to Ourselves: The Interpersonal Dimensions of Double- Consciousness." *Contemporary Psychoanalysis* 56 (2): 201–25.

Stephens, M. 2022. "We Have Never Been White: Afropessimism, Black Rage, and What the Pandemic Helped Me Learn About Race (and Psychoanalysis)." *Psychoanalytic Quarterly* 91: 319–47.

Stern, D. B. 1997. *Unformulated Experience: From Dissociation to Imagination in Psychoanalysis*. Hillsdale, NJ: The Analytic Press.

Stern, D. B. 2012. "Witnessing Across Time: Accessing the Present from the Past and the Past from the Present." *Psychoanalytic Quarterly* 81: 53–81.

Stern, D. B. 2013. "Field Theory in Psychoanalysis, Part II: Bionian Field Theory and contemporary Interpersonal/relational Psychoanalysis." *Psychoanalytic Dialogues* 23: 630–45.

Stern, D. B. 2018. *The Infinity of the Unsaid: Unformulated Experience, Language, and the Nonverbal*. New York and London: Routledge.

Stern, D. B. 2020. "Thinking Absence: A Discussion of 'The Analyst's Necessary Nonsovereignty and the Generative Power of the Negative'." *Psychoanalytic Dialogues* 30: 150–59.

Stockton, K. B. 2009. *The Queer Child or Growing Sideways in the Twentieth Century*. Durham and London: Duke University Press.

Stolorow, R. D. 2007. "Anxiety, Authenticity, and Trauma: The Relevance of Heidegger's Existential Analytic for Psychoanalysis." *Psychoanalytic Psychology* 24: 373–83.

Stolorow, R. D., and G. E. Atwood. 1992. *Contexts of Being: The Intersubjective Foundations of Psychological Life*. New York: Analytic Press, Inc.

Stolorow, R. D., G. E. Atwood, and D. M. Orange. 2002. *Worlds of Experience*. New York, NY: Basic Books.

Stolorow, R. D., B. Brandchaft, and G. E. Atwood. 1987. *Psychoanalytic Treatment: An Intersubjective Approach*. Hillsdale, NJ: The Analytic Press; York: Routledge.

Stolorow, R. D., D. M. Orange, and G. E. Atwood. 1998. "Projective Identification Begone!: Commentary on Paper by Susan H. Sands." *Psychoanalytic Dialogues* 8: 719–25.

St. Vincent Millay, E. 1917. *Renaissance and Other Poems*. New York, NY: Harper.

Suchet, M. 2015. "Entering a Space That Refuses You: Commentary on Paper by Jade McGleughlin." *Psychoanalytic Dialogues* 25: 248–55.

Sundell, M. 2003. "Francesca Woodman Reconsidered: A Conversation with George Baker, Ann Daly, Nancy Davenport, Laura Larson and Margaret Sundell." *Art Journal* 62 (2).

Swartz, S. 2019. "A Mingling of Ghosts: A Response to Daniel Butler's 'Racialized Bodies and the Violence of the Setting'." *Studies in Gender and Sexuality* 20: 165–70.

Symington, N. 1983. "The Analyst's Act of Freedom as Agent of Therapeutic Change." *International Rev. Psycho-Anal.* 10: 283–91.

Symington, N. 1996. "The Patient Makes the Analyst." *Psychoanalytic Inquiry* 16: 362–75.

Teicholz, J. G. 2000. "Chapter 3: The Analyst's Empathy, Subjectivity, and Authenticity: Affect as the Common Denominator." *Progress in Self-Psychology* 16: 33–53.

Tortorici, D. 2015. *"Those Like Us: On Elena Ferrante."* N+1. Issue 22.

Townsend, C. 2006. "Scattered in Space and Time." In *Francesca Woodman,* 6–71. Oxford: Phaidon.

Vetere, V. A. 1983. "The Role of Friendship in the Development and Maintenance of Lesbian Love Relationships." *Journal of Homosexuality* 8 (2): 51–65.

Wachtel, P. L. 2011. *Therapeutic Communication: Knowing What to Say When*. New York and London: Guilford Press.

Walter Benjamin: Selected Writings, Vol 2: Part 2. 1999. Edited by M. P. Bullock, M. W. Jennings, H. Eiland, and G. Smith. Cambridge, MA: Belknap Press of Harvard University.

Warren, C. 2018. *Ontological Terror*. Durham and London: Duke University Press.

Wilderson, F. 2020. *Afropessimism*. New York. Liveright Publishing.

Williams, P. 1992. *The Alchemy of Race and Rights*. Cambridge, MA: Harvard University Press.

Winnicott, D. W. 1949. "Mind and Its Relations to the Psyche-soma." Chapter XIX in *Through Paediatrics to Psychoanalysis*. New York, NY: Basic Books.

Winnicott, D. W. 1969. "The Use of an Object." *International Journal of Psycho-Analysis*, 50: 711–16.

Winnicott, D. W. 1971a. "Transitional Objects and Transitional Phenomena." In *Playing and Reality,* 2nd ed. New York and London: Routledge.

Winnicott, D. W. 1971b. *Playing and Reality.* London and New York, NY: Routledge.

Winterson, J. 2011. *Why Be Happy When You Could Be Normal?* New York, NY: Grove Press.

Winterson, J. 1989. *The Passion.* New York: Vintage Books.

Woodman, F. 1981. *Some Disordered Interior Geometries.* Philadelphia, PA: Synapse Press.

Woodman, F. 2006. "Seething with Ideas." In *Francesca Woodman,* 240–45. Oxford: Phaidon.

Wynter, S. 1995. "The Pope Must Have Been Drunk, The King of Castille a Madman: Culture as Actuality and the Caribbean Rethinking of Modernity." In *Reordering of Culture: Latin America, the Caribbean and Canada in the 'Hood.* Ottawa: Carleton University Press.

Wynter, S. 2015. *Sylvia Wynter: On Being Human as Praxis.* Edited by K. McKittrick. Durham: Duke University Press.

Index

Note: numbers in *italics* indicate a figure

absence: as necessary condition for vital
  life 63; in relationship to presence
  273n1, 295n1
absence-mindedness 103, 109
abstract theory 7
affective competency 45
Ahmed, S. 215, 219
Alliance Defending Freedom 223n1
Als, Hilton 271
Alvarez, A. 84, 259
Amadeus (play) 262–264
Ammons, A.R. 64
analytic: accounts 68; asymmetry 140;
  attunement 93; authority 7–9, 140–141,
  281; being 13, 252; certainty 7;
  containment 118; couple 86, 131, 174,
  256, 286; dialogue 257; endpoint 280;
  field 17, 131, 157, 255, 284; frame
  102; hour 183; ideas 282; joining 138;
  knowing 260; language 25, 39; pair
  36, 82–83, 278; process 14, 102, 293;
  relationship 37, 86, 247; scene 283;
  self 46; session 253; setup 31; situation
  88, 246; stance 137, 249; theory and
  practice 92; thinking 228; tools 131;
  training 200; treatment 204; unanalytic
  32; work 27; writers 69; writing 18, 69;
  see also psychoanalytic
analytic third, the 246, 278
anti-Black: racism 149; world 12
anti-gay groups 223n1
anti-racism 6
anti-racists 4, 156
Anzaldúa, Gloria 128, 235
Aron, L. 138–139

art: *Einfühlung* in 170n4; performance 23;
  viewer altered by and vice versa 170n4;
  transformative power of 94; when
  language fails 92; *see also* Avedon;
  Martin, Agnes; photography; Woodman
art and painting 15–19
Astor, M. 223n1
Atlas, G. 138–139
autonomy 6, 235, 270; claim of 195;
  defensive 183, 197; individual 232;
  relationship as root of 234
autotheory 70
Autotheory (Fournier) 70
autonomy 235
Avedon, Richard 92, 99–100, 114, 121;
  collage of three photographs by *99*

Barad, Karen 11
Baranger, M. 246, 283
Baranger, W. 246, 283
Barden, N. 210, 219; on gender as a verb
  210
Barthes, Roland xviii, 38, 102; *Camera
  Lucida* 2, 102; *punctum* of 2, 23, 27, 29,
  35, 38–39, 92, 109, 117, 119, 127, 129,
  137; on spectral images 105, 116n6;
  studium of 23, 26–27, 29, 116n7, 117,
  127–128
bed death 232
Benjamin, Jessica 62, 68; on alienated
  desire 232–233; *Bonds of Love* 5,
  233–235; "done to" concept of 77;
  intersubjective work by 34, 235;
  shared identification and mirroring
  complementarities of 73

Benjamin, Walter xviii, 17, 95,
107, 127
Berlant, Lauren 9, 218–219, 265–267,
287–288; on affective potentialities 291;
on crises of accommodation 186; on
disrupting fixity of identity 15; Edelman
and, disagreement with 290; on
encounter with non-knowledge 189; on
existential gap, or lack we live with 288;
on field of affective potentialities 196,
291; on force of the negative 272; on
misrecognition of self 264; on narrative
play 287; on optimism 184, 196;
phantasmatic staging of 247; as political
and cultural theorist 288; on refusal of
story 174; Sex, or the Unbearable 246,
253–254, 274n6, 276–277; on world
building 290
Bersani, L. 239
binary coupling 211
binary divide 208
binary frames 169
Bionian analysts 10; post-Bionians 262
Bionian belief 276
Bionian field theory/theorists 14, 85–86,
279–280, 285; being and knowing
in 260; critique of 247; limits of
interpretation as insight, per 282–283;
post-Bionian work, critique of 254–260,
274n4
Bion, Wilfred 2, 8–10, 137; alpha functions
and alphabetization of 280; at-one-ment
of 279; beta elements of 273n2; emotional
truth of situation stressed by 261;
Ferro influenced by 286; grids of 271;
K of 283; O 272
Black bodies 154
Black clinician 165
Black death (death of Black
people) 153
Black families, stereotypes of 230
Black feminism 119
Black gaze 153, 165
Black humanity 152
Black liberation publications 5, 234
Black lives 201
Black Lives Matter 229
Blackness 12–13
Black other 147
Black pain 151–154
Black patients 156; Fred 159–163,
164–166

Black patients/white analysts 148–149, 166
Black people in the US 94, 148; exclusion
from category of human 228; murder of
220; racism and 206
Black scholars 199, 228
Black sentient 152
Black subjection 151
Black suffering 150
Black thinkers 12
Black visual culture 149
Black women 4, 235
Black women's collective see Combahee
River Collective
Black writers 92, 147
Blanchfield, Brian 251; on force that runs
through us 253; on letting field run
through us/him 248, 275; on meadow
running though Martin 270, 272; on
sense of ground water running all along
276
blank/blanc mourning 53
Blechner, Mark: dreams of supervision 61
Blessed Sacrament 54
body modification 209–211
body as source of terror 110–112
Bollas, C. 115n2, 277
Bolognini, S. 155
borders and border-crossing 3, 128;
liminality and 124, 133; obliteration of 8
both/neither 209
breach: created by trauma 92; nonbeing
or 124; of own trauma 15; psychic 83,
88, 93, 148; scene of 16; traumatic
132–133, 146, 166; see also breach, the
breach in time 148
breach of analyst and patient, symmetry
between 141
breach of mind, breach in mind 128, 130
breach of subjectivity 140
breach, the 92–170; being left in 157;
first sign of 97–98; listening for and
from 96; Lui's recognition of 132, 137;
in mind's experience 101; patients
who live in 95; repetition of 134;
unconsciousness or 95; working in 138,
168–170
bridge theory 12
Bromberg, P. 19n2, 29, 34, 73, 96, 136
brown children 159
Brown, Michael 153–154
Bruhm, S. 211; see also misgendered self;
transgender

Bryant, Anita 212
butch/femme relationships 235
Butler, Judith 70–71, 243; Harris
    influenced by 190; on heterosexual
    women and same-sex desire 190; on
    norms with the power to craft us 178,
    219, 239; on process of unbecoming
    217; on the real and its representation
    282; on tactile impressions made on the
    body 84; on "you" separated from "I"
    192, 217, 278

Campt, Tina 149, 153, 165; hapacity of
    157; see also Black gaze
Cartesian self 7, 36
Caruth, Cathy: analysis of *Hiroshima my
    amour* 116n8, 128–130, 132–138,
    140–142; analysis of Resnais on
    Hiroshima mon amour 93, 130; on
    breach in the mind's experience 95, 101;
    on dreaming without knowing one is
    dreaming 109; Leys' critique of 116n9;
    on terror and trauma theory 112–113;
    on transmission of unrepresentable 109
case vignettes: Sarah, Troy, Christina
    83–88; see also Sarah
castration and castration anxiety 26, 231
Cerullo, Margaret 5, 227
child: battered 60; Black 153, 159, 164;
    disturbed 74; enigmatic messages
    passed onto 242; enslaved 228; figure
    or idea of 211–213, 219, 239; gender
    nonconforming 223n2; hated 264; Lacan
    on 192; loss of 191; mother as infant
    of 46; Oedipal situation of 228–229,
    231; primacy of 230; protection of 212;
    psychosocial sexual development of
    231; queer 4, 215, 218; queer raising
    of 241; sideways growing of 212, 231;
    stray 86; transgender 220; youngest 143
childhood fear 189
child self 44, 49
child sexual abuse 207
child welfare system 164
child work/child play 167, 284
Chodorow, Nancy 233–234; see also
    mothering
cis-gendered heterosexuality: female 203,
    205, 207–208; male 221; white 201
cis-heteronormative bourgeois 219
Civitarese, Giuseppe: on analyst falling
    ill at the level of the patient 134; on

asymmetry necessary to treat the patient
    259, 285; on the field contracting the
    patient's illness 23, 85; on hallucinosis
    140, 274n5, 281; on sovereignty of field
    theory 247, 284–285
clinical: accounts 68, 70; approach 24;
    career 2; case presentation 247; choices
    231–233; contexts 37; decisions
    121; encounter 248; experience 141;
    experiences 72; idea 148; imperatives
    23; implications 85; knowing 6;
    ontological clinical paradigm 10;
    outbursts 138; practice 13, 73, 94;
    process 6–7, 183; reports 34; setting
    130; situation 132; theory 227
clinical stories 10, 15–16, 37; subjectivity
    in 174; telling 16, 155, 175, 193,
    198, 204
clinical storytelling 16, 175–176, 248
clinical writing 76 176; by author of present
    work 246; belief and 173, 193
clinical work 1, 69, 119, 134, 139; by
    author of present work 159; enactive
    mode of 96; intersectionality as lens for
    149; ontological 13–15
co-excitation 49
Combahee River Collective 5, 229, 235
Cooney, Amy Schwartz 248, 276–282, 292
cooperation *see* hermeneutic cooperation
Cooper, Stephen 11; pluralistic third of 12
countertransference: of author of present
    work 24, 73, 87; defining 38; empathy
    and 155; interpretive sharing of 80;
    managing 14; sharing 259; subjectivity
    and 68; transference/countertransference
    dilemmas 28; transference/
    countertransference enactments 155;
    transference/countertransference
    as opportunity 133; transference/
    countertransference significance 78
crunch, the 36, 56, 130

Davies, J. 30, 76
dead body 163
dead father 109–110, 123, 237
dead mother 44, 46, 52, 55, 62, 75–77, 79,
    273
dead mother syndrome 134
Dead Lecturer, The (Jones) 40
deadness: liminality as distinct from
    124–125; psychic 30, 32
dead seals, dream of 56

dead, the: ashes of 121; crossings from 98; half life of 105; silence of 97; world of 115n3
death: bed death 232; life and, knowing difference between 109–111
death drive 239, 273n1
death threats 220
decathexis 53, 88, 124
De Lauretis, T. 120
Deleuze, Gilles 294
Derrida see texts
developmental mother story, alternative 237–243
developmental stories 177, 201–202, 229–231; universal 228
developmental theory 228, 229
difficult-to-reach analyst 17, 22, 25, 29
difficult-to-reach patient 16, 22, 25, 27, 29, 39
diffraction 11, 283
diffraction in the mind 293
diffractive methodology 11
disavowal 122; cycles of 267; of death 110, 113–114, 123–124; as relational phenomenon 122; of suicide 110; trauma and 113
disavowed 148, 161, 166
dissociation 59, 101; by author of her own ghosts 108; bodily awareness of absence and 114, 128; breaking through of dissociation of liminality 122–123; defining 170n3; disavowal distinct from 122; language of 122; melting of 280; splitting and 280; Suchet and Green on 124; uses of 122
drive theory 83
Du Bois, W. E. B. 151
Dumas, Marlene 17, 176, 196, 246
Duras, Marguerite 127
dying: in captivity 50; fantasies of 51; lover's (Hiroshima Mon Amour) 134, 136

Edelman, Lee 9, 287; Berlant and, debate/disagreement with 265, 274n6, 276, 290; on crises of accommodation 186; on death drive 239; on disrupting fixity of identity 15; on encounter with non-knowledge 189, 253; on existential gap, or lack we live with 288; on fetishism 289; on field of affective potentialities 196, 259, 291; on misrecognition of self 264; on nonsovereignty 277, 290;

phantasmatic staging of 247; on refusal of story 174, 183; on relationality 267, 269, 286; Sex, or the Unbearable 246, 253–254, 274n6, 276–277; on spirit and force of the negative 272; on stories to which we are being led 177
Einfühlung 170n4
Eliade, Mircea 115n3
Elliot, T.S.: "Love Song of Prufrock" 56–57
empathic 64
empathic: analyst 65n1; immersion 132; meeting 78; method 81; recognition 157; understanding 131
empathy 65n1, 131–133, 155–156; attunement and 147; countertransference and 155; expressing 78; feeling, for patient 32; identificatory 148–149; intersubjective 158; limits of 93, 127–142; potential and pitfalls of 150–153; recognition theory and 156–159; Robbins on 80–81; thinking about 136; transformational 158; white 93, 147–170, 282
empathy/interpretation 7
enactive mode 96, 246
enactive writing v, 92, 261–262, 291, 293
enactment 85, 133, 276; acting out of feeling or 138; affects, thoughts, and 155; destructive 76, 79; inevitability of 26, 35; generative 131; intense 140; involving mix-up of insides of two people 78; living in 259; negative 96, 109, 135; of primary unconscious elements 81; remembering replaced by 31; theorizing about 13; therapeutic agent of 74; writing 121; writing/reading 119; writing without 118
enactment following enactment 29
enactment story 174
enactment, the (Woodman) 107–108
enigma: Lila as (Ferrante) 197
enigma of gender 209
enigma of vision 105
enigmatic 135, 141; behaviors 95; in Ferrante 176; tears 162, 168; what is, encounters with 174, 260; woman 59
enigmatic message 19, 106, 226, 240; Ferrante 183–184, 185, 188, 198; Laplanche 106, 183, 208, 242, 268; passed onto child 240, 242; return of 265–269; translating 277

enigmatic, the 13, 15; efforts to know 252;
     making legible 120; thriving of 269;
     unconscious force of 175
envy: author of present work's mother 263;
     deadliness of 266; defining 190; desire
     turning into 182; Lenù's (Ferrante)
     183–184, 190–191; "Muteness Envy"
     (Johnson) 121; Salieri's (*Amadeus*)
     262–264; Sarah's (patient) 79; sight
     denied by 191
eulogy to author of present work's
     stepfather 94, 143–146

family/ies: alternative 231; Black 164,
     230; challenging, as exclusive site of
     development of sexuality 5; constructing
     229; conventions of 189; creating 201;
     forgotten by 53; heteronormative 228;
     foster 163; immutable forms of 178;
     institution of 227, 241; Jewish 237;
     lesbian 226; LGBTQ+ 228; loss of 162;
     more inclusive theory for 227; queer
     228, 241; separation from 239; subject
     formation beyond 175, 182, 235, 240;
     western 228; without 239
family-busting 238
family drama, Oedipal 236
family history 242
Family Policy Alliance 223n1
family romance, normative 233
family story 148
family, the: as ideological hotspot 233;
     Oedipal crucible of 234; primacy of 229
family values 219
Fanon, Frantz 147
feminism 6; second-wave 235; white 5
feminist psychoanalysis/psychoanalysts
     6, 201; refiguring of the Oedipal by
     233–236
feminists 11; Black 119
feminist theory/theorists 11, 209, 229; of
     Black visual culture 149
Ferenczi, Sandor 6, 10–11, 68, 76
Ferrante, Elena, novels of: *Neapolitan
     Quartet* 218–219; crypto-lesbianism
     in 185; displaced heterosexuality
     in 190–191; enigmatic message in
     183–184; envy's denial of sight in
     191–193; erotic gaze in 188–189; first
     use of the other in 185–188; Lenù's
     telling of Lila's story, lessons of 70,
     174–178, 193–197; love in 188; love's

turn in 189–190; psychoanalytic
     storytelling disrupting law of the gaze in
     novels of 197–198; radical relationality
     in novels of 175, 181–198; transitional
     object in 185
Ferro, Antonio 248; on asymmetry
     necessary to treat the patient 259,
     285; on avoidance of mental pain
     286; on benefits of looking to read
     feedback from characters in the field
     282; bewilderment welcomed by 283;
     Bionianism of 276; on field theory 284;
     on the field contracting the patient's
     illness 23, 85; on individual illusions
     of subjectivity and sovereignty 278;
     nonsovereignty acknowledged by
     258, 276, 285, 287; on power of the
     unrepresented 280; on projective
     identification 140; on readers'
     experience of text 292; situating of
     analyst and analysand in the field
     255–259; on transformative potential of
     storytelling 268, 287–288, 290
field theory 14, 121, 246; Barangers' 283;
     Bionian 279; changing 284; Ferro on
     284; Hartman on 258; limits of 249;
     post-Bionian 255–260
figure or idea of the child 211–213, 219,
     239
film 16; silent 121; talkie 121; *see also
     Hiroshima mon amour*
filmmaking 92
Forché, Carolyn 42, 45, 51, 57
Foucault, Michel 13
Fornier, L. 70; *Autotheory* 70
Frankenberg, R. 156, 170n2
Frankenstein 195
freedom: analyst's act of 137–148
freedom from suffering 271
freedom of choice 210
Freudian developmental narrative 218
Freudian slip 120
Freud, Sigmund 48; *Analysis Terminable
     and Interminable* 31; on analysts' need
     to cure 30; on analysts' own corporality
     and instincts 37; *Beyond the Pleasure
     Principle* 115n4; Caruth on 116n9, 130;
     on child sexuality 211; De Lauretis on
     120; Dora 42; early trauma theory 113;
     on empathy and countertransference
     155; Ferenczi and 6; grandson 105,
     115n4; Klein and 19n1; Leys' critique

of Caruth's reconceptualization of
116n9; on negation 252; Oedipus
theory of 228; Phillips on 26, 30–31;
repeating, remembering and working
through sequence of 133; repression
as understood by 132; on speaking as
articulation of wants 26; theory-making
by and clinical work of 69; warning of
transgressive transference 45
Friedman, L. 26, 31

Gabbard, G. 120
gender: evolving 216; Halberstam on 200,
234; normative developmental theory of
177; race and 5; sexuality and 156; as
"soft assembly" 199, 229; as verb 210;
as "woman" and "man" 200; *see also*
cis-gendered
gender-altering technologies 214
gender binary 6, 208–209, 211
gender dysphoria 202, 215, 220, 223n2;
rapid onset gender dysphoria (ROGD)
207–208
gender identity 190, 220
gender outliers 212
gender theory 204
gender variation 205
Gerson, S. 125
Ghent, Emmanuel 60; on dread and envy
preceding surrender 112, 190
ghost father 105
ghost pictures (Woodman) 105
ghosts: author of present work's own
ghosts 108, 112; belief in 226; death
in words killing 110; demanding 188;
entropy and 121; gaps and 139; haunting
of Woodman by 106–107; liminal
227; severing analytic writing from
18; several Oedipal theory from 236;
Woodman's tyro ghosts 103
ghostly photographs 96
Gilroy, Paul 170n1
going-on-being 3, 78
Goldberg, P. 292
Goldsmith, Kenneth 153–154
González. Francisco 209
Green, André 32, 46; on absence as
necessary condition for vital life 63;
on absence in relationship to presence
273n1, 295n1; on blank/blanc mourning
53; on co-excitation 49; on the dead
mother/dead mother syndrome 55, 75,

77, 134; decathexis 88; disputing the
idea of withdrawal as actual engagement
74; on external and internal world
consciousness 21; on the negative 252;
on pleasure of the analyst's narcissistic
investment 55; on representation of
the absence of representation 124; on
reversal of subject and object 75; on
state of alien action 101; on work of the
negative 124
Greenberg, J. vi, 19n3
Grosz, Elizabeth: on bewilderment 249;
Deleuze and 294; Martin's work
interpreted via 270–272, 294; on
medicalized bodies pliable to power
210–211; on the negative 252

Halberstam, Jack: on gender 200, 234; on
negation of the subject 178; ontology of
13; on slavery and generational legacies
of loss 239–240; on white gendered
heteronormativity 228; on women as
repositories of generational logics 238
hallucinosis 140, 274n5, 281
hapacity 157
Haraway, Donna 11
Harris, Adrienne xxii–xxiii, 6, 38; on
analyst's contribution to impasse 30,
114, 123; on female homosexuality 190;
on forbidden love 190; on gender as
"soft assembly" 199, 229; on repression
of desire as gender arrangement 189;
"You Must Remember This" 30, 32;
warnings of omnipotence by 35
Hartman, Saidiya 12, 94, 149–154, 156; on
field theory 258; Halberstam's reading
of 240; on identity produced by negation
228; on jouissance of role of witness
159; *Scenes of Subjection* 150; white
empathy and 149
Hartman, Stephen 117–121, 124, 125
Heritage Foundation 223n1
hermeneutic cooperation 256–257
heteronormative families 228; non-
heteronormative families 227
heteronormative theorizing 231
heteronormativity 177, 219; white-
gendered 213
heterosexism: white 230
heterosexist bias 234
heterosexuality: centrality of 6; cis-
gendered 207; cis-gendered white

201; compulsory 189, 219; displaced
(Ferrante) 190–191; "fixing" gender
followed by 204; inevitability of 189;
Lemma's assertion of 206, 218; as
natural order 205
heterosexual women 190, 232
Hiroshima, bombing of 142
Hiroshima mon amour (film) 93–94,
127–142; Caruth's reading of 93–94,
116n8, 128–129, 132, 141–142;
cultural blindness in 141–142; empathy
in 131–133; gift of implication in 141;
interventions that surprise 137–141;
Japanese suffering in 142; liminality in
133–134; plot of 128–129; what the
Japanese man can teach us 134–137
Hoffman, I. 68
Holder, Ann 203
home, concept of 116n3
Howe, Fanny 273
Hurly, N. 211; *see also* transgender

identity: closed 62; desire and 176;
destabilizing or revealing 106; fixity
15, 102; mistaken 50; self and 103;
self-attacking 81; shared 150; writing as
sign of 119
identity: formation 184; groups 149; politic
5; position 176
image *see* self-image
image of the child *see* figure or idea of the
child
image of the mother 264
images 93, 100, 168; art and 153, 158,
294; Avedon's 121; Campt on 153;
of Hiroshima's destruction 130; of
liminality 108; Martin's 270; spectral
105; Woodman's 105, 109, 112,
116n6
imagelessness 104
implicated 154, 164; inter-implicated 216
implication: analyst's own place of 141;
clinical 85; gift of 17, 118, 141; in
Hiroshima mon amour 141; of really not
knowing 139; vulnerability and 155, 158
individuation 185
intersectionality 5, 149, 235
intersubjective 229; communications
155; complexity 213; conjunction
56; empathy 158; exchange 6, 37;
engagement 82, 190; entanglement 113,
168; experience 82; field 167; knowing

237; object-relational dynamics 294;
process 85; process of recognition 157;
relating 24, 131–132; relationality
166; scaffolding 123; space 101, 177,
234–235; story 34, 72; system 33, 76,
109, 290; third 124–125, 234, 256
intersubjectivity 6, 182; Benjamin (Jessica)
on 233; creating 278; relational 80, 82;
two subjects required by 125
Intersubjectivists 10
intrapsychic: conflict 24, 31–33, 72, 76,
80, 85; development 230; need 35;
surfaces 83
intrapsychic, the 7

Johnson, Barbara: on aesthetics of
psychoanalytic writing 165; on
constraints and censorship in writing
15, 260; on individuation 185; "Lesbian
Spectacles" 188–189; on Lila and
Lenù's "I" and "you" (Ferrante) 183,
193; "Muteness Envy" 121–122; on
personal experience and discourse of
knowledge 69; on Williams 119
Johnston, Jill 271
Jones, Kima 153
Jones, Leroi 12, 40
Jones, Zinnia 223
Joseph, Betty 52, 74
Joseph, Gloria 4–5

Keller, C. 106
Klein, Melanie 19n1, 45, 69, 230
Knoblauch, Stephen 166
Kohut, H. 81
Kraus, R. 105

Lacan, Jacques 184, 192; concept of the
real 123, 254
LaCapra, D.: on emphatic unsettlement
109; on unsettled knowledge 133
Langer, S.: on cultural regulation 208;
on gender's wide arc 209; on fixing
(correcting) gender 204; on gender as
embodied and performed 216; on what
counts as real 223
Lanzoni, S. 170n4
Laplanche, J. enigmatic messages of 106,
183, 208, 242, 268; nonsovereignty of
277; Queer theory and 178, 235; on
pleasures of relationality 267; on repair
and subjectivity 287

Lara, Ali 293
Laub, Dori 109
Layton, Lynne 155
Lemma, Alessandra: "Trans-itory
  Identities" 176–178, 202–223; Jane's
  story as told by 176–177, 204–205,
  213–220
lesbian: credible analyst versus credible
  lesbian analyst 201; family 226; plot
  188–189; president of psychoanalytic
  institute 200; "old world" 235;
  understanding sexuality among 232; on
  women's softball team 221; see also
  LGBTQ+
lesbian fusion literature 235
lesbian identity 241
Levenson, Edgar 6–8, 10, 68
Levine, Howard: on acts of figurability 123,
  259; on representational imperative 258;
  on the unrepresented 13, 112, 259
Levine, Lauren 170n5
Lewis, Jill 5, 12
Leys, R.: critique of Caruth's
  reconceptualization of Freud 116n9
LGBTQ+: acceptance of 201; "arrested
  development" 230; clinicians 206;
  community 205; families 227; sexuality
  228; violence 200; see also homosexual;
  queer; transgender
liminal: being 113; construct 149; grief
  94; place 168; realm 127; refraction 4;
  Sarah as 70; space 26, 141, 169; state
  122, 140, 148; of Woodman's pictures
  106; zone 21
liminality 93, 100; affective experience
  of 133; of author of present work 108,
  122–124, 133; being in 113; blankness
  and 128; in Hiroshima mon amour
  133–134, 137, 139–141; interrupting
  137; metaphoric 112; of personhood
  104; shared 113; state of 135, 148;
  themes of 108; of time and space 102
literature: analytic 83; clinical 132; difficult
  treatments described in 68–69; lesbian
  fusion 235; object-relations 75; one-
  person 31, 35, 74; relational 30
Lombardi, R. 31, 33, 37, 114; somatic
  resonance of 85, 85, 255
loneliness v, 28, 86–87, 162

Martin, Agnes 16, 248–249, 253, 255;
  creative force of the negative in work

of 270; grids of 270–271; Grosz
  and 249, 253, 259, 272, 294; limits
  of representation illustrated by 293;
  negativity's potential power and art
  as the negative in work of 269–272;
  schizophrenia of 271–272; the
  unrepresentable in work of 275
masochism 32, 239; sadomasochism 32,
  47, 74
McGleughlin, Jade 114, 118, 122, 278, 283;
  After Lichtenstein 91; After Winnicott
  xxiv; "Afterwords on Technique"
  (2009) 72–82; "Afterwords on Writing"
  (2020) 67–71; "Analyst's Necessary
  Non-Sovereignty and Generative
  Power of the Negative" (2019) 246,
  251–274, 275–276, 287, 289; Benjamin
  Clementine 171; Blue Room 90; 'Do
  We Find or Lose Ourselves in the
  Negative?" (2015) 92, 95–120, 168,
  290; Dreaming Hughie Lee Smith
  224; Dreaming in a Pink Chair 225;
  Dust Ruffle 20; further thoughts on
  'Do We Find or Lose Ourselves in
  the Negative?' (2015) 117–125;
  Henry Taylor and His Painting 126;
  "Impossibility of Meaning" (2019)
  275–295; "Interlude with Life and
  Death: Eulogy to my Stepfather"(2016)
  143–146; Lost 89; "Love Letter to a
  Patient or the Raw Story" (2001) 40–65;
  PIII.1 Vital 173; PIII.2 The Swimmer
  180; PIV.1 She Knows/She Doesn't Know
  245; "Promise of Radical Relationality
  in Novels of Elena Ferrante" (2015)
  175–176, 181–198; Room 1 (one) 295;
  on sovereignty 280; "Thinking Outside
  the Oedipus Box" (2021) 177, 226–236;
  "Transgender Imagining and Danger of
  Normative Theory" (2019) 199–223;
  "Translation: Alternative Developmental
  Mother Story" (2020) 237–243; "Two
  Case Vignettes: How Sarah Helped me
  Help Troy and (Almost) Christina"
  (2014) 83–88; "When You are in the
  Cellar, am I Dead?": Understanding the
  Limits of Empathy and the Power of
  Otherness through the film Hiroshima
  mon amour"(2020) 127–142; Waiting
  66; "White Empathy" (2020) 93,
  147–170, 282
McKay, Rachel 157–158

memory: emotional 26; false 71; non-declarative 26; procedural 26; verbal or narrative 21
Michaels, Anne 18, 145, 181
misgendered self 219
Mitchell, Stephen vi, 19n3, 83, 138–139, 142
Mom, J. 246
Moraga, C. 235
Morris, Humphrey 27, 114–115, 124, 165
Morrison, Toni 165; *Sula* 292
Moten, F. 166; idea of the break 239
mother: alternative developmental mother story, 237–243; dead mother/dead mother syndrome 44, 46, 52, 55, 62, 75–77, 79, 134, 273; alternative developmental mother story, 237–243; "good enough" 178; image of 264
mothering 233; reproduction of 178, 240
Munoz, J. 242

narratives 117, 122–123; affect and 213; alternative 175; building of 202; closed 138; creating other 237; departing from 135; forward-moving 67; Freudian developmental 218; frozen 139; grounding 21; historical 18, 236; knowledge as 197; letting emerge 2; masochism as counternarrative 239; mimetic 177; Oedipal 229, 241; patient's 148; power of 286; psychoanalytic 201; repetitive 217; replacing interpretation 284; replacing symptoms 251; self-narratives 114, 128, 147; self-referential 137; stalled 131; underside of 265–269; unreliable 194; white 150
narrative action of session 246–247
narrative comments 256
narrative complexity 165
narrative device 265, 279
narrative experiment 249, 278
narrative meaning 269
narrative memory 21
narrative of peace 142
narrative organizations 256
narrative play 283, 287
narrative storytelling 93
narrative strategy 248
narrative time 262
narrative truth 15, 260
Nathans, Shelly 226–232

negation 101, 147, 252; forces of 159; Freud on 252; haunting 227; history of 229; identity produced by 228, 240; social forms of 189
negation of subject 178
negative: positive and 64, 155
negative, the 8, 15, 246–249; "Analyst's Necessary Non-Sovereignty and Generative Power of the Negative" (McGleughlin) 246, 251–274, 275–276, 287, 289; at-one-ment in 280; contact with 277; creative force of 270; creativity of 273; 'Do We Find or Lose Ourselves in the Negative?" (McGleughlin) 92, 95–120, 168, 290; experiences of 262; "Freedom to Want Passionately" (1980s) 232; further thoughts on 'Do We Find or Lose Ourselves in the Negative?" 117–125; force of 294; generative force of 149, 158, 272; generative potential of 16; generative power of 251–274; generative work of 279–281; grappling with 252–255; idea of 22–23; impossibility of meaning and 275–295; liminal space of 169, 198; living with 283; power of 275; work in 148, 259, 261; work of 271; *see also* decathexis
negative capability 257, 259, 292–293
negative capacity 137
negative enactments 135
negative therapeutic reaction 28, 72
Nelson, Maggie 71
Nestle, J. 235
Nguyen, Leanh 115
nonbeing: Black people and 12; experience of 92; metaphor of 113; phenomenological view of 34; representing 123; sense of 113; shared state of 168; state of 35, 95, 104, 112, 123–124, 290
nonbelonging 227
non-entity and entity 105
nonrepresentational 168
nonrepresentational artists 253
nonrepresented states (of being) 119
nonresponse 50
nonseeing 294
nonsensical 2
nonsovereign analyst 282, 291
nonsovereign attunement 148

nonsovereignty or nonsovereign 13, 158;
acknowledging 290; analyst's 15, 24,
138; analyst's necessary nonsovereignty
xxii, 16, 251; "Analyst's Necessary
Non-Sovereignty and Generative Power
of the Negative" (McGleughlin) 246,
251–274, 275–276, 287, 289; existing
in the field as nonsovereign 281; Ferro
on 285; idea of 9–10; the negative
and 248; potential of 275; shared 292;
willingness to live in 290; working
from 249
nonsovereignty of self 242

object 18; absent 134; all-bad 33; art and
272; bad 267; erotic 111; Fred as 162;
internal 17, 30, 49, 118; libidinal 240;
loss of self and 123; love 183; others/
objects 122; patient as 248; self as 3;
subject and 15; subject reduced to 153;
surveillance of 175; transitional 183,
185; who is 68
object choice 207; sexual 229
object development 84
objectification 81
objective and subjective 99
objective form of psychoanalytic writing
23, 24, 71
objective positivist stance 277
objectivist thinking 36, 70; one-person 83
objectivity 68, 119; narrative 176
objectless existence or state 21, 86,
124, 252
object loss, primary 53
object of desire 104
object of gaze, patient as 178
object of study, self as 136
object relating 113, 192
object relational: approach 10, 24; framing
78; history 208; stance 79; supervisor
80; theory 76
object relations 19n2, 217, 256–257, 287
object relationship, unconscious 69
object relations perspective, relational
73–75
object use 192
Oedipal family drama 178
Oedipal negotiation 230
Oedipal, the 184; feminist psychoanalysts
refiguring of 233–236
Oedipal theory 176, 228
Oedipus 227, 229

Oedipus box, thinking outside 177,
226–236
Ogden, Thomas 2–11, 19n1, 64, 85; on
absence 124; on individual as object
136; on intersubjective third 256; on
unconscious thinking 264
Olds, Sharon: "The Space Heater" 54
Oliver, Mary 55
omnipotence: checks on 146; clinician's
or analyst's 30–31, 35, 43, 79–80, 99;
Lenù (Ferrante) 285, 192, 195; phantasy
of 229, 231, 236; self-productive 22; of
white imaginary 230
omnipotentiality 209
omnipresence, of liminal state 124
ontological challenge to notion of discrete
self 249, 278
ontological clinical work 13–15
ontological psychoanalysis 6, 11, 94, 277
ontological sensibility 7, 128
ontological, the 1, 2–4; the epistemological
and 9
ontological thinkers 10
ontological way of working 140
ontological writing 15–18
ontology 12–13; untamed 13
ontological turn 9
orange aura 100, 122
Orange, D. M. 10, 33–34
orange (fruit) 181
origins: fogging of distinction and 247,
262; rethinking 241
origin scenes 242
origin story: better 219; psychoanalytic
202, 228; thinking with others 4–6
others: thinking with 4–6; surveillance
of 252
other, the: being with 286, 293; first use of
(Ferrante) 185–188; recognition from
and by 6, 152, 181–182; recognizing
other (the therapist) 234–235; self, other
and space created by analytic pair 83;
self–other normative development 273,
295n1; suffering 62

Panagia, Davie 293
parental: anxiety 212; care 185; couple
230–231, 233, 243; failure 88; loss 168
passion: "Freedom to Want Passionately"
(McGleughlin) 232; mad 55, 75;
Winterson on 48–49
Passion, The (Winterson) 22

performance: listening as 175; self-conscious acknowledging of 179; telling as kind of 17
performance art 23, 92
performance not one's own 251, 275
performance of wanting 26
performative 19, 152, 237
performative "I" 255
performative writing 23, 261; stumbling on 260–262
phallus 181, 231
Phelan, Peggy: on belief and clinical writing 193; on blind spots within the theoretical frame 175, 177; on imagelessness 104; on non-entity and entity 105; on photography 105; on seeing what we know 71, 282; on self-identity 266; on self-image 270; on self-seeing 268; on surveillance of the other 252; on the unmarked 15, 258; on Woodman's death and meaning of death in work of 108
Phillips, A. 26, 30–31
photographer/model 121
photographs: Avedon 99; Benjamin on 107; ghostly 96; intimate 48; Martin's photography of Woodman's photographs 106; negative of 109; punctum in 27, 38, 115n5; studium in 26, 115n5; Woodman 92–93, 96, 103–109, 120, 123, 142n2; see also Avedon
placeholder 266–267, 289, 292
Pogue Whyte, [Kathleen] 12
poles: sovereign and nonsovereign 248–249, 277; three (self, other and space created by analytic pair) 83
Poletti 70
politics of sensation 293
Powell, D. 12
projective identification 47, 76, 140, 257, 284; projective counter identification 30
Prosser, J. 214
Proust, Marcel 103
psychoanalytic: antipsychoanalytic 107; authors 207; canon 23; clinicians 215; communities 199; concept of subjectivity 9; critics 107; discovery of transference 26; encounter 10; frame 238, 249, 285; idea 4, 11, 133, 290; innocence 206; instinctual unconscious 127; language 289; language of subjectivity 277; logic of the real 282;

models of development 177; moment of free association 57; narrative 201; origin story 202, 228; presuppositions 216; principles 201; relationships 149; stories 173–174, 176, 218; story, of subjectivity 241; storytelling 197–198; supervisor 160; telling, as art 17; theorists 235; term (subjectivity) 254; theorizing 277; theory 229, 233, 236; theory of gender development 222; thinkers 156; thought 177; training 22, 99; treatment, of transgendered people 203; valuing of logic 254; witness to trauma 96; work 6; writers 117, 147; writing 17, 24, 93–94, 148, 165, 248, 252, 261
Psychoanalytic Dialogues 226
psychoanalytic technique as understood through Hiroshima mon amour see Hiroshima mon amour
psychoanalytic theory, normative 174, 176, 221
punctum 2, 23, 27, 29, 35, 38–39, 92, 108, 117, 119, 127, 129, 137

queer 70; child 4; gender queer 199; Lenù (Ferrante) as potentially described as 190
queer activists 201
queer analyst 4, 200, 205; "normalcy" offered to 227
Queer Art of Failure (Halberstam) 178
queer bodies and minds 206
queer child/ren and young people 4, 211, 213, 215, 218, 220; anti-queer 219; new generation of 233; suspiciousness of 230
queer community 204
queer contexts 222
queer couples 231
queer families 228, 241
queer liberation 6
queer lives 238
queer minds 241
queerness 177, 218, 243; as defiance 238
queer patients 242
queer project 240
queers: author of present work as 227, 230; gender 199; new generation of 233; Oedipus as child of 241; women and 240
queer theory and theorists 11, 209–210, 229, 235, 253
queer way of seeing 18

race: analysts paired with patients of same
race 160; critical race theory 11; cross-
race storytelling 154; gender and 5;
intersubjective recognition warped by
157; kinship and 229; racial trauma and
141; racism and 92; radical social divide
of 94; white analysts treating patients of
different race 147–149
race relations, in the US 151
race theory 166
racial trauma 141
racism: analysts' own 158; anti-Black
149; anti-racism 6; constraints of
169; exposing 154; field's history of
206; heterosexism and 230; power
imbalances and 141; race and 92;
structural 228; trauma of 148, 166;
trauma of, in the US 147
Racker, Heinrich 68; concordant
identification of 49
Rankine, Claudia 149–150; *The White
Card* 153
rapid onset gender dysphoria (ROGD)
207–208
Raymond, C. 105
recognition: of absences 114–115; of
betweenness 278; of Black pain 151,
228; breakdown of 73; as citizens 151;
of continuation of own life 110, 134;
creative 123; empathy and 131, 155; of
experiential gap 124; family ideology
and 227; Fred 159, 166–168; of girls by
their fathers 233; of impossibility 288;
Lenù's desire for (Ferrante) 184; Lenù
failure to recognize Lila as separate or
real person (Ferrante) 192–193, 197;
Lenù's withdrawal of (Ferrante) 186;
misrecognition in discussant responses
276; misrecognition of self 9, 254;
mutual 47, 83, 125, 220; of mutuality
120; of need, by analyst 30, 53; of no
truth 101; of Other 152; of patient 219;
from powerful other 6, 181–182; of
present absence 96; of queer families
241; of sovereignty 281; of strangeness
133; of suffering other 62; surveillance
and 282; of transgender people 201;
of trauma 95, 135; unconscious 130;
of unrecognizable 166; of what versus
where 184
recognition theory 149, 156–159
recognizer 94

recognizing: by analyst 68; of analyst, as
being separate from client 72
recognizing look 219
recognizing other (the therapist) 234–235
relational intersubjectivity 80, 82
relationality: empathy and 155;
intersubjectivity and 158, 166; intrinsic
249; learning and 6; nonsovereign 265,
269; non-sovereign selves as encounter
with 254; radical, in the novels of Elena
Ferrante 175–176, 181–198; relating
and 24; sensual pleasures of 267;
subjectivity and 176; trauma and 111
relational object relations perspective
73–76
relational self-psychological perspective
76–79; self-psychological-relational
approach 24
repeating, remembering and working
through sequence 133
repetition 19, 183, 248; concept of 133;
destructive 131; enduring 267–268;
inevitable 17, 266; generativity and 272;
work of 215
repression 108, 124; of desire 189; of
message 184; of personality 30; of
trauma 132
Resnais, Alain 92, 93
Rich, Adrienne 57
Robbins, Michael 31–33, 74; case for
qualitatively different mind 79–82
RODC 212
ROGD *see* rapid onset gender dysphoria
Rothko, Mark 253
Rozmarin, Eyal 152, 243
Rukeyser, Muriel 41
Russell, Paul 68; on affective competency
45; on concept of the repetition 133; on
"the crunch" 36, 56, 130

sadomasochism 32, 47, 74
Saketopoulou, A. 6
Sarah 21–24, 41–42, 44–47, 49–50, 53,
55–56, 58–61, 64–65, 67–70, 72–82,
83, 252
schadenfreude 192
schizophrenia: Agnes Martin 271–272;
paranoid-schizoid positions 69
schizophrenics 97, 162
Schutz, Dana 154
Searles, Harold 31, 36, 53, 68, 74
seeing what we know 71, 282

self-attack 28; vicious 81
self-awareness 220
self-contempt 55
self-creation 170n1
self-defined subjectivity 219
self-development 33
self-destructive beliefs 80
self-determination 206
self-disclosing 17
self-division 276
self-effacing 183
self-emancipation 170n1
self-experience 84, 125, 136
self-fulfilling loop 258
self-identity 266
self-image 71, 196, 270, 282
self-knowledge 9, 254
self-loathing 50
self-narratives 114; looping 128, 147
self–other normative development 273, 295n1
self-psychological-perspective, relational 76–79
self-psychological-relational approach 24
self-psychological theories 132
self-psychological "selfless" stance 34
self-realization 210
self-referential: knowledge 141–142; narrative 137; view 193
self-representation 96, 120, 123
self-revealing 176, 183
self-seeing 268
self-serving 195
self-shattering masochism of jouissance 239
self-states 33, 73–75; alien 130; emerging 96; other 103; shifting 29, 85, 104, 105; wild affective 32
self-sufficiency 264
sexual abuse 87; child 207
sexual abuse team 159
sexual agents 235
sexual assault 154
sexual body 218
sexual experience, pretend 191
sexuality 5, 156; child and childhood 211; crisis of 234; desire and 232; gender and 177, 199, 212, 220, 233; identity and 238; Lenù's (Ferrante) 188–191; LGBTQ 228; marriage shame and 237; masochism as counternarrative of 239; mind and 176, 182; queer 211;

subjectivity and 184; unconscious 268; womanhood and 196; see also heterosexuality; homosexuality; queer; transsexual
sexualization 183
sexual object choice 229
sexual orientation 221, 231
sexual outliers 212
sexual subjectivity 5, 238
Shaw, P. 22
Signorelli 118–119
Smith, Stevie: "Not Waving but Drowning" 64
Smith, Zadie 141; gift of implication of 17, 118, 141; on mind/body affect 123; review of Signorelli 118–119
Society for Evidence- Based Gender Medicine 223n1
soma 9; psyche-soma 216
somatic: anlage 33; discharge 13; elements 36, 46, 85–86; experience 86; manifestation 288; mind 86; resonance 86, 255; reverie 109; rubbing 111; sensations 53
South Africa 18
sovereign discrete subject 278
sovereign mastered self 289
sovereignty 9; assuming 283; certainty and 217; Cooney on 277; disrupting 15; implicit 14, 247; Lemma's 214; McGleughlin on 280; Mitchell's 139; problem of 284; risk of 284; sense of 279; Stern on 277–280; unconscious 282; see also nonsovereign; poles
speaking as articulation of wants 26
spectral character of suffering 152
spectral images 105, 116n6
Spivak, Gayatri 117
Steiner, John 32, 46–47, 74–75; Psychic Retreats 46–47
Stephens, Michelle 12, 147
Stern, Donnell 115n2, 274n4; on analyst's retreat to knowing 286; on being with the other 286, 293; on impossibility of meaning 286; on living in negative capacity 286; on McGleughlin 278, 283, 292; on the negative 279; on power of the unrepresented 279–280; on psychic destabilization 283; on sovereignty 277–280; "unformulated experience" of 273n2, 276, 280
Stolorow, R. D. 76

Stolorow, Brandchaft, and Atwood 88, 115
Stolorow, Atwood, and Orange 10,
    33–34, 56
studium 23, 26–27, 29, 116n7, 117,
    127–128
subjectivity: agency and 234, 240;
    analyst's 6, 16, 68–69, 131; author of
    present work's 32, 78, 88, 109; baby's
    9; concept of 9; conceptualizing 140;
    doomed 182; establishing 156, 208;
    Ferrante's claims regarding 183–184;
    gaps in 95, 261; identity and 252;
    individual 159, 253–254; inexpressible
    aspects of 174, 198; inscription of
    121; interior 210; lack propelling 192;
    Lila (Ferrante) 192; limits of 104;
    narrating 260; nonsovereignty and 248,
    256; otherness and 132; patient's 16;
    process of 120; reader/observer's 17;
    self-defined 219; sense of 102; separate
    140; sexual 5, 232, 238; sovereignty
    and 276–279; story of 242; theories of
    229; timelessness of 262; unconscious
    277; unconscious core of 268; using 36,
    154; white 151; women's 232; *see also*
    intersubjective; intersubjectivity
subjectivity of the seeing "I" 173, 193, 196
sublime: post-modern 22
sublime, the 272
Suchet, Melanie 120, 122–124
suffering: Black 150–152; of analyst 68;
    Lila's (Ferrante) 187–188; of patients
    38, 80, 162; possible 162; race and 157;
    relief of 30–31
suffering other 62, 155
surveillance of the other 252
Swartz, S. 17, 236
Symington, N. 137

Teicholz, Judy 65n1
texts 207; anchoring 202; conservative 200;
    reader's involvement with 16
the analytic third *see* analytic third, the;
    third, the
the negative *see* negative, the
the Oedipal *see* Oedipal, the
the ontological *see* ontological, the
third: intersubjective 30–125, 234, 256;
    vital or live 125
third, the 246, 278; interrupting liminality
    137
thirdness 73

Till, Emmett 154
Townsend, Chris 103–104
transference 7, 102, 247, 283; being in
    3; interpreting 281; psychoanalytic
    discovery of 26; reversal in 32,
    75; "taking the transference" 26;
    transference/countertransference
    dilemmas 28; transference/
    countertransference enactments 155;
    transference/countertransference
    as opportunity 133; transference/
    countertransference significance 78;
    transgressive 45
transference theory 140
transformation 272; channel toward 37,
    114; creative 13; disruption leading
    towards 129; goal of 265; *Hiroshima
    mon amour* and 132; portrait of 99;
    possibility of 128, 268; route towards
    86, 257, 260
transformational dreaming 283
transformational empathy 158
transformational field, shared 140
transformational process 150
transformative potential of storytelling 268,
    287–288, 290
transgender acceptance 176
transgender adolescents 207–208
transgender community 204, 206
transgender identification 210; Jane 214
transgender imagining 199–223
transgender people 206–207; death
    threats against 220; persecution of
    209; rights of 200, 208; softball played
    with 221–222; "Trans-itory Identities"
    (Lemma) 176–178, 202–223
transgender practitioners 202

unbelonging 4
uncanny, the 82, 273
undrawn patient 84, 259
unexpected, the: making room for 255–260
unmarked, the 15, 252, 254–255, 258, 270
unrepresentability 267, 273n2
unrepresentable, the 109, 253, 266
unrepresented 112, 123; represented/
    unrepresented 169; unknowable and 183
unrepresented experience 136, 254, 259
unrepresented mental states 83–85, 275,
    281; generative work of the negative
    and 279–281; growth impeded by 279
unrepresented states 13, 15, 32, 251

unrepresented, the 252; power of 280;
    working with 255
unseen 77, 151–152, 270
unseen absence 146
unseen death 141
unseen, the 242, 252–253

vertigo 13; "Analyst's Necessary Vertigo"
    (McGleughlin, 2011) 21–24; "Analyst's
    Necessary Vertigo" (McGleughlin,
    2008/2011) 25–40; "Love Letter
    to a Patient or the Raw Story"
    (McGleughlin) 40–65; necessary 16
vulnerability: accountability and 153;
    analytic 13; analyst's 6, 9, 16, 155, 158,
    255, 258, 269, 278, 281–282, 284;
    authenticity implied by 70; of author
    of present work 28–29, 46, 54, 93,
    160, 165, 168; feelings of 28–29, 46;
    generativity and 272; issues of power
    and 94, 148; Lenù's (Ferrante) 194;
    Lila's (Ferrante) 186–187; Martin's
    248; psychic 157; showing 4

white empathy 93, 147–170, 282
whiteness 12; Blackness and 149;
    disassociated 155; disavowed meanings
    of 157; ideological gaze of 166; pain of
    163; specific 164; system of 156
whiteness machine 162

Wilderson, F. 12
Williams, Patricia 119
Winnicott, Donald W. 2–3, 8, 10; child
    play 159; "entitled to remain alive"
    assertion by 286; going-on-being of
    3, 78; "good enough" mother of 178;
    object relating to object use 192;
    psychoanalytic thinkers after 156; on
    psychotherapy overlapping between
    patient and therapist 160; real use
    of the other 197; on recognition and
    subjectivity 140; on relationality 19n3;
    subjective object of 185; on transitional
    relating 113; unintegration of 103; After
    Winnicott xxiv
Winnicottian 16; transitional space 233
Winterson, Jeanette 47–49, 52, 54, 115n3
witness 94, 102; bearing 105, 115; inability
    to 152; jouissance of role of 159;
    psychoanalytic 96
witnesses: fellow sufferers and 157;
    observers as 168; viewers as
    153, 165
witnessing 282; act of 152; being witnessed
    and 168; surveilling and 282
witnessing interruption 128
witnessing trauma 101, 113
Woodman, Francesca 96; death and
    meaning of death in work of 107–108
Wynter, Sylvia 199, 201–203